Don't be a statistic! WOMEN'S HEALTH ██████████ *to protect yourself against the common* ████████████████, *and products that could endanger your life.*

- 20 million American women have had a hysterectomy, and 600,000 more have one each year. At the current rate, one in three women will lose their uteruses by age 60—and yet more than a quarter of these operations are unnecessary.

- Of the 10 million American women who have had at least one cesarean section, 3 million have had c-sections that were unnecessary, and millions more have had automatic and largely unnecessary repeat c-sections with all subsequent deliveries. Almost half a million more unnecessary cesarean deliveries are performed each year.

- 2 million American women have had silicone gel breast implants surgically placed in their chests, causing hundreds of thousands of injuries, some extremely disabling.

- 600,000 American women have been prescribed Accutane, a large proportion without justification. This drug has caused hundreds of severe birth defects and coerced thousands of women into an abortion for fear of delivering a severely affected child.

- 13 million American women are currently using the birth control pill. More than 100,000 are getting a pill which is too strong, and millions are unaware of the recent studies linking long-term use of the Pill to an increased risk of breast cancer in women under 45.

- More than 10 million postpartum American women have been prescribed lactation suppressing drugs (to stop breast milk production) such as Parlodel, estrogens, or other hormones because they did not want to breast-feed after childbirth. These drugs, which experts and even the FDA agree should never be used for this purpose, can cause heart attacks, strokes, blood clots in the lung, or severe high or low blood pressure. 800,000 more women are prescribed these drugs each year.

- At least 10 million postmenopausal American women have been prescribed long-term hormone replacement therapy to prevent osteoporosis or heart disease even though many of these women are not at especially high risk for either of these diseases. Many women are unaware of the increasingly clear evidence that long-term use of these drugs causes a 50 to 100 percent increase in breast cancer.

- Mammography, proven to be an important way of detecting breast cancer at an earlier stage in women 50 or older, is not routinely obtained by more than 30 million American women (at least 85 percent of the women in this age group) who could benefit from this important diagnostic test. For most women 40 to 50, the evidence supporting yearly mammograms is less clear.

WOMEN'S HEALTH ALERT

SIDNEY M. WOLFE, M.D.
and the Public Citizen Health Research Group

with Rhoda Donkin Jones

What Most Doctors Won't Tell You About Birth Control, C-Sections, Weight Control Products, Hormone Replacement Therapy, Osteoporosis, Breast Implants, Tranquilizers, Hysterectomies, And Other Medications, Procedures, and Conditions That Could Endanger Your Life

Addison-Wesley Publishing Company, Inc.

READING, MASSACHUSETTS   MENLO PARK, CALIFORNIA
NEW YORK   DON MILLS, ONTARIO
WOKINGHAM, ENGLAND   AMSTERDAM   BONN
SYDNEY   SINGAPORE   TOKYO
MADRID   SAN JUAN

This book is meant to educate and should not be used as an alternative to proper medical care. The authors have exerted every effort to ensure that the information presented is accurate up to the time of publication. However in light of ongoing research and the constant flow of information it is possible that new findings may raise questions about some of the information presented here.

Many of the designations used by manufacturers and sellers to distinguish their products are claimed as trademarks. Where those designations appear in this book and Addison-Wesley was aware of a trademark claim, the designations have been printed in initial capital letters (i.e., Parlodel).

Library of Congress Cataloging-in-Publication Data

Wolfe, Sidney M.
    Women's health alert : what most doctors won't tell you about
  birth control, C-sections, weight control products, hormone
  replacement therapy, osteoporosis, breast implants, tranquilizers,
  hysterectomies, and other medications, procedures, and
  conditions that could endanger your life / by Sidney M. Wolfe
  and the Public Citizen Health Research Group, with
  Rhoda Donkin Jones.
      p. cm.
  Includes index.
  ISBN 0-201-55041-5
  1. Gynecology, Operative—Popular works.   2. Gynecologic
  drugs—Popular works.   3. Women—Drug use.   4. Women—
  Health and hygiene. I. Jones, Rhoda Donkin.   II. Public Citizen
  Health Research Group. III. Title.
  RG104.W65   1990

Cover design by Linda Kosarin
Text design by Joyce C. Weston
Set in 11-point Garamond by DEKR Corporation, Woburn MA

23456789-AL-9321

Contents

This book is dedicated to our mothers, sisters, daughters and all other women who provide the inspiration to do the research, to summarize the findings, and transfer the power of this information. To Them. And to Suzanne and Patrick without whose love and understanding the book would not have been possible.

Acknowledgements

I. Medical Advisers

The following physicians, with expertise in various areas, gave generously of their time to read and make helpful suggestions about the chapters which fell into their area of expertise.

Mammography

John Bailar, M.D., Ph.D., McGill University School of Medicine, Office of Disease Prevention and Health Promotion, Department of Health and Human Services

Silicone

Richard Grossman, M.D., FACS, private practice plastic surgery, Sherman Oaks, California

Douglas Teich, M.D., Internal Medicine, Washington, D.C.

Hysterectomy

Paul D. Stolley, M.D., Professor of Medicine, University of Pennsylvania, School of Medicine

Robert C. Reiter, M.D., Department of Obstetrics/Gynecology, University of Iowa Hospitals and Clinics

Lynn J. Soffer, M.D., M.S., specialty in general internal medicine, Washington, D.C.

C-Sections

Lynn D. Silver, M.D., MPH, Rio de Janeiro, Brazil, specialty in pediatrics. Dr. Silver was the principal author of an earlier Health Research Group report, *Unnecessary Cesarean Sections: How To Cure A National Epidemic*, upon which the c-section chapter was based.

Bruce Flamm, M.D., Assistant Clinical Professor, Obstetrics/Gynecology, Kaiser Permanente, Riverside, CA

Norbert Gleicher, M.D., Obstetrics/Gynecology, Mt. Sinai Hospital, Chicago, IL

Birth Control Pill

Paul D. Stolley, M.D., MPH, Professor of Medicine, University of Pennsylvania, School of Medicine

Robert Hoover, M.D., Ph.D., Chief of the Environmental Epidemiology Branch, National Cancer Institute, Bethesda, Maryland

Ida Hellander, M.D., Public Citizen Health Research Group

Tranquilizers

Fredric Solomon, M.D., Psychiatrist, private practice, Washington, D.C.

Alan Stone, M.D., Internal Medicine, private practice, Washington, D.C.

Lactation Suppressants

Philip Corfman, M.D., Obstetrics, Fertility and Maternal Health Drugs, Food and Drug Administration

Douglas Teich, M.D., Internal Medicine, Washington, D.C.

Hormone Replacement Therapy

Paul D. Stolley, M.D., MPH., Professor of Medicine, University of Pennsylvania, School of Medicine

Robert Hoover, M.D., Ph.D., Chief of the Environmental Epidemiology Branch, National Cancer Institute, Bethesda, Maryland

Weight Loss

Michael Newman, M.D. physician in private practice of internal medicine, Washington, D.C. and attending physician, George Washington University Medical Center

Arthur Frank, M.D., Internal Medicine, private practice, Washington, D.C. specializing in weight reduction

Tobacco

Michael Newman, M.D., physician in private practice of internal medicine, Washington, D.C. and attending physician, George Washington University Medical Center

Mark Manley, M.D., MPH, Smoking, Tobacco, and Cancer Program, National Cancer Institute, National Institutes of Health

II. Other Public Citizen Staff

Phyllis McCarthy for her exceptional organizational skills, limitless know-how, preparation of the manuscript, proofreading and editing suggestions

Ingrid VanTuinen for preparing the updated data on state and hospital c-section rates which is in Appendix A

Durrie McKnew for spending long hours in the library checking references

Patti Goldman, attorney, for reviewing the entire manuscript

Joan Steiber, attorney, for reviewing the entire manuscript and for making helpful suggestions

III. Addison-Wesley Staff

Nancy Miller, Editor; Sandra Hutchinson, Production Coordinator, Lynne Reed, Production Design Coordinator; Johanna Van Hise, Editorial Assistant.

We would also like to thank the women who shared their experiences—sometimes very painful—with us in the hopes that other women could become more aware and more cautious.

Preface

by Rhoda Donkin Jones

INITIALLY I had some reservations about writing this book—not from any quandary over the importance or relevance of what's here, but because these pages are filled with bad news. It is not a reassuring or comforting book. It's not very easy going. So who will want to read it?

As a woman, I see we make bad decisions about our health, but often they are decisions we don't want to be talked out of. The medical, cosmetic, drug, tobacco, and alcohol industries spend billions convincing us that we can and should change ourselves, and they have been very successful. We want to be wowed by the good news that fad diets are easy and everlasting. We are reassured when a physician says that surgery is the answer. We want to believe that a pill that relaxes us can't be so bad and certainly that a pill which prevents pregnancy is nothing less than a Godsend.

In our rush to feel better or simply feel different about ourselves, we are capable of losing our common sense. Where is our common sense when we decide it must be safe to install foreign objects into our breasts so that we can spend our adult lives being bustier than nature intended? Where is our common sense when we renew drug prescriptions for years—say tranquilizers or hormones—without stopping to investigate if perhaps the pills are doing more harm than good?

While I was writing this book women repeatedly told me their biggest mistake was trusting an ad, or even the opinion of one doctor. In some cases the worst health care decisions of their lives were simply the result of not questioning medical authority.

We should. Even when we don't want to. We should always get second, even third opinions. We should have more than one pathologist read test reports. We should ignore advertising. We should read information that doesn't gloss over important issues.

Women's Health Alert doesn't pretend to be easy reading or what you want to hear. It is not written to be read at one sitting or even as your book-of-the-month. It is not an encyclopedia or self-help guide and it is not nearly the complete list of things we should be cautious about. Use it as a decision-making tool, perhaps better read when you need it—as a balance—a voice appealing to the kernel of caution we all owned as kids and some of us lose as women.

Since finishing the book I realize my reservations were unfounded. We as women do want to be talked out of bad health care decisions, but we need sound information first. I hope *Women's Health Alert* will be your guide.

Introduction

Sidney M. Wolfe, M.D.

THIS book is about overkill—about everyday health care practices that unnecessarily harm perfectly healthy women, either physically, emotionally, or both, all in the name of good medicine.

The topics covered here are household subjects, familiar to any woman between ages 15 and 75. In your lifetime, the chances you will experience at least one of the medications, other products, procedures, or conditions we discuss are very high. While there is something in here for everyone, there are, unfortunately, many more medicines, other products, and surgical procedures about which women would benefit from being alerted. These 12 were chosen because the Health Research Group has been involved in efforts to better regulate or to eliminate the use of each of them. Our perspective on these issues may surprise you. We won't be repeating the opinions you will get from most of your physicians. In most cases we will give you information that mainstream medical thinking completely leaves out.

We estimate that of the 100 million American women 15 or older, at least 85 million have used one or more of the products discussed in the book or have had one or more of the operations—cesarean section, hysterectomy, or silicone gel breast implants. During every new year, millions more women, told largely about the good news but not the bad, are sold on these goods or services by the companies which produce them or by the doctors who do the operations.

Since starting the Health Research Group 19 years ago I have watched doctors' and drug companies' enormous appetite for dumping hormones and other drugs into women's bodies. I have been awed at surgeons' seemingly endless capacity to cut into women's bodies, removing "useless" uteruses through millions of unnecessary hysterectomies, surgically delivering "perfect babies" through cesarean sections, and deforming women's breasts by implanting silicone devices inside their bodies.

This inexhaustible capacity to cut and medicate women in this country comes, in part, from a cultural view that women's natural biological processes are treatable illnesses.

Menstruation, pregnancy, childbirth, and lactation, for example, are all normal female reproductive functions which have been occurring since the days of Adam and Eve. But a series of paths, paved initially with good and legitimate intentions, have led to the commercialization of treatment for each of these normal female functions, ultimately in order to sell as many millions of dollars of operations (cesarean sections) or goods (tampons, birth control pills, or lactation suppressing drugs) despite the emergence of evidence in each case of serious but avoidable risks to women.

Put another way, if treatments are too vigorous or aggressive to treat women who are, in most cases, entirely healthy, there is a strong risk of causing more harm than good and turning healthy women into sick or dead women. For example:

- Tampons are used by millions of women, but in their super-plus absorbency (12–15 g absorbency) are also super risky for toxic shock syndrome. Millions of women will, when informed, trade off some extra absorbency for a decreased risk of this preventable disease.

- Birth control pills, although a very effective contraceptive, would be used with lower amounts of estrogen and by fewer women if the needless risks of higher dose pills, including the risk of breast cancer, became known.

- Lactation suppressing drugs, which should never be used, and cesarean sections, half of which are unnecessary, are the other two examples of dangerously exploiting and commercializing normal reproductive functions. Five more of the topics discussed in *Women's Health Alert* concern products which are sold in part either to improve women's self-image or to cope with the change-of-life or menopause.

■ Hormone replacement therapy was originally "pushed" on women to treat the acute symptoms of the menopause and to allow them to remain "feminine forever." While estrogens were later shown to prevent some broken bones, mainly in women over 70 with osteoporosis, there is now clear evidence that estrogens can also cause cancers of the uterus and breast.

■ Silicone gel breast implants have now been surgically implanted in over two million American women, 85 percent of whom had these bags of sticky silicone implanted purely for cosmetic reasons. Silicone gel breast implants routinely leak, occasionally break, frequently harden, can cause serious immune disorders and may cause cancer. But doctors (from the largely male subspecialty called plastic surgery) and women's perceptions of men's attitudes about those parts of their bodies have convinced these women that if they only had larger or more shapely breasts, they would lead a happier and much more satisfying life.

■ Weight Loss and Dieting. Whereas obesity poses serious health risks, millions of women who are not significantly overweight (but who do not look as thin as the often underweight-looking models who grace print and TV ads) try an unending succession of largely ineffective and sometimes dangerous products or processes that promise the "thin world." As discussed in the chapter on dieting, about one-half of all women are currently on a diet, far more than the number who are actually overweight and more than the proportion of men who are now on a diet.

■ Cigarettes. There is no question that smoking is a serious and all-too-common addiction. In the process of their monstrous recruitment of women into the ranks of those who smoke, the cigarette death merchants successfully exploit women's self-image as "having come a long way," looking or wanting to look sexy, or use other attributes which the ads imply are more likely to come true for smokers.

- Accutane. There are approximately 5,000 women a year of childbearing age in the United States who have severe cystic acne which has not responded to less dangerous treatments. For these women, the use of the very effective but birth defect-causing drug, Accutane, may well be appropriate. However, although women are but a small fraction of people with this severe kind of acne—it affects men about 5.5 times more commonly than women—women are prescribed the drug just as often as men. About 50,000 to 60,000 women of childbearing age are prescribed the drug each year. This has resulted in hundreds of severe life-threatening or fatal birth defects and thousands of induced abortions in women who are under-standably frightened when they become aware that the fetus they are carrying has a high risk of having such problems.

The sexism in American and other societies places much more emphasis on a woman's appearance than on a man's and, as a result, the medicalization and commercialization of image-fixing women's bodies flourishes. Those who promise bigger breasts through silicone and surgery, Accutane-clear skin, thinner bodies, sex and success through smoking, and femininity forever with hormones are exploiting women.

These ways of manipulating women's bodies are largely a recent phenomenon. Only in this century has it been possible to medicate or surgically alter female biological processes which have been occurring since the beginning of human reproduc-tion. Certainly the Pill has given women invaluable power over their own reproductive decisions, a freedom that cannot be underestimated. Cesarean section deliveries have saved infants and mothers who would otherwise have died. In some cases hysterectomies have been the only solution to women with reproductive cancers.

But where women's health care is concerned, we have simply gone too far and we continue to go farther at the great expense of healthy women. The Pill has never enjoyed greater popularity, and now women in increasing numbers will be taking hormones beyond their reproductive years and well into old age as replacement therapy. Despite our great societal need to see hormones as the panacea for the reproductive burdens of being female, taking them in any form has risks that are understated by almost everyone.

There is no practical limit in this country when it comes to female reproductive surgery. In the United States we perform many more cesarean sections than are done in countries with much lower infant mortality rates, so the notion that we are saving babies through our excessive use of c-sections is simply false. We perform many more hysterectomies than other industrialized nations, despite insignificant differences in uterine cancer rates between the U.S. and other countries. Do we do this to save lives? The answer, most of the time, is clearly no. These are examples of medical practice and habit, not medical necessity.

Certainly implanting silicone gel breast prostheses has never saved a life, and yet thousands of women today are eagerly awaiting their chance to have this operation. Implants are one of the most popular cosmetic surgeries today, and that is largely because no one, not even some of the major health magazines, has described the severe medical consequences of these lethal time bombs.

When women agree to a hysterectomy, seek surgery for breast implants, or decide to continue taking hormones throughout their reproductive life and beyond, there is an implicit trust that what they are doing is both necessary and safe. This is clearly and tragically not so, despite information women depend on to make their health care decisions.

In 1990, expenditures in the United States for advertising were approximately $132 billion, an amount greater than the gross national product of all but a few countries in the world. Many billions of these dollars were spent in pushing and promoting the products discussed in *Women's Health Alert*. Largely missing from these slickly made accentuations of the positive is anything which even hints of the negative, the bad news.

The false, misleading, and incomplete information which

companies and doctors disseminate for the 12 topics which are discussed here guarantees that a large proportion of these 100 million women will not be in control and may unwittingly and unwillingly subject themselves to surgery, to needlessly dangerous drugs or medical devices, believing that the benefits outweigh the risks. As a result, they may die preventable deaths or suffer serious preventable injuries, to say nothing of wasting billions of dollars or more.

Women's Health Alert is a book whose main purpose is to change the balance of power between 100 million women and the doctors, hospitals, drug companies, medical device companies, and tobacco companies who sell them tens of billions of dollars of surgery, drugs, and cigarettes each year. Accurate and complete information, such as that provided here, can empower you to make decisions based on what is in your own best interest.

HOW TO USE THIS BOOK

This book is not meant as a replacement for your doctor or as a definitive answer for what you should do, with the exception of cigarettes, lactation suppressants, appetite suppressants, and silicone gel breast implants, all of which we strongly advise against ever using. For the other topics covered in the book, the idea is to supplement and help to balance out the often benefit-tilted/distorted information obtained from many doctors or from the commercial sources which inform them or directly inform you.

By reading about the issues discussed in this book which affect you, many of you will be much more aware and more able to negotiate a better decision as to what you should do, often in conjunction with your doctor or, in the case of an over-the-counter product such as tampons, on your own. Being informed will help you to defend the various parts of your body from the commercially-driven assaults which the purveyors of health goods or services might otherwise make to your detriment. Read and use in good health!

PART I

Procedures

Mammography, Silicone Gel Breast
Implants, Hysterectomy, Cesarean Section

MAMMOGRAPHY

In Women Without Symptoms or Risk Factors, Routine Screenings Should Clearly Begin After Age 50

In the United States in 1990, an estimated 150,000 new cases of breast cancer will be diagnosed in women, and 44,000 women will die of the disease.

- For women past age 50, mammography is the best means of detecting early breast cancer but it is not routinely obtained by 30 million women (85 percent) in this age group. However, the evidence for the benefits of routine annual screening in women who are under age 50 (and have no increased risk factors for breast cancer) is not clear. In these (asymptomatic) women, repeated routine mammograms produce a high incidence of false positives. A false positive is when a person qualified to read films says that there is (or may be) cancer and this opinion turns out to be wrong. These incorrect readings may inflict a great deal of emotional pain and unnecessary medical procedures on young women.

- There is a wide variation in radiation dose (tenfold) and image quality between mammography practices because no federal standards exist which specifically target quality control for mammography equipment.

Recommendations

- Annual clinical breast examination (manual exam by a trained individual) should be done on all women aged

40 and above.

- A clinical exam and mammography is recommended every one to two years for all women beginning at age 50 and concluding at around age 75 unless pathology is detected. Most studies have not shown a clear benefit in routine mammography screening in women aged 40 to 49.

- For the special category of women who are at high risk because their mothers or sisters have had premenopausally diagnosed breast cancer, annual clinical breast exams and mammography are recommended at an early age.

- Patients should be referred to mammographers who use low dose equipment and adhere to high standards of quality control. You can obtain information about which mammographic facilities in your area are accredited by contacting your state's division of the American Cancer Society or by calling the National Cancer Institute at 1-800-4-CANCER. (Note: Both of these groups recommend routine mammography screening starting at age 40 or even earlier.)

*O*NE in 11 women will be diagnosed as having breast cancer, but fortunately it remains a relatively rare disease in women under age 50. The sooner most cancers are discovered, the better. Early detection means better chances of surviving an often fatal disease. Screening for breast cancer is the best means of detecting the disease early, but unfortunately the perfect screening method or technology hasn't been found. The use of x-ray mammography has improved the diagnosis and treatment of breast cancer, but there are also serious drawbacks to this procedure. There is little disagreement that regular screening of women who are past 50 years old saves lives.

Over the past few years there has been a great deal of debate over the value of routine mammography for women who have not yet reached age 50. One problem is that the risk of having breast cancer is less for younger women.

In any case, the evidence to date is unclear as to whether routine mammographic screening in women between ages 40–49 adds even modest health benefits. Even these must be weighed against considerable costs and risks.

HOW SHOULD YOU BE SCREENED FOR BREAST CANCER?

The three screening tests usually considered for breast cancer are clinical examination of the breast (manual exam done by a trained individual), x-ray mammography and breast self-exam. None of these is infallible. The accuracy of clinical breast exams depends a lot on the experience and skill of the examiner, and the characteristics of the breast being examined. A well trained practicing physician or health professional who takes time to do a good breast exam can be very successful in finding even small lesions. Studies have shown that physicians' detection rate is as high as 87 percent.[1] Studies have also shown that training women to do their own breast exam improves the accuracy of that test significantly and also reduces the number of times women mistakenly believe they have breast cancer.[2]

Mammography (an x-ray of your breast) can find and locate a suspicious lump in the breast so it can be removed and looked at under a microscope. In women of any age with suspicious lumps that have been detected through physical exam, it may be used as an additional test to decide whether a biopsy (surgical removal of a small bit of breast tissue) is necessary.

It is also useful as a routine test in populations of women where the incidence of breast cancer is high, namely older women (over 50) and in younger women who have risk factors. (See chapter on birth control pills for discussion of "high risk".) The incidence of breast cancer in this country goes up with age (from 28 per 100,000 at age 30 to 195 per 100,000 at age 50).[3] This is one reason that regular screening will correctly detect something serious after age 50. In fact, mammography testing in women over 50 picks up existing cancer 87 percent of the time, only missing cancers 13 percent of the time.[4] Furthermore, in this age group, when the test suggests cancer, the chances are much better that it will be accurate. In other words, if you are over age 50, you might question a negative x-ray a little, but you can be very sure of a positive x-ray.

MAMMOGRAPHY FOR WOMEN UNDER AGE 50

However, when a mammogram is used to screen otherwise unsuspicious breasts in women under age 50, it isn't very accurate. In fact, it correctly detects dangerous lesions only 56 percent of the time.[5] Furthermore, when done routinely in asymptomatic women, abnormal mammograms are very likely to be wrong—they are usually not indicative of cancer. Only about 10 to 12 percent of young women with positive mammograms have cancer.[6] In most young, asymptomatic women, most of the nodules found by x-ray are not dangerous and need no surgical attention.

Unfortunately, when something looking like a lump shows up on the x-ray film, too often unnecessary surgery follows, and with it extreme anxiety, extra medical costs, and ultimately distrust of x-ray screening by the time (age) women benefit from it the most.

No study of women under 50 has yet shown reduced death rates from breast cancer for those who have had screening mammograms. Therefore, the only reason to have a mammogram under age 50 is for use in specific cases where abnormal findings such as lumps are present and x-ray is needed for confirmation, or if there are increased risk factors.

It is the consensus of experts that women who have genuine signs or symptoms which suggest cancer are candidates for mammography, regardless of their age, if this test is needed to determine the next steps in the diagnostic process.

However, good evidence exists that routine screening of women who are younger than 50 provides only modest health benefits which must be weighed against large costs.

- Too many women receive false positives.
- Too many mammographers don't do the palpation or don't do it well.
- Too many times cancer is missed.
- Excessive exposure to radiation. This is more serious in younger women than in women over 50. Ten years of routine screening with mammography in the decade between 40–49 carries a small but real risk of radiation-induced cancer.
- High monetary costs in extra and unnecessary visits to the doctor for tests, unnecessary surgery and other medical procedures.
- Tremendous unnecessary anxiety

SCREENING AFTER 50

A U.S. government-sponsored Preventive Services Task Force differed sharply with the advice given by the American Cancer Society and the National Cancer Institute, both of which recommend routine mammography for women 40 to 49. This task force found that:

Most studies have not shown a clear benefit from mammography in women aged 40–49. Studies that will provide important information on this topic are in progress. In the meantime, it is unclear whether the effects on breast cancer mortality achieved by screening women aged 40–49 are of sufficient magnitude to justify the costs and potential adverse effects from false-positive results that may occur as a result of widespread screening. Until more definitive data become available, it is reasonable to concentrate the large effort and expense associated with mammography on women in the age group for which benefit has been most clearly demonstrated: those aged 50 and above.[7]

Virtually all experts agree that women who are at least 50 years old and are asymptomatic will benefit from regular breast cancer screening that combines mammography and careful physical examination. The benefits at this age outweigh the costs, which include the price, inconvenience, and exposure to low doses of radiation.

While it is true that radiation can increase the risk of breast cancer, patient radiation exposure from mammography equipment has been reduced by as much as 50 percent over the last several years.[8] Perhaps more reassuring is that the risk from radiation-induced breast cancer is lowest among women who are exposed later in life, as they would be with mammography. So for older women, for whom the radiation risk is the lowest and the chance of detecting cancer is highest, the benefits of a properly performed mammogram outweigh the risks.

Women over 50 should be encouraged to get clinical breast exams along with routine mammograms. It is estimated there are now between 5,000 and 6,000 mammography units in the United States. However, women should be aware that mammography facilities do not all offer the same quality and skill in performing mammograms.

According to recent data, the radiation dose you may be exposed to can vary by a factor of 10, and image quality of the picture of your breast can also vary significantly between units.[9]

In fact, an accreditation process carried out over the past several years flunked almost one-third of the mammography practices evaluated. According to data collected by the American College of Radiology (ACR) Mammography Screening Accreditation Program, as of February 1990, of the 1,438 units evaluated, 443 failed the first attempt at accreditation.[10]

Dr. R. Edward Hendrick, chief of the division of radiologic sciences at the University of Colorado in Denver, has been involved in the ongoing accreditation process. He writes:

At the heart of the observed variations in image quality and breast dose is the lack of standardized quality control practices in mammography sites within the United States. The majority of mammography units that are in hospitals undergo annual inspection of x-ray-producing equipment by a physicist as part of an ongoing quality assurance program. . . however, more than 50% of mammographic screening sites are located outside of hospitals and therefore are not necessarily subject to mandated annual inspections. To my knowledge, no accurate statistics exist on the fraction of mammography units located outside of hospitals that are evaluated annually.[11]

When you go for a mammogram, try to go to a facility that has been accredited. You can find them by calling your state's division of the American Cancer Society or by calling the National Cancer Institute at 1-800-4-CANCER.

ASK QUESTIONS

It is important that the facility's personnel be properly trained and that up-to-date equipment be used so that images produced will be of the highest quality. The better the quality of the image, the better the chance of detecting cancer if it is present and of not finding a false positive. High quality images also help avoid unnecessary levels of radiation exposure.

Here are some questions for you to ask about a facility before getting a mammogram:

1. Do your x-ray technologist and radiologist have specific training in mammography?

Technologists perform the exam and they are responsible for properly positioning the patient, operating the equipment and developing the film. Radiologists are medical doctors who interpret the results of the mammogram. Both technicians and radiologists need special training to get the best images with the least possible radiation and to interpret those images properly.

2. Is the mammography equipment "dedicated"?

In technological parlance, "dedicated" means that the

equipment is designed specifically for mammography, providing the best mammograms with as little radiation as possible.

3. **How often is your mammography equipment inspected and calibrated?**

When was the last time? Is a copy of the inspection report available? The equipment should be inspected at least annually.

WHAT HAPPENS DURING A MAMMOGRAM?

The patient usually stands during the procedure and the technologist positions the breast on a horizontal support above the x-ray film. Compression of the breast by a device called a "paddle" is necessary for proper positioning. With some equipment, the technologist uses the paddle manually to compress the breast. It stays in position while the picture is taken. After the exposure, the compression is released. In the newer equipment, the technologist compresses the breast only partially before going behind the machine where there is a button allowing automatic completion of compression. After the x-ray is taken, the compression is automatically released, minimizing the discomfort time. The newer equipment may be more uncomfortable than the older style, but newer devices provide higher quality images.

Although there may be some discomfort while the breast is compressed, there shouldn't be a great deal. Proper compression is crucial to a high quality mammogram with the lowest radiation dose possible.

1. Fletcher SW, O'Malley MS, Bunce LA. Physicians' abilities to detect lumps in silicone breast models. Journal of the American Medical Association 1985; 253:2224–8.

2. Hall DC, Adams CK, Stein GH, Stephenson HS, Goldstein MK, Pennypacker HS. Improved detection of human breast lesions following experimental training. Cancer 1980; 46:408–14.

3. Cancer Statistics Review 1973–1987, National Cancer Institute 1990.

4. Edeiken S. Mammography and palpable cancer of the breast. Cancer 1988; 61:263–5.

5. Ibid.

6. Wright CJ. Breast cancer screening: A different look at the evidence. Surgery 1986; 100:594–8.

7. Report of the U.S. Preventive Services Task Force. Guide to clinical preventive services: An assessment of the effectiveness of 169 interventions. Williams & Wilkens, Baltimore 1989, p. 43.

8. Willis J. Progress against breast cancer. FDA Consumer May 1986; 8.

9. Galkin BM, Feig SA, Muir HD. The technical quality of mammography in centers participating in a regional breast cancer awareness program. Radio-Graphics 1988; 8:133–45.

10. Personal correspondence with Dr. R. Edward Hendrick.

11. Hendrick RE. Standardization of image quality and radiation dose in mammography. Radiology 1990; 174:648–53.

SILICONE GEL BREAST IMPLANTS

Time Bombs Ticking

Even after 25 years on the market, silicone gel breast implants have never been proven safe in women who expect to have them inside their bodies for a lifetime.

- Over two million women already have breast implants and over 100,000 or more additional women each year decide to have the surgery. Up to 40 percent of them will eventually suffer painful hardening of their breasts, sometimes requiring repeat surgery or other painful procedures to help alleviate the problem.

- Repeat surgery for other complications—including deformities, infections, and implant failures—is also common.

- The silicone gel bags used in many implant models are known to rupture or leak, causing silicone to disperse into the woman's body.

- A growing number of women with implants develop mysterious and debilitating allergic reactions to the silicone, including swollen joints and scleroderma, an often fatal disorder in which the body's connective tissue hardens.

- Most of the implants contain silicone gel which has been proven to cause highly malignant tumors in test animals.

- While human cancer studies on silicone gel breast implants are incomplete at present, it is clear that implant devices often interfere with the routine mammography screening for breast cancer, thus possibly increasing the number of breast cancers not detected until dangerously late stages.

- In 1989 the Food and Drug Administration, in summarizing studies on breast implants, wrote: "FDA has weighed the probable risks and benefits to the public from the use of the silicone gel-filled breast prosthesis and believes that the studies present evidence of significant risks associated with the use of the device. These risks must be addressed by manufacturers of the device."

  So far, they have not.

Recommendations

- We strongly advise against the use of silicone gel breast implants.

- Women who have implants should see their primary care doctor regularly (at least once a year) to be checked for the possibility of various medical problems which implants can cause.

- If you are getting a mammogram and you have breast implants, make sure your doctor, the x-ray technician and the radiologist all know about your implants. The accuracy of the exam depends on this.

*N*EXT to nose reshaping and liposuction, breast augmentations have become the most popular plastic surgery in this country. In the past several years, 100,000 or more women each year in the United States went to surgeons to get their breasts enlarged. While some have the operation immediately following a mastectomy, the majority—85 percent—simply want bigger breasts. Today, more than two million women already have breast implants, and each day 300 more women get them.

Most breast augmentations involve some form of silicone gel breast implant, which amounts to a rubbery silicone capsule with jelly-like silicone inside. There are a variety of different models (see box). The surgery isn't cheap. The operation typically costs over $3,500 including surgical fees and anesthesia. One national survey estimated that the cost of breast augmentations jumped almost 20 percent in 1988.[1] Obviously, when it

---

Breast Implant Models

There are a variety of different breast implant models. Silicone is used in both the outer shell and the inside of most implant devices.

- *Silicone gel-filled implants* have rubber-like silicone shells which contain silicone gel.
- *Silicone gel-filled implants with polyurethane coating* also have a rubbery silicone shell and the gel inside, but the entire capsule is coated in polyurethane foam.
- *Inflatable saline-filled implants* are made of the rubbery silicone shell; during surgery the physician fills the shell with salt (saline) fluid.
- *Double lumen implant* has a rubber-like silicone shell with an inner chamber containing silicone gel and an outer chamber that is filled with fluid during surgery. The Reverse Double Lumen implant has an inner chamber filled with saline fluid and an outer chamber containing silicone gel.
- *Adjustable reconstructive implant* is intended primarily for mastectomy patients who lack sufficient skin for placement of the implant, but it is occasionally used for breast augmentation. This implant has an outer silicone shell which is filled with saline fluid during surgery. Over time, a detachable tube is used to slowly inflate the implant with more saline.

is done for purely cosmetic reasons, most insurance companies won't help out.

MONICA'S STORY

The cost doesn't bother Monica, 27, a legal secretary in Washington D.C., who believes she will like herself better in a larger bra size. The divorced mother of a three-year-old, Monica believes herself to be a cautious, reflective person after having gone through a painful marriage. She is setting money aside with every paycheck to be able to afford her surgery in several months. She wants implants, she says, so she can look better in a two-piece bathing suit. Furthermore, she complains, big hips and big busts run in her family and she feels nature "cheated" her by relegating her to a B cup.

She trusts that medical science, government regulators, and the product manufacturers have done what they are supposed to do to ensure the safety of products she uses. Unfortunately, medical science is still testing silicone gel implants, federal regulators are still waiting to decide what kind of tests need to be done to see if the implants are safe, and manufacturers are making millions of dollars on these products in the meantime.

Not knowing all this, Monica is looking around, and she sees people like her friend Erika, who after two years has had no problems with her implants. "She looks great and I know her husband loves them even though he'd never come out and say that."

Monica understands that the implants she wants should last for perhaps 50 years or more, and that no one knows what happens much past 10 years. "I'm aware there are some risks," she says, but "I believe that whatever can go wrong can be corrected."

Sadly, Monica is dead wrong.

In recent years the bad news about silicone gel breast implants has surfaced and evidence of silicone's extremely dangerous effects on the body are now more than anecdotal. The millions of women in this country walking around with breast implants do not realize these devices have not been adequately tested by the manufacturers for safety in humans, nor approved as safe by the FDA. The data needed to determine safety is just now being amassed from the women themselves, women who unwittingly have participated in what scientists now call "two decades of human experimentation."[2]

In 1986, accumulated evidence, in the form of sick women, finally forced manufacturers to change the guarantee on their products' labels to reflect risks not previously disclosed by the company.[3] And because of these after-the-fact warnings, many companies have been dragged into court in a growing number of lawsuits around the country.

Unfortunately, more than 100,000 women each year continue to trust that breast implants are safe, simple, and affordable and choose to have the operation.

Here's the bad news coming from women who have had silicone gel breast implants:

- Up to 40 percent are finding that their new breasts harden up in as little as six months, leaving them deformed and often in severe pain. The condition is called "capsular contracture" because an internal scar forms around the implant and actually contracts like a hand squeezing a water balloon. The hardening and the pain are the result of this process. This condition frequently requires repeated surgery or painful nonsurgical treatment. It cannot be prevented from recurring. In a written document issued by the FDA in 1989, the agency stated: "The number of repeat surgeries that a patient may face in a lifetime to release contracted fibrous capsules is unknown. FDA believes that the risks associated with repeat surgeries for treating capsular contracture are significant."

- A growing number of women are showing up in the offices of rheumatologists, dermatologists, and internists with a variety of serious autoimmune diseases, ranging from crippling arthritic conditions to incurable connective tissue disorders, such as scleroderma. It is suspected that these disorders result from a silicone-induced disturbance of the immune system, leading the body to reject some of its own tissues as "foreign." According to the FDA, "Immunological sensitization may be a serious risk associated with the implantation of a silicone gel-filled breast prosthesis."[4]

- Virtually all silicone gel implants routinely "bleed" or ooze silicone gel, even with their outer shells completely intact. The phenomenon of "gel bleed" implies that the implants are causing the equivalent of repeated small injections of silicone into the bodies of women wearing them. According to the FDA:

  Silicone gel bleed through the intact envelope of breast implant is a serious risk associated with implantation of all silicone gel-filled breast implants, regardless of design. Gel bleed may result in deposition and migration of free silicone in the body leading to capsular contracture, silicone granuloma [an abnormal tissue reaction caused by a foreign substance], lymphadenopathy [enlarged lymph nodes due to a reaction to silicone] and other unknown systemic toxic effects.[5]

- Hundreds if not thousands of these implants rupture or develop large leaks spewing irretrievable amounts of silicone into the chest and beyond. So-called "migrating" silicone has been found in tissue throughout the bodies of affected women, and the health hazards of this free floating chemical are still being uncovered.

- Silicone gel has been found by its own major manufacturer (Dow Corning) to be a carcinogen (cancer-causing substance). These studies found that silicone gel caused highly malignant soft tissue cancer in laboratory animals. In an internal memo analyzing the company data, an FDA official stated that "while there is no direct proof that silicone causes cancers in humans, there is considerable reason to suspect that it can do so."[6]

- It is clear that implants can interfere with x-ray detection of breast cancer (mammography), which can result in delayed treatment for women in the early stages of the disease. Delayed treatment means reduced chances that treatment will work.

Addressing this problem the FDA wrote, "It is estimated that out of the more than 1 million women in the United States who have undergone augmentation mammaplasty, 100,000 (10 percent) will develop or already have developed breast cancer. [This figure results from assuming, for the sake of argument, that breast implants do not cause breast cancer; it is the same as the percentage of "normal" women who get breast cancer.] With the present evidence that silicone implants mask radiographic tumor detection [mammography], a significant number of these cancer patients may have worsened prognoses, once the cancer is [later] detectable by other means, such as by palpation [manual breast exam]."[7]

New techniques are being developed that improve the accuracy of mammography in women with breast implants. However, unless the technician and the radiologist are alerted to the fact that a woman has them, the exam will be done as though she doesn't. It is very important that both the x-ray technician who handles the equipment, and the radiologist who reads the picture, know that implants are involved.

KAREN'S STORY

The most damning evidence against silicone gel breast implants does not come from well designed scientific trials intended to protect consumers, because those were never done before these devices went on the market 25 years ago. The bad news is coming from people like Karen, who believes she is the living example of all that can go wrong.

In Karen's case, the implants were inserted during the same surgery that removed large amounts of precancerous breast tissue. Eleven years after her first breast implant, Karen now has scars from 10 breast surgeries that criss-cross her chest like train tracks. Two sets of implants have ruptured, scattering silicone into her body. And today, far worse than the scars across her chest, are the debilitating symptoms she endures of so-called "human adjuvant disease." This term is a relatively new one used to describe a series of problems uniquely linked to human silicone poisoning. Unfortunately, the disease has been named long before it can be treated.

In 1978 when Karen's surgery was performed, plastic surgeons were enamored of the "improved" breast implant prostheses on the market. Since they were first introduced in the early 1960s, implants with thinner outer shells had gotten softer to the touch. Plastic surgeons were among those lobbying manufacturers to liquify gel bag contents and make the bag itself thinner, so the result would be more lifelike. By 1978 they looked and felt more like real breasts than their bulkier predecessors.

Ironically, for many women with implants, the effort to engineer an artificial lifelike breast was wasted, because up to 40 percent of the time, their artificial breasts hardened up anyway soon after an implant was inserted.

The human body treats any artificial implant as a foreign object, no matter how soft or smooth. In cases of capsular contracture a woman's immune system mounts an all out attack on the object, but because it cannot be ejected, the body forms a collagen layer to wall it off. In some women this wall of scar tissue contracts over time. This shrinking scar capsule eventually compresses the implant, causing pain and deformity. As the capsule continues to contract over time, it pushes the implant into different positions and many patients complain, for instance, that one breast assumes a position higher than the other.

The scar tissue can be removed surgically or it can be "broken up" manually by the plastic surgeon, the so-called "nutcracker technique." Karen remembers the procedure well.

> The doctor tucked in his tie and the nurse held me down and I knew something was going to happen. Then he took both hands and applied extreme pressure and I thought my ribs were breaking because I heard a crackling sound.

I screamed and cried. He let me rest, then he did the other side.

The procedure broke her implants (she realized later) and her breasts hardened up again in two months.

Most women are told that their breasts could harden up and choose to have the surgery anyway. Product labeling years ago warned of this foreign body reaction, but did not include more detailed information about the outcome of women who suffer from it and the treatment it requires. In 1979 warning labels barely hinted of the problem that was already being experienced by women and would plague hundreds more in years to come. "Some patients, for unknown reasons, develop spherical contracture around the implant, post-op. This can cause discomfort, firmness and undesirable shape of the breast(s)."[8]

The treatment for capsular contracture seldom corrects the problem permanently, which often leads to multiple surgeries. After Karen's breasts hardened up again she had surgery to remove the tough scar tissue that had re-formed around her implants. It was from that point on that her general good health began to deteriorate. At first she developed lumps, under her arm, along her neck, and in her groin. Then they multiplied. "Back then I always wondered if the lumps had anything to do with my implants, but I was always told that since I had no breast tissue left, I had nothing to worry about. I didn't even need a mammogram," she recalls.

In 1989 the FDA would summarize for the scientific community what Karen intuitively suspected about her own experience.

In humans, numerous reports described silicone granulomas or lymphadenopathy in distant organs such as axillary lymph nodes, liver, kidney and even the brain which demonstrate silicone migration in patients that underwent augmentation mammaplasty 5–20 years earlier. . . . It may be assumed that silicone migration is a possible risk associated with silicone implants in general.[9]

Karen got sicker. Fatigue was constant, she lost weight and developed chest pain so severe that she had to quit work. The lumps persisted, and once again, her breasts hardened up. She returned to her plastic surgeon who "broke up" the scar tissue inside her breasts by manually squeezing and rotating them. Soon after a mammogram confirmed what she already suspected—that both implants had been ruptured.

After new implants were put in, the second set also failed. During each surgery, whatever free floating silicone that could be found was removed, but no one thought that all the free silicone had been retrieved. As months passed, Karen would experience what doctors now believe to be her body's immune system fending off droplets and clusters of a foreign substance—silicone—which had migrated throughout her body.

At her worst, just before final removal of her implants, Karen describes her condition this way:

> The skin on my arm had broken down, and my fingers were infected. The whites of my eyes were yellow. I had a fever and I was spitting up blood. My hair was falling out and it seemed that everything that could bleed, bled. I was so tired I could hardly walk.

When Karen finally had her implants removed she was not surprised, but still horrified at what the surgeon told her he had found. "There was so much old and new silicone in my chest he couldn't begin to get it all. It was like oil on rocks all over the place, he told me."

IMPLANTS FREQUENTLY RUPTURE

One breast implant company's own product label, as early as 1977, acknowledged that the bags could break:

> the silicone elastomer envelope of these products has a low tear strength and is thin to achieve desired prosthesis

softness and mobility. For these reasons, the envelope may be easily cut by a scalpel or ruptured by excessive stresses, manipulation with blunt instruments or penetration by a needle . . . should the silicone envelope be ruptured, [the company] cannot guarantee reliable gel containment and the prosthesis should be replaced.[10]

In other words, the company seemed to be claiming it wasn't responsible for what might happen if their gel bags broke, or somehow lost their contents into the bodies of women. It would be a problem that women themselves would have to live with.

In fact, experience had already shown that implants can rupture for a variety of reasons besides the thickness of the shell or accidents with a scalpel. Everyday life can strain them, including physical stresses such as manipulation, vigorous exercise, and trauma. As mentioned above, capsular contracture and manual treatment for it are both causes of implant rupture.

Rupturing gel bags became so common that even popular magazines made light of women who suddenly discovered something had "popped" and it wasn't their beads. Appallingly, even the plastic surgery community found the popping phenomenon humorous. In a 1977 edition of *Plastic and Reconstructive Surgery* a physician wrote:

Then, suddenly about one year ago, one could hear an occasional faint pop from afar, from the east. Soon the intensity increased until it sounded like the old 4th of July celebrations. What could it be? Anon, the mail informed us that large numbers of plastic surgeons, seemingly, were busily popping the fibrous capsules which formed around breast implants . . .[11]

The FDA did not consider the popping problem amusing in 1989 when it reviewed the evidence of its frequency and health risks.

The rates of implant rupture may vary according to the chemical composition and material design of the device, length of time of implantation, site of implantation, methods of postoperative management, incidence of capsular contracture, life-style of the recipient or other factors. It has been shown that rupture of the implant may result in the deposition and distant migration of silicone gel in the body with possible toxic effects.[12]

THE GEL BLEED PHENOMENON

Women were also never told, and are still not routinely told, that even silicone gel within an intact envelope routinely leaches into the body. The permeability of gel bags has been known about since the mid-1970s and silicone gel has been known to "bleed" or ooze even under the implant's own weight.[13] The possibility that gel bleed is responsible for capsular contractures and other complications is still being researched.

According to the FDA:

Silicone gel bleed through the semipermeable envelope of the breast implant is a serious risk associated with implantation of all silicone gel-filled breast implants, regardless of design. The rate of gel bleed may vary according to the chemical composition and material design of the device. The rate of gel bleed into the tissues through the envelopes of the so-called 'low-bleed' implants is unknown. . . . Gel bleed may result in deposition and migration of silicone gel in the body, via the blood and lymphatic system, with possible toxic effects. Neither the chemical forms of silicone which leach into the breast tissue nor their metabolic fates are known.[14]

MYSTERIOUS IMMUNE DISORDERS

In the early days, when Karen's medical problems first began, her symptoms mystified her physicians. A gynecologist told her to forget about her implants, they were safer than her own (then removed) breast tissue. A plastic surgeon referred her to a psy-chiatrist, who diagnosed her problems as hysterical, and self-induced. While Karen was met with distrust and outright disgust as she sought help, the problems she was having were not unknown to medical science.

In fact, the occurrence of connective tissue diseases in women with augmented breasts has been recognized for the past two decades. Cases of these disorders or other unclassifiable rheumatic syndromes following breast implants or silicone in-jections have appeared in many prestigious medical journals.[15] Now dozens of cases of these connective tissue diseases, chronic arthritis, or autoimmune disorders following breast augmenta-tions have been reported, including the debilitating connective tissue disorder, scleroderma, which is often fatal.

In its analysis of these risks, the FDA wrote:

> In recent years, a growing number of reports have raised questions about the relationship between silicone and var-ious autoimmune diseases, such as 'human adjuvant dis-ease' and connective tissue syndromes. Although published epidemiological studies did not clearly establish the cause-effect relationship, investigations with larger numbers of subjects are needed to rule out the possibility that silicone implants may induce one or more connective tissues dis-ease syndromes, particularly scleroderma and related dis-orders.[16]

It is estimated that there are many more as yet unreported cases of scleroderma. This is in part because implant patients are not followed by plastic surgeons for long periods. The la-tency period has ranged from 2 months to 25 years, with most cases occurring 10 to 15 years after the procedure. Most women have long since lost contact with the surgeon who first put in their implants.

Furthermore, these disorders are still rare enough that gen-eral medical practitioners may miss the connection between immune symptoms and 10-year-old implants. Unfortunately, even if more doctors are making the connection, medical insight leading to improved treatment has lagged behind. As one pathologist put it, "we are in the Dark Ages in terms of understanding this disease. We have not reached The Enlightenment yet."[17]

SILICONE'S QUESTIONABLE HISTORY

Much of the early use for injected silicone liquid was to augment soft tissue contours.[18] It was injected directly into the face, for instance, to correct forehead wrinkles, depressions or deformities of the face, to reconstruct chins, or to fill in smallpox and acne scars.

Silicone caused real excitement in the plastic surgery community because, compared to other liquid compounds such as paraffin and lanolin, it seemed to incite less of an inflammatory reaction in animals and humans. Nearly 350 times thicker than water, silicone seemed "cohesive," that is it stayed roughly where it was injected. Plastic surgeons considered this substance, which seemed to produce few side effects, to be relatively "inert" and thus the "ideal implant material."[19]

However, as long ago as the early 1960s, animal tests showed that mild inflammatory responses to silicone had something to do with the dose administered. Even one of the early proponents of liquid silicone injections, researcher Dr. Thomas D. Rees, saw evidence that large amounts of silicone were dangerous.

> A systemic response was only observed with massive subcutaneous injections or following intraperitoneal administration. In these rodents, vacuoles suggestive of silicone were scattered throughout the reticuloendothelial [immune processing] system, the liver, spleen, ovary, renal glomeruli and adrenal. In the baboon and mouse only, vacuolated, red and white blood cells were recovered from the peripheral blood but only following repeated injections.[20]

This showed early evidence that when confronted with large amounts of free floating silicone, the immune systems of test animals carried bits of silicone throughout their bodies.

In 1968 another researcher put it this way:

The very property which makes silicone an excellent surface lubricant causes the silicone to disappear from the
slide preparation when a biopsy is taken from a silicone
injected area. Hence, we do not know if the estimated 20
percent of silicone which leaves the site of injection goes
to the liver, kidneys, lungs or other organs. The metabolism
of injected silicone and method of excretion, if any, continues to remain a mystery.[21]

With so much doubt about the safety of silicone liquid, the
FDA in 1965 prohibited its use by injection for breast augmentation and severely restricted injected liquid silicone for other
cosmetic treatments. Reports have since shown that liquid silicone migrates in humans as well as animals.[22] There have been
reports of tumor formation in the foot after the injection of
silicone in the leg, and tumors found not only in the breast but
in the wall of the abdomen after (illegal) breast augmentation
with injectable silicone liquid.[23]

While liquid silicone injections thankfully lost their popularity, the dangers of silicone gel still remain vastly underrated
by most of the plastic surgery community. Plastic surgeons were,
of course, quick to applaud silicone gel breast implants when
they were first introduced to the cosmetic surgery market in the
1960s. A few years after the first gel bag was implanted, the
popular press was already endorsing this wonderful new innovation, that, like so many others in our cosmetic history, would
make women more feminine.

Writing in the *Boston Herald Traveler* in 1969, Dr. George
C. Thosteson offers advice to a reader. A 20-year-old woman
laments her small breasts and wonders if she should try silicone
injections to increase her bust size. The doctor warns her against
injections, but recommends she look into this new "suitably
shaped sack which contains the silicone. . . . The silicone does
not come in direct contact with tissues and the sack makes the
material stay in the shape and position desired."[24]

Another writer who decried the use of silicone injections

calling them "Cleopatra's needles" was ready in 1968 to put in his vote for silicone gel bags. "This method of mammary augmentation has proven extremely successful."[25]

It would be five years or so after these enthusiastic endorsements, in the early 1970s, that "human adjuvant disease" would first be described in medical literature, and that the term "gel bleed" would creep into outcome studies. Ten years later, sales of silicone gel prostheses would climb into a top position in the multi-billion dollar cosmetic surgery industry.

THE CANCER CONNECTION

Silicone gel implants could increase the amount of cancer in two ways: the properties of the chemical itself could be carcinogenic or the solid mass introduced to the body could promote ongoing tumor formation. To assess the implant's cancer risk, long-term studies (at least 15–20 years) would have to be undertaken, carefully following the occurrence of cancer in some of the thousands of women who get implants, and comparing this rate to similar women without implants. Amazingly, 25 years after silicone implants were first marketed, no such study has been done.

The largest clinical study of breast implants' cancer risk to humans was done by plastic surgeons and epidemiologists hired by an implant manufacturer. The study followed 3,111 women who had cosmetic augmentation from the records of 35 plastic surgeons in the Los Angeles area for an average of 11 years. The study reported no higher rate of development of breast cancer in women with implants.[26] Speaking in November 1988 before a panel of experts studying the safety of breast implants, one of the study's authors said, "Let me assure you that the risk is no greater than many of the hazards of every day life."[27]

However, the study was seriously flawed. Patients were followed for an average of 10 years, which is nowhere near the latency period (time between exposure to a cancer-causing substance and the diagnosis of cancer) of most human cancers. For example, radium, a known human carcinogen, causing bone sarcoma, has a latency period of 23 years at high doses, 35 years at low doses. Others include: vinyl chloride (liver cancer), 21 years; nickel (lung cancer), 24 years; hardwood dust (nasal cancer), 40 years; asbestos (lung cancer), 30 years. Thus, studying the effects of silicone for an average of only 10 to 12 years was grossly insufficient and hardly reassuring.

Furthermore, the study was criticized by the FDA, which concluded:

> This study has not contributed greatly to our understanding of the relationship between breast implants and the risk of breast cancer. . . . Based on these results, and the fact that silicone can migrate to other sites, the authors should have addressed this issue by including cancers at other sites, instead of limiting their study to only breast cancer."[28]

Animal studies have been more disturbing. An unpublished two-year rat carcinogenicity study which was done by the Dow Corning Company, the major manufacturer of silicone gel, attempted to determine whether silicone gel caused cancer in laboratory rats. The researchers studied three groups of animals, each including 50 males and 50 females. The first group (controls—not receiving silicone) developed none of the malignant fibrosarcoma tumors eventually seen in the silicone treated animals. The second group was implanted with silicone gel used pre-1976 and the third group with silicone gel used in current implant models. These animals received amounts of silicone comparable to the human "dose." Of note, 23 percent of all gel-treated animals developed fibrosarcoma, a soft tissue tumor, not found in the control group. Many of these silicone-induced tumors spread to distant organs.[29] Finally, 85 percent of these tumors caused the death of the animals bearing them.[30]

Despite having designed it to see if silicone gel caused cancer in rats, this study was discounted by Dow Corning as being "uniquely a rodent phenomenon. Therefore, that it [the animal evidence] is of no human health consequence as solid-state cancer in man has not been documented."[31]

One of the leading independent researchers in the field, Dr. Nir Kossovsky of U.C.L.A., responded the way many others in the cancer research community did.

It's hard for me to discount the animal data. We have philosophically accepted animal data as reasonably good models—particularly when we use numerous different species and with implants you can use just about any species and come up with a tumor. It's hard for me to conceive of a scenario where a human being is uniquely immune to a phenomenon that affects almost every other species.[32]

IMPROVING THE FEMALE BODY IMAGE

The real and well documented risks of getting breast implants should deter women from getting them just to go up a bra size, look better in a bikini, or take another step toward body perfection. There does, however, remain a small percentage of women, up to 15 percent, who have the operation to reconstruct their breasts following partial or radical mastectomy. The availability of artificial substances to replace surgically removed breast tissue was considered a significant medical breakthrough in the 1960s when mastectomy patients were first offered reconstruction. Today, many still consider it the only alternative that makes the radical treatment of breast cancer tolerable. For this group, breast reconstruction involves different considerations.

Illustrating this point, breast cancer patient Rosemary Locke testified before a panel of medical device experts at an FDA hearing in 1988:

We have resumed active lives, we wear the same clothing we did before breast cancer . . . when I get dressed in the morning and I look in the mirror, I am not constantly reminded that I may die. Our concern is that if you ban silicone implants, many women will delay diagnosis and treatment because they fear disfigurement. For many, quality of life is almost as important as life itself.[33]

The quality of life issue is more questionable for the vast majority (85 percent) of breast implant patients who receive them strictly for cosmetic reasons. Augmenting small breasts is a decidedly cultural phenomenon, practiced much more in this country than anywhere else in the world. While most women in the U.S. who undergo breast surgery for nonmedical reasons want their breasts enlarged, it is quite the opposite in France. According to interviews with French surgeons, French doctors perform three to four times more breast reductions than augmentations. Furthermore, because American women want bigger breasts, their plastic surgeons usually use a prosthesis about one and one-half times the size of those used in France.[34]

Not only is surgical breast augmentation a uniquely American fetish, but the 1990s may prove to be a more avowedly and longer lasting breasty era than were the 1950s, when we last idealized curvaceous feminine figures. Market analysts, fashion designers, and anthropologists agree that big bustlines came back in the 1980s after a couple of decades of mingling sex roles and our passing interest in androgyny. "In the 60s and 70s the tubular body and small breasts were the body image that helped women feel they could be taken seriously as they competed for careers against men," says Dr. Ann Kearney-Cooke, a Cincinnati psychologist who specializes in body image problems in women. "It was an era when motherhood lost prestige and with women's bodies deemphasized their ultimate symbol of mothering and nurturence, namely their breasts."[35]

Now, the value of motherhood is back, but unlike the 1950s, the importance of childrearing and family is reemerging amongst women who are well established in their careers. The result is that once again big busts are the preferred body type and the image for which many in this new generation of women strive. While some women chafe at the notion that women's bodies are (once again) being reshaped to correspond to the whim of the times, cultural anthropologists say now it's women themselves who are promoting big busts.

Market analyst and anthropologist John Lowe links it to what he calls the "baby on board" generation of working women who are discovering in their 30s that nurturing and childbearing are as important as success in the workplace.

> It would be hard to think of a group that has achieved more penetration of career goals than women have in the last two decades and I think having achieved that success there is a tendency to be less concerned about making it in a man's world by imitating men. Women are essentially re-discovering their femininity and obviously breasts empha-size gender differences.[36]

Fashion historian Laura Sinderbrand agrees that after years of modeling themselves after men, women are secure enough in the workplace to show off their femininity. "Women have decided that equality is not looking like men. It's being able to have the feminine body accepted in its own right." Fashion, as always, has responded. "Designers have produced busty clothes in the past and they haven't caught on," says Sinderbrand. "Now they are. This time it's what women want, even more than men, I think."[37]

WHOM SHOULD YOU TRUST?

As she eagerly awaits her appointment with the plastic surgeon, Monica remains a believer. Anything this permanent, this impor-tant, this popular, has to be safe. Isn't there a stamp, or a seal somewhere that proves they're safe, like the kind you find on hair dryers and vacuum cleaners?

Amazingly, these products that will rest inside Monica's chest supposedly for the rest of her life have no stamp of ap-proval, no safety seal, nothing. Silicone gel breast implants have been on the market since the early 1960s but they still have yet to be tested by stringent federal standards for safety. Why? Be-cause the government waited for 14 years for the standards to be established.

In general, regulation of the $14 billion a year medical device industry has had a short and inadequate history. It wasn't even until 1976 that medical devices were subject to any form of scrutiny by the FDA before being placed on the market. Prompted by problems with the Dalkon Shield (an intrauterine device), Congress passed the Medical Device Amendments of 1976. These amendments established a framework for regulating all medical devices, from tongue depressors to heart valves, including standards and pre-market testing. In other words, from 1976 on, most medical devices which presented significant health risks were supposed to be tested for safety in humans before they went on the market, not after.

By 1976, however, hundreds of thousands of women were already wearing breast implants, and unfortunately, the passing of these consumer protection laws has done little to ensure the safety of those receiving them in the last 14 years. The Amendments lumped medical devices into one of three "classes" which defined how stringent their safety review process would be. "Class I" included things like tongue depressors and didn't require any testing, only labelling. "Class II" included things like suction pumps and theoretically all devices placed in this category did require performance standards. Any device put in "Class III" would be subject to the most stringent pre-market safety testing. Some life-supporting devices, for example, would technically be classified there.

Silicone gel implants were designated Class II devices in 1978 and, under pressure from plastic surgeons and silicone implant manufacturers, they remained in that category, although no performance standard was ever developed until 1988, when the FDA finally assigned the devices to the most stringent Class III category.

> FDA classified the silicone gel-filled breast prosthesis into class III because insufficient information exists to determine that general controls would provide reasonable assurance of the safety and effectiveness of the device or to establish a performance standard to provide such assurance. FDA has weighed the probable risks and benefits to the public from the use of the silicone gel-filled breast

prosthesis and believes that the studies . . . present evidence of significant risks associated with the use of the device. These risks must be addressed by manufacturers of the device.[38]

But what has this meant to women? By not requiring stringent and specific safety testing as early as 1976, the government has basically allowed silicone manufacturers to profit from untested and unsafe devices and ultimately women have become walking test sites. Even though the FDA reclassified implants in 1988, all silicone prosthesis manufacturers still have at least until the end of 1991 to submit safety data justifying the continued marketing of their implants.

THE CASE OF THE DISAPPEARING IMPLANT

Meanwhile, as the FDA awaits persuasive evidence from gel bag manufacturers that their product is safe in human bodies, women by the thousands continue to assume that research stands behind the implants that they read about in popular magazines. Monica's biggest concern is capsular contracture. She worries that it will hurt to have it fixed and doesn't want repeat surgeries, so she's shopped around a little. She easily found a surgeon who will implant the prosthesis specifically designed to reduce the hardening problem. She has decided on silicone gel implants with a covering made of polyurethane foam.

For the past few years these have been in vogue in parts of Canada and in southern California and may account for 20 to 25 percent of the U.S. market in breast prosthesis.[39] Soft but tough, polyurethane implants have been sold as the answer to everyone's worries. Not only do they reduce hardening, they are also less likely to pop.

In fact, leading researchers are calling these products possibly more unsafe than their silicone elastic covered predecessors. "Polyurethane is insane," said one. "Just bloody stupid."[40] The foam shell was designed to disrupt the formation of fiber forming cells or fibroblasts which lead to the hard scarring surrounding breast implants. Unlike the smooth surfaces of silicone gel bags themselves, the foam creates a lattice effect which is supposed to confuse fibroblasts, interfering with the formation of concentric layers of scar tissue, which may contract.

The result is less scarring, because these foam implants create a steady state of inflammation which preempts scarring. This continuous inflammatory response is caused by the slow disintegration of the foam inside the chest. Tests show that polyurethane breaks down in heat, ultraviolet radiation, enzymatic attack, oxidation or mechanical stress during use.[41]

The fate of the "outer shell" is already being seen by scientists. Over time there are going to be thousands of microscopic pieces of it around the implant whether they are in the capsule or in the surrounding breast tissue and they are not going to go away. These pieces of plastic are staying within the body and no one knows in the long run what will happen to the women wearing them.

In women's bodies, the foam readily breaks down under the sort of enzymatic activity that inflammatory cells are extraordinarily efficient at generating. Again, after thousands of women have had these implanted, the FDA released their opinion of these implants:

> Data in experimental animals showed that polyurethane coated silicone implants degrade within 6 to 12 months after implantation. Risk characterization of the degradation of polyurethane implants in humans has not appeared in the open literature although polyurethane foam was expected to degrade within one to two years.[42]

After this disintegration of the foam, little bits of free floating polyurethane particles are dispersed—each evoking its own little inflammatory reaction. These foam particles tend to be small enough to be eaten up by cells and carried all around the chest wall or perhaps carried off by the lymph system. "Neither the chemical form of the polyurethane which disintegrates within the body, nor its distribution or its metabolic fate are known."[43]

In the end, after an estimated two to four years of this

dissolving process and the outer coat has sufficiently broken down, the silicone gel bag is exposed. Women are then left with all the problems that have been documented with the gel-filled bags, plus the scattered polyurethane everywhere.

Possibly the nastiest aspect of this product is there is no turning back. Because of its fragmentation, retrieving the prosthesis is virtually impossible and women are left with the possibility of a future cursed with chronic inflammatory reaction, infection problems, pain, and other immune responses.

THE "GIFT" THAT TURNED INTO A NIGHTMARE

On a chilly fall day in 1989, Susan, 43, entered the hospital one more time. She was to undergo her sixth breast surgery, and, she prayed, her last. After years of pain and deformity, she wanted her silicone gel breast implants out of her chest. For good. No replacements, no treatments, no more drugs.

On the way to the hospital she recalled the reason she had decided on implants in 1972—and it seemed like a cruel joke. New, fuller breasts had been a gift to herself, one she assumed was completely safe. She had read an advertisement about breast implants in the newspaper and all the news sounded good: the procedure was uncomplicated, and she would be in and out the same day. Simple, safe, affordable. "It was exactly the same feeling as having an empty corner in your living room and going out and putting a chair there," she recalled. "As easy as that."

But it was never easy. Her breasts were never right after surgery. Within several months they hardened up and "stuck out of my chest like two tennis balls." One was lower than the other. They were painful. She had problems with massive bruising and nerve damage. All these "technical failures" with her implants were resolved with repeated surgeries and drugs over the years that followed. But having "breasts that never looked or felt human" could not be remedied. In the end, it was not the cosmetic disappointment that convinced Susan to have her implants removed. She was terrified of becoming a medical statistic.

After a year of agonizing about what to do, she finally

decided to risk "looking awful," as her doctors convinced her she would, and have her implants taken out for good.

"I decided it would be better to be healthy and look bad, than sick and look busty," she said.

Four months after the surgery, Susan says she "feels like a ten-year-old." She is flat chested but not shriveled and unattractive as she feared she would be after having her implants removed. "If I had known I would feel like this I would have had those horrible water balloons taken out years ago."

Susan is also sure of physical improvements that go beyond the way she looks. She says hip and knee joint pain is gone, as are the headaches she endured in the last few years she wore implants.

She also says she feels incredibly lucky. After 17 years of repeated surgeries, constant pain, awkward, artificial, and deformed-looking breasts, it's over. But she's cautious, very cautious about predicting her future health, and she is adamant that women who wear implants are being deeply wronged. "I never consented to being part of a medical experiment and now I know that's exactly what I and thousands of other misguided women have been."

IMPLANT INFORMATION AVAILABLE

Anyone who wants information about implants can write:

> The Command Trust Network, Inc.
> Post Office Box 17082
> Covington, Kentucky 41017

This consumer group was formed to help women make better decisions about having breast implants put in or, if already in, coping with the complications.

The Public Citizen Health Research Group has a clearinghouse for plaintiffs' attorneys who are engaged in litigation against silicone gel breast implant manufacturers. For information about the clearinghouse, write:

Health Research Group
Silicone Gel Clearinghouse
7th Floor
2000 P Street N.W.
Washington, D.C. 20036

1. Kirchner M. How much have your colleagues raised their fees? Medical Economics 1989; 66:109.

2. Talcott T., consultant, chemical engineer, contract researcher and former employee of Dow Corning. Interview with author, October 1989.

3. McGhan Medical Corporation. Product information on mammary implants, 1988.

4. FDA. 515B Regulation Preamble, 1989 draft, pg. 3 & 10.

5. Ibid, 8.

6. Memo entitled "Analysis of Dow Corning Data Regarding Carcinogenicity of Silicone Gels," from Dr. M.E. Stratmeyer, Acting Chief, Health Sciences Branch, Center for Devices and Radiological Health, FDA to Director, Office of Science and Technology, Center for Devices and Radiological Health, August 9, 1988.

7. FDA, op. cit., 24.

8. Dow Corning Corporation. Product label on Mammary Implants, October 1979.

9. FDA, op. cit., 9

10. Heyer-Schulte Corporation. Product information on Gel-filled Mammary Prostheses, February 1977.

11. McDowell F. Pop goes the breast! Capsule or Implant? Beginning or End? Plastic and Reconstructive Surgery 1977; 59:836–7.

12. FDA, op. cit., 22.

13. Barker DE, Retsky MI, Schultz S. "Bleeding" of silicone from bag-gel breast implants and its clinical relation to fibrous capsule reaction. Plastic and Reconstructive Surgery 1978; 61:836–41.

14. FDA, op. cit., 23.

15. van Nunen SA, Gatenby PA, Basten A. Post-mammoplasty connective tissue disease. Arthritis and Rheumatism 1982; 25:694–7; Baldwin CM, Kaplan EN. Silicone-induced human adjuvant disease? Annals of Plastic Surgery 1983; 10:270–3; Okano Y, Nishikai M, Sato A. Scleroderma, primary biliary cirrhosis and Sjogren's syndrome after cosmetic breast augmentation with silicone injection: case report of possible human adjuvant disease. Annals of the Rheumatic Diseases 1984; 43:520–2; Kumagai Y, Shiokawa Y, Medsger TA, Rodnan GP. Clinical spectrum of connective tissue disease after cosmetic surgery. Observations on 18 patients and a review of the Japanese literature. Arthritis and

Rheumatism 1984; 27:1–12; Fock KM, Feng PH, Tey BH. Autoimmune disease developing after augmentation mammoplasty: report of 3 cases. Journal of Rheumatology 1984; 11:98–100.

16. FDA, op. cit., 10.

17. Personal interview with Dr. Douglas R. Shanklin, Professor of Pathology, Obstetrics and Gynecology at the University of Tennessee, October 1989.

18. Wegener, EH. The problem of correction of forehead wrinkles. Med.Kosmetrik. 1957; 5:136–7.

19. Rees TD, Ballantyne DL, Coburn RJ. Liquid silicone therapy—A decade's experience. In Principles and Techniques of Human Research and Therapeutics, Vol. II, F. Gilbert McMahon. Futura Publishing Co., Inc.: Mt. Kisco, New York, 1974, 169–81.

20. Ibid.

21. Norling EP. Cleopatra's Needle. Medical Bulletin, Orange County, California, October 1968.

22. Parsons RW, Thering HR. Management of the silicone-injected breast. Plastic and Reconstructive Surgery 1977; 60:534–8.

23. Ortiz-Monasterio F, Trigoss I. Management of patients with complications from injection of foreign materials into the breasts. Plastic and Reconstructive Surgery 1972; 50:42–7.

24. Thosteson GC. Her figure lacks firmness. Boston Herald Traveler, January 9, 1969.

25. Norling, op. cit.

26. Deapen DM, Pike MC, Casagrande JT, Brody, GS. The relationship between breast cancer and augmentation mammaplasty: an epidemiologic study. Plastic and Reconstructive Surgery 1986; 77:361–7.

27. Statement of Dr. Gary Brody, representative of the American Society of Plastic and Reconstructive Surgery, before General and Plastic Surgery Devices panel meeting, Food and Drug Administration, November 22, 1988.

28. Memo entitled "A review of the article entitled 'The Relationship Between Breast Cancer and Augmentation Mammaplasty: An Epidemiologic Study,' authored by Deapen DM et al." from Epidemiology Branch, Food and Drug Administration to Melvin Stratmeyer, July 25, 1988.

29. "Analysis of Dow Corning Data Regarding Carcinogenicity of Silicone Gels," op. cit.

30. Memo entitled "Review of toxicity data for silicone gel" from Robert L. Sheridan, Office of Device Evaluation, Food and Drug Administration to Arthur R. Norris, National Center for Toxicological Research, Food and Drug Administration, July 28, 1988.

31. Ibid.

32. Kossovsky N., of UCLA. Interview with author, October 1989.

33. Locke R. Testimony before General and Plastic Surgery panel, FDA Hearings, 1988, op. cit.

34. Payer L. Medicine & Culture; Varieties of Treatment in the United States, England, West Germany, and France. Henry Holt and Company: New York, 1988.

35. Kearney-Cooke A. Interview with author, October 1989.

36. Lowe J. Interview with author, October 1989.

37. Sinderbrand L. Interview with author, October 1989.

38. FDA, op. cit., 21.

39. Ibid., 19.

40. Kossovsky, op. cit.

41. FDA, op. cit., 18.

42. Ibid., 18–19.

43. Ibid., 25.

HYSTERECTOMY

The Myth of Cures by Cutting

At the current hysterectomy rate, one in three women in this country will lose their uteruses by the time they reach age 60.

- The most common problems for which women get hysterectomies can often be treated successfully by nonsurgical means.

- Even though most hysterectomies are done because of uterine fibroids, this is not a dangerous condition and often doesn't require treatment of any kind.

- Up to 15 percent of women who get hysterectomies need repeat surgery for complications related to the original operation. Nearly half experience complications ranging from high fever to urinary problems as a result of surgery.

- Many women complain of impaired sexual functioning after hysterectomy.

- Nearly 90 percent of all hysterectomies are done for benign diseases, in many cases ones that will go away— or not impair health—without treatment of any kind.

- If American women had hysterectomies at the same rate as women in the United Kingdom and Denmark, there would be only one-half as many done, 300,000 fewer women each year.

- We estimate conservatively that, in the United States, at least one-quarter of all hysterectomies done a year, or 150,000, are unnecessary.

Recommendations

Hysterectomy should be the solution of last, not first, resort except in very specific instances. These include invasive cancer and rare emergencies where removing the uterus can save your life.

- If you have fibroids (which account for 30 percent of all hysterectomies) and no symptoms or problems such as infertility, you probably do not need any surgery. Have regular exams to make sure the fibroids are not growing rapidly.

- If you suffer from relentless pain in your pelvic area and your physician immediately recommends a hysterectomy, shop for a new physician. You should be given a battery of tests and offered other alternatives first before being advised that surgery is necessary.

*O*VER the last three decades the uterus has become a favored target of surgical abuse. Twenty-five years ago, hysterectomy was the most common surgical procedure in this country. In 1975, one-third of all women in the United States reaching age 60 no longer had a uterus.[1] The prevailing gynecological attitude could be summed up in the words of one often quoted gynecologist Dr. Ralph C. Wright: "After the last planned pregnancy, the uterus becomes a useless, bleeding, symptom-producing, potentially cancer-bearing organ and therefore should be removed."[2]

Today, the legacy of the "useless uterus" lives on. Hysterectomies have now become the second most common surgery in the United States, second only to cesarean section (see pages 73–111). In the 1990s, as was the case in 1975, one in three women will have had a hysterectomy by age 60. The vast majority of women undergoing hysterectomies are between 20 and 49, typically in their early forties.[3]

The number of hysterectomies is too high, even though over the past 10 years there has been a decrease in the total number, from a high in 1978 of 725,000 to approximately 600,000 currently. This has occurred despite an increase in the size of the total population of women "at risk" (all women age 15 and beyond).

While these figures might seem encouraging, the disturbing fact is that many hysterectomies—at least 25 percent—are extremely questionable, if not clearly unnecessary. The operation has always played an important role in treating cancer, but only about 10 percent of hysterectomies are done for cancerous growth.[4] The vast majority of hysterectomies are not done to save lives. They are "elective," attempts to conquer problems like abnormal bleeding, pelvic pain, benign tumors, and overall discomfort or inconvenience.

In the United States we have roughly twice the rate (number per 100,000 women) of hysterectomies as Denmark and the United Kingdom, and more than three times the number in Sweden and Norway.[5] Could it be that women in this country have diseased reproductive organs at a rate two or three times that of women in Europe?

Data from 1987 show that a woman under 45 living in the western part of this country is twice as likely to get a hysterectomy as a woman living in the Northeast.[6] In fact, the rate can vary dramatically between cities in the same area. The number of women in San Diego getting hysterectomies is so high, one commentator joked at the absurdity of it. "What do you call a woman in San Diego who still has her uterus?" Answer: "A tourist."

Unfortunately, what isn't comical is the fact that many women are losing perfectly healthy organs for no good reason and some will suffer both short-term and permanent consequences. In many cases there are a variety of safe and effective alternatives to this radical surgery. Even though the risk of dying from complications of hysterectomy is low—one per 1000[7]—because of the vast numbers of women undergoing hysterectomy that risk translates to over 600 women a year who will die from the surgery. As we will see later, a litany of other physical and emotional consequences are much more frequent. Furthermore, as many women will assert, removing the uterus doesn't always guarantee a solution to the problems. In fact, much of the time hysterectomies create problems that didn't exist before surgery.

WHAT IS A HYSTERECTOMY?

A hysterectomy is a relatively simple procedure that involves cutting away the uterus. It doesn't typically take more than an hour and a half and is most often done through a six to eight inch midline incision running down from the navel or across the lower abdomen below the pubic hairline. This is called an abdominal hysterectomy. The operation can also be done through the vagina, which is called a vaginal hysterectomy. These are done less frequently than in the past. One study showed that women undergoing vaginal hysterectomies experience fewer complications than women having abdominal surgery. However, vaginal hysterectomies do involve a higher risk of injury to the bladder.[8]

For either vaginal or abdominal hysterectomy there are several kinds of operations including:

- Total hysterectomy, which usually means cutting away the uterus and the cervix (mouth of the womb).
- Subtotal or partial hysterectomy, the removal of the uterus, leaving the cervix behind.
- Oophorectomy, the removal of an ovary.
- Bilateral oophorectomy, in which both ovaries are excised.
- Bilateral salpingo-oophorectomy, the removal of both ovaries and the fallopian tubes.

BEYOND THE "BABY BAG": YOUR UTERUS HAS A LIFELONG ROLE

Even if you don't want children, have had your last pregnancy, or have reached menopause, your uterus plays an important role as a living, functioning organ.

You may have been told that only your ovaries act as hormone producers but, as might be expected, the ovaries do not act alone as regulators of female fertility. The uterus also plays an important role in the complex process of receiving and circulating sex hormones. It acts as a receptor site for estrogen and progesterone.

It has been acknowledged for a long time that the ovarian function is more than reproductive. Hormones produced in the ovaries seem to reduce the amount of cholesterol in the blood and help with calcium absorption. Thus ovaries play a role in long-term prevention of heart disease and osteoporosis (see pages 193–222). Research has shown that women with surgically removed ovaries may have more than twice the risk of developing coronary heart disease, compared to women who have not had the surgery.[9]

Anatomically, the uterus rests in a central position among a variety of other pelvic organs, helping to keep them in place. One possible result of removing this pear-shaped organ is a "vault prolapse," which basically means your vagina falls out of position. The vagina, once held up by the uterus, no longer has a secure suspension system after a hysterectomy. The result may be very unpleasant, can occur years after the surgery, and can be very difficult to treat successfully.

Following hysterectomies women have reported the loss of sexual desire, weaker orgasms, loss of pleasure from penetration, fewer sexual fantasies, slower arousal, and sometimes even aversion to being touched.[10] One study showed that between 33 and 46 percent of women complained of reduced sexual responsiveness after hysterectomy when ovaries were removed also.[11]

Women have also reported the opposite, feeling no loss of pleasure and only "liberation" from anxiety about pregnancy. Obviously sexual response is highly individual, but the fact that removal of the uterus may have an effect on your sex life is another important reason why the organ belongs with you for your lifetime, if possible.

WHEN HYSTERECTOMY IS NECESSARY

We are devoting most of this chapter to the kinds of medical conditions which are more likely to result in questionable hysterectomies. However, there are cases where removal of the uterus is the best and only option.

Hysterectomy for Cancer

Women with invasive cancer of the uterus, ovaries, cervix, or fallopian tubes should have a hysterectomy, unless some other treatment (radiation or chemotherapy) is more appropriate. Cancer of the nearby organs (such as the bladder or large intestine) that also involves the reproductive organs is another valid reason to have a hysterectomy. This operation should be planned both with a gynecologist and an oncologist (cancer specialist) who can review all treatment options.

Emergency Hysterectomy

If the uterus ruptures during childbirth, during an abortion, or during some other operation (such as dilation and curettage—D&C) a hysterectomy may be needed immediately to prevent the woman from bleeding to death.

Trauma to the pelvic area, like a gunshot wound, a stabbing, or some other laceration might also require removal of the damaged uterus.

Finally, severe infection of the uterus and fallopian tubes, particularly when associated with peritonitis, ruptured abscess (pus collection), and shock may necessitate emergency hysterectomy.

ELECTIVE HYSTERECTOMIES

There are other situations where you might be told you need a hysterectomy; in some cases it may be a sound solution to your problem and in some cases not. Most of the time your condition will fall into the categories below, which constitute 90 percent of all hysterectomies performed in this country. These include:

- fibroids· (benign growths along the wall of the uterus)
- pelvic pain (or milder discomfort)
- abnormal bleeding (and inconvenience)

These distinctions are somewhat arbitrary, because there is a great deal of overlap between symptoms and diagnosis. In fact, one of the reasons it is hard to pinpoint why the hysterectomy rate is very high in this country is that physicians regularly lump symptoms and diagnoses together, and it is somewhat unclear which, if any, justify the removal of this precious reproductive organ.

Having fibroids is not, in itself, a reason to have your uterus removed. Neither is pelvic pain or abnormal bleeding. However, depending on the training, habit, or temperament of your gynecologist, you may be told the only adequate treatment is to take your uterus out. Determining other possible sources for your symptoms takes time and patience. Alternative treatments for pain or bleeding may not be as appealing as an alleged surgical quick fix, so if your physician's underlying attitude is that the uterus isn't worth keeping anyway, removing it will be a short cut, but an irreversible one.

Fibroids: Doing Nothing Is Often Enough

Uterine fibroids account for 30 percent of all hysterectomies done in this country. Most of the time when hysterectomies are done for removal of fibroids, they are done on young women between ages 35 and 54.[12]

Fibroids are abnormal masses of the smooth muscle tissue that often form within the uterus. They are also called "fibroid tumors," "myomas," or "leiomyomas," and they can be soft, hard, small as a pinhead, or larger than a grapefruit. They are almost always benign. Less than 1 in 1,000 are found to contain a sarcoma, a type of cancer, usually cured by hysterectomy.[13] It is estimated that up to 50 percent of all women have fibroids at some point in their reproductive lives.[14]

Many women never know they have fibroids. Small fibroids which dot the uterus may create no symptoms at all and may only be discovered through a routine exam. They may also be detected through ultrasound. Indeed, much of the time even large fibroids do not bother the women who have them or pose any risk. There is no reason to do anything about fibroids that don't bother you.

If fibroids begin to grow rapidly, they may need to be removed, but if the growth is slow, they may not. If a biopsy reveals that the tissue suggests cancer, a hysterectomy may be necessary. But monitoring and tissue testing should be performed first, for a hysterectomy is not automatically necessary. One of the most common reasons that women are told they must have a hysterectomy for fibroids is that the uterus is so large that the gynecologist cannot feel the ovaries and so can't be sure that there are no ovarian tumors. Although this sounds logical, this reasoning is nonsensical and should not be used to justify hysterectomy for two reasons:

1. Newer vaginal ultrasound has made examination and measurement of the ovaries simple and safe, even in cases of large uterine fibroids.
2. Gynecologists do not routinely recommend surgery to obese women, even though they cannot feel their ovaries through the thickness of the abdominal wall.

If you do have symptoms from your fibroids, these might include the following:

■ abnormal bleeding
■ abdominal swelling
■ infertility
■ pelvic or back pain

- constipation
- severe menstrual cramps

All of these symptoms, however, can also occur without any fibroids.

Commonly, hysterectomies have been done when any of the above occur with fibroids, or when they have reached a certain size, even without symptoms. It is important to keep in mind that you can have some of these symptoms, and some small fibroids, but that doesn't necessarily mean that the fibroids are causing your problems. Too often, physicians automatically conclude that your symptoms and fibroids are related and rush to take your uterus out only to discover later that the pain you experienced was due to an irritated bowel or a gastrointestinal problem. Fibroids are not always, or even most of the time, the culprits.

Women should question any doctor who immediately suggests a hysterectomy for fibroids, with or without symptoms, before other more conservative measures are exhausted. These include:

- nonnarcotic mild analgesics (painkillers) for pelvic pain or menstrual cramps
- discontinuing the use of estrogen pills such as Premarin (estrogen causes enlargement of fibroids)
- fiber supplements for constipation
- simple surgery such as a D&C.

On the other hand, very large fibroids can be painful. They can push on the bladder, bowel, or nerves, causing severe pelvic pain. They can cause vascular alterations in the uterine lining, dilating the blood vessels and resulting in abnormal bleeding. If you suffer from painful or bleeding fibroids, you might want to consider myomectomy, a surgical alternative to hysterectomy, which involves removing the fibroids and leaving the uterus behind. Traditionally, this approach has been reserved for women who want to preserve their fertility, or for women who are having problems conceiving due to fibroids. However, myomectomy should be offered to many more women.

Myomectomies are more complicated, require more surgical skill, take longer, and are bloodier procedures than hysterectomies. This means they present a slightly greater risk of transfusion to the patient. For these reasons many gynecologists shy away from myomectomy, especially for patients they define as "older," meaning near menopause or beyond. Gynecologists who are unskilled at doing myomectomies may convince the patient the procedure is dangerous.

Gynecologists may also tell women with fibroids not to have a myomectomy because there is a chance of regrowth, although this occurs less often in older than younger women. In fact, this only recurs to a degree requiring treatment 10 percent of the time.[15] Many women who want to save their uteruses are willing to take the chance they will have to be operated on again for new fibroids in the future. However, if your gynecologist doesn't like doing myomectomies, you will probably not be offered that option. Remember, neither myomectomy nor hysterectomy is appropriate treatment in most cases of fibroids.

In sum, many women do not need surgery of any kind for fibroids. You may need to have a hysterectomy in the following cases:

- If your fibroids are clearly the cause of chronic bleeding that doesn't respond to D&C or hormonal tablets and restricts your activity or results in chronic anemia that cannot be corrected with iron.

- If your fibroids are accompanied by severe pain that doesn't respond to analgesics, and other sources of pain have been ruled out.

- If your fibroids are growing rapidly (doubling in size in a six month period of time) and have reached a size greater than a uterus at three months pregnancy (larger than a grapefruit).

Before agreeing to a hysterectomy for your fibroids, you should have had a D&C first if you've been bleeding. This is minor surgery which involves scraping the inside of the uterus to obtain a biopsy. You should also have been through an extensive work-up to rule out other sources of pain and/or bleeding and gotten a second opinion. Also, ask about getting a myomectomy.

Remember that fibroids tend to shrink after menopause when estrogen levels drop. Beware of any doctor who says you need a hysterectomy because your fibroids are bound to grow larger. That's not necessarily true.

The Mysteries of Pelvic Pain

There are two kinds of pelvic pain for which tens of thousands of hysterectomies are done annually.

- Pain that can be traced to disease.
- Pain that can't be traced to any pathology.

The latter type of "chronic pelvic pain" (CPP) remains mysterious and frustrating to patients and physicians alike. It's a problem for which thousands of healthy uteruses are removed each year in the U.S. We will show that recent studies have revealed important new evidence that hysterectomy for chronic pelvic pain may be unnecessary 80 percent of the time.

When Disease Causes Pelvic Pain: There are several common disorders of the reproductive organs besides fibroids that can cause pain. A huge number of hysterectomies are done for the reasons listed below:

- Endometriosis
- Adenomyosis
- Chronic pelvic infection

In cases where pain can be traced to a pathological uterine cause, hysterectomy may be a final solution, but not before pain management has been attempted, other medical and nonmedical means of suppressing the disorder have failed, and a complete investigation into the possibility of nongynecological sources has been done.

According to new guidelines published by the American College of Obstetricians and Gynecologists,[16] hysterectomies for chronic pelvic pain should never be performed until the following have been tried and proven unsuccessful:

- Evaluation of all of the following possible sources of pain:
  - urinary
  - gastrointestinal
  - musculoskeletal (back, hips, etc.)
- Therapeutic trial of at least one of the following:
  - diuretics
  - nonsteroidal antiinflammatory drugs
  - oral contraceptives
  - induced amenorrhea

Endometriosis and adenomyosis: Nationally, next to fibroid tumors, the second most common benign condition that results in a hysterectomy is endometriosis, over two-thirds of these occurring in young women aged 25 to 44.[17] Endometriosis is a condition where tissue normally found within the uterine lining (endometrium) grows elsewhere. Most often these transplanted growths occur within the pelvic cavity, on the fallopian tubes, ovaries, even on the surface of the bowels. They can, however, be found as far away as the lungs, thighs and chest.

Despite the fact that it is commonly regarded as justifying a hysterectomy, in most cases endometriosis is not a painful condition. One recent study of women undergoing routine tubal ligation showed that the number of women with endometriosis in a group of women with pelvic pain was exactly the same as in a group without pain.[18] When a woman suffers from pain and a few spots of endometriosis are found, gynecologists are often quick to connect the two. Before a hysterectomy is done, an exhaustive search for other causes of the pain should be done, and other treatment should be attempted.

Bridgett, 52, suffered constant pain in her lower abdomen and had a hysterectomy after her physician identified a small patch of endometriosis on her uterus. After the operation, her pain continued and it was later found to be a bladder problem that required further surgery. Endometriosis was not the cause of her pain. The hysterectomy was unnecessary.

Endometriosis, however, can be painful in some instances. It can cause pain throughout the lower back and the entire pelvic area that intensifies during periods and while having intercourse. Endometriosis can also cause infertility; in fact, 15 to 25 percent of all infertile women have endometriosis,[19] but many women who are fertile also have endometriosis.

It is important that a clear diagnosis of endometriosis is made before a hysterectomy is even considered. This is done most effectively using a laparoscope, which is a small lighted tube that is inserted through an incision beneath the navel.

Having a hysterectomy for endometriosis should still be the treatment of last resort after attempting pain management and other non-surgical and surgical approaches, such as laser treatment. Recent analysis of more than 27 separate studies involving almost 1200 women with pain associated with endometriosis between 1958 and 1986 revealed that simple, inexpensive, and relatively safe medical treatment such as progesterone tablets or birth control pills were effective in relieving symptoms in 86 to 95 percent of all cases.

One caution: the response rate from these drugs was identical to that obtained with the use of Danazol (88 percent), which is far more expensive and has many unpleasant side effects (including weight gain, acne, facial hair growth and possibly depression) and which appears to increase cholesterol levels to potentially dangerous levels.[20]

Trying these routes first is especially useful for women who are near menopause because, like fibroids, endometriosis is estrogen-dependent and will probably dry up after menopause.

Adenomyosis is a condition which used to be called "internal endometriosis" because with this disease the endometrial lining grows abnormally inside the uterus, invading the surrounding muscle walls and causing the organ to grow bulky and large. Some women with this abnormality have no symptoms at all, although some other women experience pain and heavy bleeding.[21] If you have adenomyosis and have few if any symptoms, or symptoms that respond to simple medical therapy, hysterectomy is not necessary.

Infections: Persistent infection of the reproductive organs (chronic pelvic inflammatory disease—PID) which fails to improve despite long-term antibiotic treatment can be an appropriate reason for a hysterectomy. PID is usually caused by a sexually transmitted infection. It can be a debilitating and maddeningly persistent disease which may not be detected until it has spread from the uterus to the fallopian tubes, where it becomes more dangerous and harder to treat. If oral antibiotics don't clear up the infection, it may be that it has progressed to a point where this route of antibiotic administration is not effective. In some cases, hospitalization will be required in order to administer intravenous antibiotics. Your physician may recommend a hysterectomy if repeated infection has created scar tissue that is responsible for chronic pain. The number of hysterectomies for PID could probably be reduced if optimal antibiotic treatment were used earlier in the course of the disease and if more couples who have not been together exclusively for a long time practiced barrier contraception.

Chronic Pelvic Pain: The perplexing problem called chronic pelvic pain (CPP) remains a huge gray area because by definition the problem can't be pinpointed to a specific disease.

Unfortunately, too often the "solution" is a hysterectomy, where a completely healthy uterus is removed. Nationally, about 10 to 19 percent of all women have hysterectomies for CPP,[22] even though it is known that when laparoscopy (a test to detect conditions such as endometriosis) is done before the operation it often shows no abnormality. This should simply never happen. "When you don't see anything there, it doesn't make much sense to take out normal tissue," says Dr. Robert Reiter, a gynecologist from the University of Iowa who has researched CPP for the past decade.[23]

Reiter and others recently studied 250 women who suffered from CPP and had been told they needed hysterectomies despite normal laparoscopy. (20 percent of the study group had already had hysterectomies and the pain did not abate.) Through an exhaustive investigation of each case, researchers found that 50 percent of the women in the whole group had identifiable reasons for the pain which had been missed. Astoundingly, 80 percent of the origins of pain were nongynecologic.[24] These maladies included irritable bowels, bladder problems, abdominal wall pain, and other problems of nonreproductive pelvic organs. In other words, most of these women who had been told they needed hysterectomies clearly did not.

The other 50 percent were found to have psychogenic (psychological) pain disorders, related to previous sexual trauma, stress disorders, and depression. A large number of women in the study (significantly more than in the group of women without pelvic pain) had been the victims of early sexual molestation and other traumatic sexual experiences which had never been discussed in previous interviews with physicians. "What is tragic about this is that the doctor, even with the best intentions, doesn't realize that the last thing in the world a women needs is to have another assault on her sexual organs," says Reiter, "as if the original trauma were not enough. These are people who continue to pay and pay, because, as our research shows, they continue to experience multiple physical symptoms which keep them returning to doctors, searching for physical explanations."[25]

The new guidelines mentioned earlier included the suggestion that a psychological evaluation be performed before a hysterectomy is done for CPP. This, researchers say, is the stumbling block for many physicians.

Because of lack of training or fear of alienating or insulting patients, the physician remains reluctant to consider possible psychogenic causes of pain. Moreover, these patients are characteristically resistant to any nonsomatic explanation or treatment for their pain. As a result, and largely out of frustration, patients and physicians are apt to consider 'definitive' surgical therapy, which usually involves removal of a grossly and histologically normal uterus and adnexa [ovaries and fallopian tubes].[26]

Uterine Prolapse

Prolapse, or "dropped womb," accounts for 16 percent of all hysterectomies, with over one-third of these occurring in women 55 years old and over.[27] Uterine prolapse occurs when the ligaments that suspend the uterus stretch, causing the organ to fall or descend. It is commonly regarded as a consequence of pregnancy.

There are many instances of prolapse that are minor, where the womb has descended into the vaginal canal, but not yet through the vaginal opening. It is important to understand that if you don't have any discomfort (even if the cervix protrudes through the vagina slightly), you don't need to get a hysterectomy for prolapse.

When the uterus descends further, it can emerge from the vagina. Symptoms can include lower abdominal pressure that increases as the day passes (especially after long periods of standing), lower back ache, and pain during intercourse. Severe prolapse can also result in the uterus pressing against other pelvic organs such as the urethra, rectum, and small intestine.

Operations that reposition the uterus by shortening the ligaments and reattaching them have been done for years and are still done today by some physicians, but results have been mixed. The surgery is highly desirable because it saves the uterus, but it can fail if the ligaments become stretched out again.

Some women can avoid surgery by using a "pessary," a rubber doughnut-shaped device that is manually inserted into the vagina in much the same way as a diaphragm. It must be fitted and inserted by a physician and must be removed periodically for cleaning. Unfortunately, as one gynecologist put it, "the art of pessary fitting is a dying one in this age of quick fix surgery. While physicians used to be trained in it, they really aren't anymore."[28]

Stress Urinary Incontinence

Stress urinary incontinence is diagnosed in people who involuntarily leak urine as a result of "stress," which can result from such everyday activities as coughing, laughing, sneezing, walking, running. The leakage usually occurs in spurts and isn't triggered by any warning or desire to urinate.

Stress urinary incontinence is not uncommon in women who have had a couple of children. For years, physicians have told women that while they are inside doing a bladder suspension (to correct the incontinence) a hysterectomy should be done too. The idea was that because the uterus sits right behind the bladder, removing it would remove further stress on the bladder. However, there has never been a shred of evidence to support this practice, and in fact a recent study has proven otherwise.[29] Stress urinary incontinence should rarely, if ever, be "treated" by hysterectomy.

It is important to know that just because you lose urine doesn't mean it's an anatomical problem that needs corrective surgery. A lot of women have a form of bladder spasm that may be treatable with inexpensive, safe, and effective antispasmodic medication.

Before you have any surgery for incontinence, you should first be tested for a "fallen bladder" to make sure your problem is indeed anatomical and not something else. Even if the problem is anatomical, it does not need to be corrected surgically if it is a minor problem to you and controllable by such simple measures as emptying your bladder regularly and wearing a minipad. Other possible causes of incontinence should also be explored. These include some diuretics, beta-blockers, high blood pressure drugs, mind affecting tranquilizers or sleeping pills, antidepressants, and anti-infectives (urinary tract).[30]

Abnormal Bleeding

Nearly one-fourth of all hysterectomies done in the U.S. are done to control abnormal, prolonged bleeding.[31] As with pain problems, many women with severe bleeding problems will never have a diagnosis of abnormal tissues, and yet their bleeding is enough to disrupt their lives. Before a hysterectomy is done in these cases, all conservative measures should be exhausted. According to the 1989 guidelines put out by the American College of Obstetricians and Gynecologists, the following steps should be taken first:

- physical exam to rule out cervical or uterine pathology that could cause the bleeding
- laboratory tests to detect abnormality of the uterine lining, or malignancy of the cervix[32]

You should be examined to rule out the following possible causes of bleeding:

- foreign object like an IUD or a tampon
- polyps, adhesions, fibroids in the uterus
- ovarian cysts
- cervical infections

None of these situations calls for an immediate hysterectomy. Treatment with hormonal therapy should be tried first. Removing benign growths such as cysts and polyps can sometimes relieve symptoms. Very often a D&C will take care of abnormal bleeding, and treating infections and anemia are also important.

Women who have continuous heavy menstrual bleeding, enough to require extra protection lasting 10 to 15 days, may be diagnosed as having "intractable, dysfunctional uterine bleeding." It is believed that this is caused by some sort of derangement of the endometrium's normal responsiveness to hormones. Again, hormonal treatment should be tried before hysterectomy. If more than one D&C doesn't correct the problem, and you have been fully tested for any other potentially correctable disorder, then a hysterectomy might be the only solution. Obviously, this alternative is only for women who are not interested in having children.

Endometrial Hyperplasia: A common cause of irregular and prolonged bleeding is an abnormal overgrowth of the uterine lining, known as endometrial hyperplasia. This is rarely a valid reason for a hysterectomy because in most women it can be managed medically.

Actually, the term endometrial hyperplasia is used to describe a variety of kinds of overgrowth: hyperplasia, cystic hyperplasia, adenomatous hyperplasia with atypia, adenomatous hyperplasia with mild atypia, and adenomatous hyperplasia with severe atypia. Most investigators legitimately feel that unless the condition involves adenomatous hyperplasia with severe atypia—the one kind of abnormal overgrowth which could mean premalignancy—hysterectomy is not necessary. All other kinds of endometrial hyperplasia can be treated medically and don't require surgery. There is some controversy over surgical treatment for cases of adenomatous hyperplasia with mild atypia.

Endometrial hyperplasia occurs most frequently among women in their 20s and 30s and is generally attributed to excessive estrogen, which causes an overstimulation of the endometrium. It also occurs commonly in menopausal or postmenopausal women who are using estrogens. A diagnosis of endometrial hyperplasia is best made from a uterine biopsy or a D&C.

If you are told you have this condition, you should not be advised that you need a hysterectomy. Endometrial hyperplasia is not cancer and rarely if ever leads to cancer. Fewer than one percent of women with endometrial hyperplasia develop cancer.[33] This problem can often be treated successfully with a D&C or by stopping the use of estrogens.

When deciding whether a hysterectomy is needed for endometrial hyperplasia, you may run into the problem of different viewpoints over what constitutes severe hyperplasia. If you get this diagnosis, or any diagnosis of a precancerous form of endometrial hyperplasia, it is very important that you have your laboratory report viewed by more than one pathologist. A second opinion is critical, especially when you are considering radical surgery or a hysterectomy.

If you have an advanced form of endometrial hyperplasia which has become cancer, a hysterectomy may save your life. In all cases, if a malignancy is found in your uterus, the uterus must be removed.

Ovarian cysts: Ovarian cysts should not be confused with ovarian cancer. There are several different kinds of ovarian cysts, most of which are a part of normal fertility and ovarian function. These do not require surgery. Furthermore, most nonfunctional or abnormal cysts, even when extremely large, can be removed from the ovary, leaving a healthy, functioning ovary behind. Removal of the ovary is not necessary unless the cyst has damaged it beyond repair.

Sometimes cysts collect fluid or blood and need to be aspirated. But for women over 40, often the best thing to do with a cyst is to wait and see if it shrinks by itself. In many women they will eventually disappear and not require treatment of any kind. If your bleeding or pain continues, stay in close touch with your gynecologist.

Cervical Dysplasia

Someday you might have a Pap smear that detects abnormal cells on your cervix. A Pap smear is a painless scraping of the cells around your cervix, and it is instrumental in detecting cervical cancer. However, if this test reveals cervical dysplasia, venereal warts, or carcinoma in situ (CIS) you do not need a hysterectomy.

There are other safe, simple, and effective treatments for these conditions which can eradicate them completely, including cryosurgery (freezing tissue), and laser surgery (vaporizing tissue).

Cervical dysplasia is diagnosed when microscopic changes have occurred in the tissue of the cervix. This condition does not automatically evolve into cancer, but it can in some women if left untreated. CIS is a severe form of dysplasia which is almost 75 to 97 percent curable if treated promptly by a minor surgical procedure called cervical conization, laser therapy, or cryotherapy.[34] Unfortunately, despite the availability of minor surgery to appropriately treat CIS, hysterectomy remains the most common treatment.

While it is uncommon to have symptoms from CIS or cervical dysplasia, you may experience:

- breakthrough bleeding (in between periods)
- bleeding after menopause
- bleeding after intercourse
- bleeding after a pelvic exam
- increased, foul smelling vaginal discharge

If left unchecked, CIS may turn into invasive cancer. When this happens the cancer cells have developed in the deeper layers of the cervix where they have come in contact with blood vessels and the lymphatic system. To prevent the spread of CIS early detection and treatment is important. If you have invasive cervical cancer, your only choice is a radical hysterectomy. In this case, it may save your life.

Other Reasons Not to Elect a Hysterectomy

There are a host of other "reasons" why gynecologists perform hysterectomies when they shouldn't. At the top of the list is sterilization, basically using hysterectomy as a form of birth control. If a woman wants to be sterilized permanently, a tubal ligation is quite effective and has far fewer complications.[35] Doctors claim that having a hysterectomy for sterilization will benefit you by preventing cancer of the uterus. But the risk of dying of cancer of the uterus (including the cervix) is comparable to the risk of dying as a result of a hysterectomy.[36] Diagnoses that really just amount to menstrual disorders, so-called "pelvic congestion," excessive menstruation, and severe cramping, also should never be an excuse to take out your uterus. Severe menstrual cramping in many cases can be handled with medication.

COMPLICATIONS FROM HYSTERECTOMY

As we stated earlier, the chance that you will die from getting a hysterectomy is low, about 1 per 1,000, but the risk of other complications is significant. In a report published in 1984, it was found that 40 out of every 1,000 hysterectomy patients required hospitalization for complications in the two years following their hysterectomies. According to the report, "although women visit their physician less frequently with gynecologic problems after surgery, they visit more frequently for psychological problems, urinary tract infections, and menopausal symptoms."[37]

A hysterectomy is major surgery. Therefore, it carries with it all the risks of major surgery including those associated with anesthesia, blood clots, hemorrhaging, and transfusions, namely: high fever, secondary infection, nerve damage, and in the case of abdominal surgery, digestive disruption. When this operation is recommended for a condition that is annoying but not dangerous, a woman should seriously consider the danger of surgery before agreeing to it.

For a closer look at the problems, consider the fact that between 8 and 15 percent of women getting hysterectomies need blood transfusions (this rate may be much higher depending on the skill of the surgeon). Transfusions carry the added risk of contracting blood-borne diseases such as hepatitis. Nearly one-third of hysterectomy patients suffer high fevers after surgery. Between one and three percent will need a second operation.[38] After leaving the hospital, 13 to 15 percent return to a doctor within a month because of bleeding, infection, pain, or other complications. Overall, nearly half of women having an abdominal hysterectomy and one quarter of those having a vaginal hysterectomy will have at least one complication.[39]

Even in the absence of major complication, recovery after a hysterectomy takes five to seven weeks. Subsequently, a number of women have emotional and psychiatric problems, such as depression. These problems are fairly common and they can be severe.[40]

"I never expected to feel like this," says Sharon, 37, who had a hysterectomy six months ago for fibroids. Sharon has two children and says she expected to feel only relief from her painful periods and no hesitation whatsoever about losing her uterus. "I guess I will describe it as a sense of being old, too soon. I don't feel vibrant. I feel like something very important is missing now. It's depressing. I can't help wondering if there was some other way to take care of my problem."

For premenopausal women, an unnecessary hysterectomy, often accompanied by the removal of ovaries, causes the symptoms of early menopause which may incur the risks of hormone replacement therapy (see chapter on "Hormone Replacement Therapy.")

WHY SO MANY HYSTERECTOMIES?

Whether or not a woman undergoes a hysterectomy seems to depend most of all on where she lives and on her doctor's attitude toward surgery. From 1980 until 1987, if you lived in the southern or western United States you were almost twice as likely to get a hysterectomy than if you lived in the Northeast. Women in the Midwest were usually somewhere in between.[41] Even more striking findings came from a study of two communities in New England. Women living in one area were four times as likely to have a hysterectomy as those living in another area; the differences could not be explained by differences in health or in access to doctors. The authors of this study concluded that the most likely explanation for this was the judgment and preferences of physicians.[42]

With so much variation in the hysterectomy rate, the obvious conclusion is that many should have been avoided. It has been recognized for a long time that there is confusion and a lack of agreement within the medical community as to the acceptable reasons for this radical surgery. There have been very few studies which have offered objective justification for many of the generally accepted reasons for hysterectomies. One, however, reported that in 48 percent of the hysterectomies reviewed, the accuracy of the preoperative diagnosis could not be evaluated.[43] In other words, even experts couldn't tell whether the hysterectomies in question were justified. When rigorous preoperative diagnostic standards for hysterectomy were implemented in a five-year-long study at one large hospital in this country, the hysterectomy rate dropped by 24 percent.[44]

Without question, the importance of the uterus, beyond its obvious role in reproduction, remains undervalued. In the 1990s the notion of the useless uterus still shapes the decisions of both physicians and patients. Hysterectomy is still seen as the panacea for many ills and in the absence of rigorous attempts to save these organs, many are routinely taken out.

Physicians tend to resort to what they are trained to do when faced with a problem they do not understand. In cases of chronic pelvic pain, for example, since the pain can't be traced to a specific abnormality, and most gynecologists aren't trained in psychological interviews, psychogenic sources for the pain are seldom even suggested. Most of the time nongynecological sources of pain aren't considered either. A hysterectomy is the likely solution because "it is the path of least resistance."

And what are the consequences for doctors who resort to surgery? They're paid handsomely, about $3,000 for each procedure in 1988.[45]

Furthermore, the doctor is rewarded with a sense of having done something. "Wait-and-see" approaches or less dramatic surgical attempts to address complicated gynecological problems may only be met with distrust and impatience from women. The abuse of this surgery may be perpetuated by women themselves who are much too influenced by doctors and even well-intended relatives and friends into believing their uteruses have become obsolete. In searching for reasons behind the extraordinary hysterectomy rate in this country, uninformed patient demand is at least partly to blame.

1. Pokras R. Hysterectomy: past, present and future. Statistical Bulletin, Metropolitan Life and Affiliated Companies, October–December 1989; 70: 12–21.

2. Payer L. Medicine & Culture. Henry Holt and Company: New York, 1988, 130.

3. Pokras, op. cit.

4. Ibid.

5. McPherson K. International differences in medical care practices. Health Care Financing Review Annual Supplement. 1989; 9–20.

6. Pokras, op. cit.

7. Dicker RC, Greenspan JR, Strauss LT, Cowart MR, Skally MJ, Peterson HB, DeStefano F, Rubin GL, Ory HW. Complications of abdominal and vaginal hysterectomy among women of reproductive age in the United States. American Journal of Obstetrics and Gynecology 1982; 144:841–8; Wingo PA, Huezo CM, Rubin GL, Ory HW, Peterson HB. The mortality risk associated with hysterectomy. American Journal of Obstetrics and Gynecology 1985; 152:803–8.

8. Dicker et al., op. cit.

9. Colditz GA, Willett WC, Stampfer MJ, Rosner B, Speizer FE, Hennekens CH. Menopause and the risk of coronary heart disease in women. New England Journal of Medicine 1987; 316:1105–10.

10. Doress PB, Siegal DL. Ourselves Growing Older. Simon and Schuster: New York, 1987, 298.

11. Zussman L, Zussman S, Sunley R, Bjornson E. Sexual response after hysterectomy-oophorectomy: recent studies and reconsideration of psychogenesis. American Journal of Obstetrics and Gynecology 1981; 140:725–9.

12. Pokras, op. cit.

13. Buttram VC, Reiter RC. Uterine leiomyomata: Etiology, Symptomatology and Management. Fertility and Sterility 1981; 36:433–45.

14. Entman SS. Uterine leiomyoma and adenomyosis. In Novak's Textbook of Gynecology. 11th Edition. Williams & Wilkins: Baltimore, 1988, 443.

15. Buttram, op. cit.

16. The American College of Obstetricians and Gynecologists. Quality Assurance in Obstetrics and Gynecology. Guidelines issued May 1989, 31.

17. Pokras, op. cit.

18. Walker E, Katon W, Harrop-Griffiths J, Holm L, Russo J, Hickok LR.

Relationship of chronic pelvic pain to psychiatric diagnoses and childhood sexual abuse. American Journal of Psychiatry 1988; 145:75–80.

19. Wentz, AC. Endometriosis. In Novak's Textbook of Gynecology, op. cit., 304.

20. Reiter RC. Medical Management of Endometriosis. Postgraduate Obstetrics and Gynecology 1987; 7:1–6

21. Bird CC, McElin TW, Manalo-Estrella P. The elusive adenomyosis of the uterus—revisited. American Journal of Obstetrics and Gynecology 1972; 112:583–93.

22. Reiter RC, Gambone JC. Demographic and historic variables in women with idiopathic chronic pelvic pain. Obstetrics and Gynecology 1990; 75:428–32.

23. Reiter RC. Interview with author, February 1990.

24. Reiter RC, Gambone JC. Nongynecologic somatic pathology in women with chronic pelvic pain and negative laparoscopy. Journal of Reproductive Medicine 1990, in press.

25. Reiter, interview, op. cit.

26. Reiter and Gambone, Demographic and historic variables in women with idiopathic chronic pelvic pain, op. cit.

27. Pokras, op. cit.

28. Reiter, interview, op. cit.

29. Langer R, Ron-EL R, Neuman M, Herman A, Bukovsky I, Caspi E. The value of simultaneous hysterectomy during Burch colposuspension for urinary stress incontinence. Obstetrics and Gynecology 1988; 72:866–9.

30. Wolfe SM, Fugate L, Hulstrand EP, Kamimoto LE. Worst Pills, Best Pills: the older adult's guide to avoiding drug induced death or illness. Public Citizen Health Research Group: Washington, D.C., 1988, 43–4.

31. Pokras, op. cit.

32. Quality Assurance in Obstetrics and Gynecology, op. cit., 33.

33. Symposium: conservative or aggressive management of early CA. Contemporary OB/GYN 1984, 253–74.

34. Jones HW. Cervical intraepithelial neoplasia. In Novak's Textbook of Gynecology, op. cit., 643–78.

35. Whitelaw RG. 10-year survey of 485 sterilisations; Sterilisation or hysterectomy. British Medical Journal 1979; 1:32–3.

36. Bunker JP, McPherson K, Henneman PL. Elective hysterectomy. In Bunker JP, Barnes BA, Mosteller, F. Costs, Risks, and Benefits of Surgery. Oxford University Press: New York, 1977, 262–76.

37. Roos NP. Hysterectomies in one Canadian province: a new look at risks and benefits. American Journal of Public Health 1984; 74:39–46.

38. Dicker et al., op. cit.

39. CDC also cites a high rate of hysterectomy complications. Medical World News, December 7, 1981:21–6.

40. Notman MT. In: Bunker JP. Elective hysterectomy: pro and con. New England Journal of Medicine 1976; 295:264–8; Barker MG. Psychiatric illness after hysterectomy. British Medical Journal 1968; 2:91–5.

41. Pokras, op. cit.

42. Wennberg J., Gittelsohn A. Variations in medical care among small areas. Scientific American 1982; 296:120–34.

43. Lee NC, Dicker RC, Rubin GL, Ory HW. Confirmation of the preoperative diagnoses for hysterectomy. American Journal of Obstetrics and Gynecology 1984; 150:283–7.

44. Gambone JC, Reiter RC, Lench JB, Moore JG. The impact of a quality assurance process on the frequency and confirmation rate of hysterectomy. American Journal of Obstetrics and Gynecology 1990; 163:545–50.

45. Rinaldo D, Corporate Health Strategies, Westport CT. Communication with author February 9, 1990.

CESAREAN SECTION

How to Avoid Being Part of a National Epidemic

Today one in four women who pass through the doors of a labor and delivery suite will undergo major abdominal surgery. The national rate of cesarean section (c-section) quadrupled from 5.5 percent of all deliveries in 1970 to 24 percent in 1986, and rose again slightly in 1987 and 1988. In 1984, researchers estimated that if the increases continue unabated, the United States cesarean rate could climb to an incredible 40 percent by the year 2000.

- Fifty percent of the 967,000 cesarean sections done in the U.S. in 1988 were unnecessary, a toll of 483,000 surgeries exposing women to the risk of postoperative infections and a maternal death rate which may be two to four times higher than for vaginal delivery.

- Cesarean section is not the fast, painless, and convenient "Hollywood" delivery that some believe it to be. It is a painful, major abdominal operation, associated with infection or other significant injury or complication in 5 to 40 percent or more of the women on whom it is performed.

- While cesarean sections can save infant lives in specific instances, the excessively high rate of cesareans has not lowered the rate of newborn death. Good prenatal care and economic and social supports for pregnant women are far more important in the prevention of newborn death, by helping babies to be born at term and with normal weight.

- Simple, proven changes in clinical practice could have

a profound impact on the c-section rate. By following a consistent policy of encouraging vaginal birth after a previous cesarean section, approximately 237,000 c-sections could have been safely avoided in 1987. A recent study in California, the largest ever in the world, found that 74 percent of almost 6,000 women with a previous cesarean section who tried to have a vaginal delivery were successful in doing so. Using proven, safe methods for turning breech babies around in utero, another 65,000 cesareans could have been avoided. Both of these interventions involve virtually no added risk to mother or child.

Recommendations

For an expectant mother, the most important information needed to avoid unnecessary cesarean surgery is full knowledge of the cesarean "track record" of available doctors and hospitals. (See Appendix A) Much more than the size of your pelvis or the health of your baby, the factor which is most likely to decide how you deliver your baby is the practice style of your obstetrician and the hospital's policy toward c-sections. If you have had a previous c-section, enrolling in a LaMaze class at the beginning of your next pregnancy will reduce the chance of your being talked into an automatic repeat c-section.

*T*HE average American woman expecting a child is increasingly unlikely to deliver her baby the way nature intended. Instead, one in four pregnant women who walk through the doors of a hospital will have a cesarean section. For years controversy raged in the United States over whether the increased use of cesarean sections represented a gross and excessive danger to mothers, a new and more convenient way of delivering normal babies, the guarantee of a perfect baby, the root of the decline in infant deaths, or a knee-jerk response by physicians to problems of malpractice. At one point an academic article went so far as to suggest that all women be offered a cesarean at their due date.[1] However, the truth is that cesarean section, while at times a life-saving intervention for both mother and child, is a cause of significant harm to mothers and provides no additional benefits to infants when performed for other than certain well-defined medical reasons. Today, we are beginning the long road back from this epidemic of unnecessary surgery.

C-SECTIONS: A METEORIC RISE IN POPULARITY

Cesarean section is a major surgical operation in which the abdominal wall is cut open, followed by an incision in the uterus or womb. The infant and placenta are removed through the uterine incision, and both the uterus and the abdominal wall are closed. It is similar in surgical scope to taking out an appendix or gall bladder, in that it involves entering the abdominal cavity and modifying an organ. In the distant past, when women would die if they were unable to deliver an infant vaginally, cesareans were performed as a last-ditch effort to save the mothers' lives. They were almost universally fatal, due to infection, hemorrhage, or other complications. Antiseptic surgical technique began to be used at the end of the nineteenth century, and led to far more women surviving the operation. In the twentieth century improved and more antiseptic surgical techniques, antibiotics, and the ability to perform safe blood transfusions all combined to make cesarean sections far safer.

After the 1950s, as families began to have fewer children, women became pregnant later in life, and the likelihood of a mother dying in childbirth diminished, the focus of obstetrical innovation shifted towards improving infant outcome. Cesarean section began to be used as one approach to improving infant health in certain defined situations. Appropriate uses of cesarean section have undoubtedly contributed to decreasing maternal deaths and improving infant outcome. Yet obstetricians remained almost universally cautious in their use of cesarean section through the 1960s,[2] being well aware of the serious hazards associated with any major abdominal surgery. In 1970 the national cesarean rate (the percent of all deliveries performed by cesarean section) was 5.5 percent,[3] slightly below the rate today in several European and Asian countries.

However, after 1970 there was a virtual explosion in the use of cesarean delivery. Whereas in 1970 only 1 in 20 women delivered surgically, by 1988 that rate had more than quadrupled to one out of every four, or 24.7 percent. In 1987 and 1988 the rate of growth slowed slightly for the first time in years. However, cesarean section is the most common major surgical operation in a hospital today, surpassing such procedures as tonsillectomy, hysterectomy, hernia repair, and gall bladder removal. In 1988, based on live births only, an estimated 967,000 cesarean operations were performed.[4] In 1984, researchers estimated that if the increases were to continue unabated, the U.S. cesarean rate could climb to an incredible 40 percent by the year 2000.[5]

This rapid rise in c-section rates should be of great concern to potential mothers and fathers as well as physicians and health planners. There are several distinct dangers and disadvantages which a woman faces when she has a c-section. The benefits and risks of cesarean section are reviewed below.

THE MYTH THAT OUR HIGH C-SECTION RATE LEADS TO FEWER NEWBORN DEATHS

In defense of the rising c-section rate, many obstetricians point to the decline in United States perinatal mortality rates over the past 15 years. (Perinatal mortality rates measure what percentage of babies die after 28 weeks of pregnancy or before seven days after birth.) Some claim that this increase in infant safety is mainly attributable to the increased c-section rate. However, the decline in perinatal mortality rate is not due to such a simple cause and effect relationship. Several other factors have contributed to the decline, such as improved prenatal care, better educated and better nourished mothers, and extraordinary advances in care of the premature or ill newborn. The greater importance of these latter factors in reducing infant deaths is demonstrated in Europe, where most countries have perinatal mortality rates equal to or lower than our own, while resorting to cesarean section far less frequently. For example, the National Maternity Hospital in Ireland has reported a drop in its perinatal mortality rates from 36.5 to 16.8 per 1,000 infants from 1970 to 1980 while the United States perinatal mortality rates dropped from 29.3 to 17.7 per 1,000 infants. However, during this time the Irish c-section rate rose only slightly from 4.2 percent to 4.8 percent, while the United States c-section rate dramatically escalated from 5.5 percent to 16.5 percent.[6] It has never been clearly determined how much each individual factor has contributed to the drop in perinatal mortality, but it is not likely that the increased use of cesarean section is a major factor.

While the use of c-sections in certain situations has undoubtedly contributed to an increase in survival and well-being of newborns, data from Europe and Japan show that c-section is definitely not the sole or even the primary reason for better infant health. Indeed, Japan, with the extremely low cesarean rate (7 percent), has the lowest infant and perinatal mortality rate anywhere. Brazil, in contrast, has the dubious distinction of having one of the highest cesarean rates in the world, 32 percent, while failing to resolve basic problems of extremely high infant and perinatal mortality.[7] Many countries have been able to lower their infant and perinatal mortality through reducing the proportion of babies born with low birthweight, a goal with which the United States has recently had limited success.

THE FOUR CLINICAL CULPRITS CAUSING UNNECESSARY CESAREAN SECTIONS

C-sections are performed for a variety of reasons. In some of these conditions, such as placenta previa (a relatively uncommon condition where the placenta is blocking the opening from the uterus), a c-section can be the only safe method available to deliver a baby. There are dozens of other possible situations

Table 1. International Cesarean Rates

Country	Year	Cesarean Rate As % Del.	Perinatal Mort. % Del.	Infant Mortality % Del.
Japan	1985	7	8.7	6
Netherlands	1985	10	9.9	8
Norway	1985	12	9.4	8
Denmark	1985	13	8.1	8
Canada	1984–5	19	8.8	9
United States	**1985**	**23**	**10.8**	**10**
Brazil	1981–6	32	n/a	68(1984)

Source: [8]

which may arise during a delivery and necessitate a c-section. However, matters are greatly simplified when we analyze the causes for the recent increases in the c-section rate. National statistics indicate that there are only four medical diagnostic categories which have been major contributors to the increase in c-sections from 1980 to 1985.[9] These four categories account for 98.3 percent of the increase. In order of greatest contribution they are:

1. **Repeat c-sections**—women who have had a previous c-section are almost automatically given repeat c-sections. This diagnosis contributed 48.4 percent of the increase from 1980 to 1985.

2. **Dystocia**—this is the medical name for labor that is progressing abnormally. The most common medical diagnosis used within this group is fetopelvic disproportion (FPD), also known as cephalopelvic disproportion, which means that the baby is too large to fit through the mother's pelvis. This diagnosis contributed 29 percent of the increase from 1980 to 1985.

3. **Fetal distress**—which is a general term meaning that the baby is not getting enough oxygen, its heart rate is erratic, or

something else seems to be wrong. This diagnosis contributed 16.1 percent of the increase from 1980 to 1985.

4. Breech deliveries—where the baby is positioned to come out with buttocks or feet first, rather than head first, making the delivery more difficult. This diagnosis contributed 4.8 percent of the increase from 1980 to 1985.

Because these diagnoses contribute significantly to the increasing c-section rate, this chapter will focus on their causes and possible solutions. A number of other causes have been proposed as contributing to the c-section rate, including rising public expectations for the "perfect baby," increased revenue for hospitals and physicians, and the fear of malpractice suits. We will also review these causes and their contribution to the cesarean problem, using data from across the country.

As outlined above, four clinical diagnoses have been associated with over 98 percent of the rise in the cesarean section rate between 1980 and 1985. We will briefly discuss each of these here.

Repeat Cesarean Section: The Slow Demise of "Once a Cesarean, Always a Cesarean"

At age 36 Nancy gave birth to her third child, an eight-pound, eight-ounce boy. (The examples of patients cited in this chapter are compilations of experience rather than individual experiences.) It had been a normal pregnancy, a rapid labor and thankfully, she had to push for only half an hour before Christopher was born. Her joy at the arrival of her son was compounded by the way he came—her first vaginal delivery. Nancy's first baby had been born appropriately by cesarean section after the umbilical cord slipped out ahead of the baby's head. She was told then that she would "always have to deliver by Cesarean." When she became pregnant the second time, the obstetrician never discussed the option of a normal delivery after a previous cesarean. Nancy's second child was born by an "automatic repeat cesarean." During the third pregnancy she heard of the option of vaginal birth from a nurse friend, and changed obstetricians to someone who was fully supportive of vaginal birth after cesarean (VBAC).

Today Nancy is deeply satisfied at having had a natural delivery, with a far more rapid recovery than in her earlier deliveries. She is adamant that without her strong will and a great deal of support, she would never have been able to make the comparison and switch.

Nationally, the foremost contributor to the increase in c-sections between 1980 and 1985 was the long-standing policy of automatically repeating c-sections for any woman who had already had one. This policy is summed up in the 1916 dictum of obstetrician E.B. Craigin, "once a c-section, always a c-section."[10] Repeat c-sections constituted 35.3 percent[11] of all c-sections performed in the United States in 1987 and contributed to 48 percent of the rise in the c-section rate between 1980 and 1985.[12] This policy multiplies any other increase in the c-section rate, since it dictates that once a woman undergoes a c-section for any reason, she will continue to have c-sections for subsequent births. A vicious cycle is created, leading to a continuing escalation in the use of this surgery.

This policy was appropriate when it was first suggested over 70 years ago, because occasionally the old style of uterine scar from a previous c-section ruptured during subsequent labor, an event which would have been catastrophic in that pre-transfusion era. The old method of c-section involving a large, vertical surgical incision in the womb was the major cause of this fear. Between 1917 and the present, new, safer methods of performing c-section using a small, horizontal (low transverse) incision and stronger closure of the uterus have come into use and the danger of uterine rupture has been largely eliminated. The proper alternative to a repeat cesarean is a "trial of labor," in which a woman proceeds with normal labor while being closely monitored for complications. If it becomes apparent that she cannot deliver her baby through natural labor, only then is a c-section performed. Several large studies have demonstrated that between 50 and 95 percent of patients who have had a previous c-section can deliver vaginally through a "trial of labor" with no evidence of increased risk for the mother or the baby.[13] Reviews of almost 10,000 such deliveries revealed an average 79 percent success rate.[14] According to Dr. Luella Klein, past president of the American College of Obstetricians and Gynecologists (ACOG), "not a single mother has died in recent years because of trial of labor."[15]

Since these initial recommendations, additional work has been published establishing the safety of vaginal birth in women with more than one previous cesarean[16] and in women with an unknown scar type.[17] ACOG still recommends repeating cesarean sections for the vanishingly small group of women with previous classical (vertical) incisions. What is clear is that the catastrophic rupture feared by obstetricians is now an extremely rare event. More commonly, small separations of the uterine scar which require no treatment may occur when women undergo labor.

In contrast, women do die every year as a result of the use of anesthesia which is administered during c-section.[18] With an estimated maternal mortality rate directly due to cesarean surgery of greater than 6 and less than 60 deaths per 100,000 women undergoing cesarean section,[19] and the fact that 330,000 repeat cesarean sections were performed in 1987,[20] it follows that dozens of women (given the low total number of reported maternal deaths) die each year from the outdated policy of "once a cesarean, always a cesarean." Therefore, not only does a "trial of labor" allow more women to deliver naturally, but it is a safer alternative than a c-section.

In late 1988 ACOG issued a new and stronger set of guidelines, indicating clearly that a trial of labor should be offered all women in the absence of a new medical indication for cesarean. The new guidelines also clarified that the requirements of this policy are the same as for any good obstetric care facility—the ability to perform a cesarean section rapidly in the event of an emergent complication. The impact of these new guidelines on obstetric practice remains to be seen. Up until now, the recommendations of both the National Institutes of Health and ACOG in regard to a "trial of labor" have been largely ignored by obstetricians.

Dystocia: Who is Abnormal, the Mother, the Baby, or the Doctor?

After waiting until age 35 to have her first and very wanted baby, Jean found herself lying on a bed at midnight in the labor suite, exhausted after 18 hours of contractions. She couldn't really get up and walk around because she had a fetal monitor strapped to her stomach and she was afraid if she took it off the medical staff might miss something important. She hadn't had anything to eat or drink all day.

Finally, her doctor came in and told her that since her labor had gone on so long, it would be a good idea to have a cesarean section "to get it over with." On Jean's chart he documented the reason for his decision as "failure to progress." Jean's husband didn't have any idea what was best, but she was very reluctant to have surgery, despite her exhaustion. They decided to have another doctor come in for a second opinion.

The second obstetrician carefully studied the course of her labor and found that though long, it was within normal limits for a first birth. This physician suggested that Jean get up and walk as much as possible, take a warm shower and drink some fluids. She reassured Jean that with proper nursing care and a normal pregnancy, taking the fetal monitor off was perfectly safe.

After following this advice, Jean felt much more relaxed and optimistic and over the next few hours her labor progressed normally. At six o'clock in the morning she gave birth to a healthy baby girl and went home feeling great after two days in the hospital.

Nationally, dystocia, or abnormal progress of labor, is the second largest contributor to the dangerous rise in c-sections. It accounted for 28 percent of all cesareans nationally in 1987,[21] and contributed 29 percent of the rise in c-sections from 1980 to 1985.[22] This resulted mainly from a 42 percent increase in the reported rate of dystocia—that is, the rate at which physicians say that a woman has this problem—rather than an increased use of c-section for this diagnosis.[23] Dystocia of some sort was diagnosed in 14.1 percent of all women giving birth in 1986.

There are three factors that can contribute to dystocia: the powers (uterine activity), the passenger (the fetus), and the passage (the mother's pelvis). Real dystocia results when an abnormality in one of these three factors interferes with labor. There is no evidence to indicate that any of these factors has changed significantly over time; mothers' pelvises have not gotten 42 percent smaller nor have babies' heads gotten significantly bigger. Therefore, this large increase in the diagnosis of dystocia must be due in part to subjective factors in obstetrician judgment.

Dystocia is a catch-all diagnosis which encompasses several specific medical problems. However, there are several fundamental decisions that an obstetrician must make to distinguish among these problems. First, is the labor abnormal at all? If there is abnormal labor, is it because the baby cannot fit through the mother's pelvis or because the uterus cannot push the baby out? Distinguishing between these two possibilities has major implications for whether a mother will receive a c-section, because the situations are handled quite differently.

For example, fetopelvic disproportion (FPD), where the baby's head is too large for the mother's pelvis, is one of the major subcategories of dystocia. Unfortunately, 99 percent of all women who were diagnosed with fetopelvic disproportion were ultimately treated by a c-section in the United States in 1986, accounting for 19.3 percent of all cesareans, although many of these women may not have had true disproportion.[24] On the other hand, c-section should rarely be recommended for inefficient uterine activity, since this problem can usually be corrected through appropriate medical management. Yet, one-half of the women with the diagnosis "abnormality of forces of labor" had cesareans in 1986.[25]

Proper medical management of inefficient uterine activity and long labor includes allowing the mother to get out of bed and walk around, ensuring she is properly hydrated, and patience on the obstetrician's part to allow natural labor to take its course. Frequently women are now tied to the bed by fetal monitors, which can inhibit them from getting up and walking.

"Tincture of time" along with judicious use of oxytocin (a medication which stimulates uterine contractions) in selected cases will usually correct the problem of dystocia due to inefficient uterine activity. A recognized authority on obstetrics, Dr. Emanuel A. Friedman, Professor of Obstetrics and Gynecology at Beth Israel Hospital in Boston, and other authors have documented that about 50 percent of "arrest" disorders, where labor stops progressing for a certain period of time, resolve spontaneously without either oxytocin or surgery.[26] Others have found that only about 13 percent of mothers with "arrested labor" need to have a cesarean.[27]

It is likely that many American women said to have fetopelvic disproportion are being misdiagnosed and actually have insufficient uterine activity. As a result, they are receiving c-sections when good medical management would allow them to deliver vaginally. Friedman has stated that "more often than not [over 50 percent of] c-sections performed in the second stage of labor [for failure to progress] are not indicated."[28]

Fetal Distress

Marie, 23, was waiting in a city hospital to have her first baby. Unmarried, she was alone for this delivery after having split up with her boyfriend. She was scared and desperately hoping for a strong, healthy baby. But she also felt helpless, strapped to an intravenous drip in one arm and a fetal monitor clutching her belly as she lay flat on her back.

The labor progressed quickly and after six hours her cervix was almost fully dilated. An obstetrics intern came by and reviewed the paper rolling out of the monitor. She looked worried and showed Marie why: the graph showed a series of dips which could mean the baby was in trouble, she was told.

The next thing she knew nurses were bustling about preparing her for an emergency cesarean section. But before being wheeled off to the surgical suite, the chief resident appeared and quickly reviewed the fetal monitor's data. She looked over the information with the intern and calmly explained that the dips weren't really dangerous. Then she asked Marie to turn on her side for a while. The resident also did a test where she rubbed the baby's scalp and checked the response of the heart rate. The baby's heart responded well to the stimulation and the older resident assured Marie that she didn't need a cesarean and that all was well with the baby. Three hours later Marie gave birth normally to a strong, healthy baby girl.

Nationally, the third main contributor to the increase in c-section is the increased rate of diagnosis of fetal distress. Sixteen percent of the rise in c-sections between 1980 and 1985 was due to fetal distress. During those five years there was an increase from one to four percent in the reported incidence of fetal distress.[29] There is no evidence of declining health in fetuses or mothers in the United States during the last five years which would explain this enormous increase. One must assume, there-fore, that the cause again lies not in the changing health of the mother or baby population, but in the process of how accurately these diagnoses are being made.

What has changed in the birthing process has been the increased use of continuous electronic fetal monitoring (EFM), a technique which has gained widespread use in the last fifteen years. Although widely believed to be a more sensitive method of monitoring the fetal heart rate than the traditional stethoscope, there has been no demonstrated decrease in infant death or clear improvement in outcome between groups monitored elec-tronically and those monitored by traditional auscultation (lis-tening with a stethoscope-like instrument). The data on whether EFM decreases neurologic problems, such as seizures, in new-borns is equivocal. Yet the use of EFM has been associated with an increase in cesarean section and forceps delivery, each of which causes its own morbidity and mortality.[30] There is some more favorable suggestion that EFM is useful if limited to the high-risk pregnancies for which it was originally intended.[31]

Additionally, proper interpretation of EFM results requires

special training and experience, and the quality of this training varies enormously. Studies show that the rate of c-sections proposed as a result of EFM is inversely correlated with the amount of training or experience that a clinician has had with this technique.[32] In other words, the doctor better trained in EFM makes fewer incorrect diagnoses of fetal distress and performs fewer unnecessary c-sections as a result.

A major problem with fetal monitoring is that even if the readings look abnormal, there is only a small to moderate chance that the fetus is in true distress. In one recent German study, 17 percent of low-risk, and 35 percent of high-risk women had some alarm signals on the electronic fetal monitor. However, only four percent of all women in either group actually had distressed infants as measured by abnormalities in fetal blood. The authors compared electronic fetal monitoring to intermittent use of a stethoscope, and concluded that the electronic fetal monitor was far more sensitive, and would identify more cases of real fetal distress, both in high- and low-risk groups. However, for every infant with real fetal distress identified by EFM, three infants showed false signs of distress.[33] Of course, cesarean section is not the only solution to abnormalities on EFM. Sometimes these can be resolved with simple changes in position such as going from lying on one's back to one's side, giving fluids, or administering oxygen.

Even when one defines "real distress" as abnormalities in fetal blood pH (acid content), it is not clear what proportion of those babies would actually have long-term problems from that distress.

Because EFM is performed routinely in most hospitals, a great many false alarms are sounded. One test that can clarify the picture is fetal scalp pH testing, which measures the acid-base status of the fetal blood. This test can help differentiate between babies that are in distress and those that are not. In one study, the proper usage of scalp pH tests helped cut the rate of c-section for fetal distress in half.[34] In the German study, only 8 out of 35 fetuses identified by the fetal monitor had a problem confirmed on blood testing. Due to its invasive nature and the difficulty of performing this test, fetal scalp pH testing, is, in reality, not used very often. Although its use is on the rise, one survey showed that, at major university hospitals, three percent or less of their laboring patients undergo this procedure.[35]

Fortunately, there are new, easier, and less invasive "stimulation techniques" available which could replace most scalp pH testing. These techniques consist of stimulating the fetus by either direct pressure to the scalp or sound waves, and observing the fetal monitor for a certain increase in the fetal heart rate that indicates there is no sign of fetal distress. The combined experience of three studies on these tests showed that 99 percent of the infants with a normal, positive response to such a stimulation test had scalp pH readings that indicated they were not in distress,[36] although their EFM readings indicated otherwise. This test would let the clinician know that it is safe to continue to deliver vaginally, thereby significantly reducing the number of unnecessary c-sections for fetal distress. The simplicity and noninvasiveness of these techniques might make them more readily accepted and widely used than fetal scalp pH testing. Scalp pH testing could then be reserved for only the most ambiguous cases.

Breech Deliveries

It was Liz's third pregnancy and she just assumed everything would go as smoothly with this delivery as it had gone with her other two children, now six and three. But at seven months her doctor noticed the baby was sitting bottom down and told Liz they would have to keep an eye on this. Three weeks before her due date her doctor told her the baby was still breech, so he intended to wait until she started going into labor—to make sure the baby was fully mature—and then do a cesarean section, which he said was safer for the baby.

Liz had read enough to have second thoughts, so she asked her doctor if there weren't any other options. He explained that she could either try a vaginal breech delivery, in which case he was worried about the small increased risk to the baby, or he could refer her to another obstetrician who routinely "turned" babies from breech position to the normal head-first position in the last weeks of pregnancy. Liz opted to see another doctor, who performed the turning (version) in the outpatient clinic of a local hospital. The baby remained head down and two weeks later she had one more handsome son in a delivery that went as smoothly as her earlier ones.

A breech presentation means that the baby is positioned in the uterus with the buttocks or feet down, as opposed to the more common head-first position. While a breech position is common early in pregnancy, most fetuses spontaneously turn to the head-first position before delivery. By term, between three and four percent of infants are still in breech position if nothing is done.[37] Babies in breech position are usually normal, but babies with underlying abnormalities are also more likely to be breech. Breech deliveries have long been associated with a higher likelihood of death or injury for the baby and mother, even when the baby is otherwise normal. Breech presentation accounted for 10 percent of all cesarean deliveries in the United States in 1987.[38] About three percent of all babies were in breech position at the time of birth, and 86 percent of their mothers had cesarean sections.[39] While some vaginal breech deliveries have increased risk of trauma to the baby, this high cesarean rate represents a failure to use alternative, safer methods for the vaginal delivery of most breech babies.

The most important of these alternative methods, as mentioned above, is "external cephalic version." In this technique, after 37 weeks of pregnancy, or just a couple of weeks before the due date, the obstetrician can manually turn a baby who is in breech presentation. This maneuver should be done in a hospital setting, with medication which relaxes the uterus, but it is extremely safe. External cephalic version is successful in turning babies into the normal head-first position about 60 to 90 percent of the time.[40] When performed after 37 weeks, most infants remain head-first until the time of delivery.

A recent survey of obstetricians specializing in perinatology showed a clear consensus that external cephalic version is safe and recommended for babies detected in breech position, and 79 percent of these experts practice version.[41] Unfortunately, external cephalic version is not widely used in the United States. The mere fact that three percent of babies are listed at delivery as breech indicates that most breech babies are not being turned, since that is close to the number expected to be breech in the absence of intervention. The consistent use of external cephalic version after 37 weeks has been shown to lower the number of babies who are still breech at labor to between 0.6 and 2.9 percent of all deliveries.[42]

If a baby cannot be successfully turned by the time labor begins, the question of whether to deliver a breech baby vaginally or by cesarean is far more controversial. Experts still call for more well designed prospective studies of this issue.[43] There is some evidence indicating that premature breech babies, especially those weighing less than 3½ pounds, do worse if delivered vaginally. For full-term infants who weigh between 5.5 and 8.4 pounds, there is reasonable evidence that a vaginal delivery is a legitimate alternative to cesarean section, although birth trauma such as injuries to the nerves of the shoulder still occur at a low rate. Most of these injuries resolve with time. The benefits of avoiding these injuries to the baby through cesarean section are tempered by the risks of surgery for the mother, so there is no completely "right" answer.

ARE CESAREAN SECTIONS SAFE?

Safety is always a relative concept. A cesarean is a safer alternative for women—a tiny fraction of all women getting c-sections— who would otherwise die in labor, or for a baby who would be significantly injured, but in most cases, where the benefits are less clear, cesarean surgery holds significant risks for both mother and child.

Death in childbirth is fortunately a rare event in the United States today, occurring in approximately 251 women in 1987. There are 6.6 maternal deaths for every 100,000 live births.[44]

Nonetheless, cesarean surgery itself is conservatively associated with an increase of between two and fourfold in the likelihood of death in childbirth.[45] While this is extraordinarily lower than the 85 percent maternal death rate of cesarean section in Great Britain and Ireland in the mid-1800s,[46] it still carries a far greater risk of death than does vaginal delivery. This increase holds even for women undergoing elective repeat cesarean sections. Death rates vary among states from year to year, and are related to both the health of mothers and to the quality of anesthesia and obstetric care. In Massachusetts, one of the states with the lowest hospital death rates overall in the nation,[47] cesarean delivery (and not the underlying medical problems of the mother) has been estimated to be directly responsible for 5.8 deaths for every 100,000 women so delivered.[48] In contrast, in Georgia cesareans were held directly responsible for a maternal death for 59 women of every 100,000 delivered by cesarean.[49] Overall deaths (deaths related either to the surgery or to the mother's underlying condition) in women having cesarean section have ranged from 22.3 per 100,000 cesareans in Massachusetts to 105 per 100,000 in Georgia.[50] If, as we estimate, approximately 483,000 unnecessary cesareans were performed in the United States in 1988, as many as 100 women or more (since less than half of maternal deaths are in mothers delivered by cesarean, and only some of these were unnecessary operations) are likely to have died directly as a result of this unnecessary surgical procedure each year.

While death is a rare occurrence after a cesarean section, there are other extremely common complications of cesarean surgery. The most common problem is infection, particularly endometritis (infection of the womb), which occurs in 6 to 18 percent of women; urinary tract infection, which occurs in one to seven percent of women[51]; and infection of the surgical wound, in one to seven percent of women.[52] These infections are often associated with longer hospital stays, pain, and poor wound healing.

A cesarean section's increased risk of abnormal blood-clotting is well known.[53] These can be blood clots in the extremities, or the more dangerous pulmonary embolus, which can block blood flow to the lungs.

The surgery itself may result in injuries to the surrounding organs. Injuries to the bladder (0.3 percent), ureters (which carry urine from the kidneys to the bladder; 0.1 percent), and bowel can also occur.[54] Repeat cesareans are associated with a higher incidence of trauma because of scarring from the previous surgery. Overall, between 4.2 and 18.9 percent of women undergoing cesareans have some immediate complication of surgery, such as injury to organs, lacerations, difficulty in removing the infant, or excessive bleeding requiring transfusion.[55]

Another adverse effect of cesarean section may be a higher rate of infertility following the surgery. One study found a roughly threefold increase in infertility following cesarean section in women with no previous history of infertility, from 2.2 percent in women delivering normally, to 6.4 percent after a cesarean.[56] This area requires further research, but argues strongly against performing cesareans lightly in women who desire additional children. Yet it is precisely in the group of women having their first infants that unnecessary cesareans for dystocia are generally performed.

In addition, a c-section can take a psychological and emotional toll on the mother, causing her to experience a whole range of emotions including depression, loss of autonomy, feelings of powerlessness, lowered self-esteem, as well as guilt for experiencing such negative feelings, at a time that should be joyful.[57]

Nancy, the mother of an eight-year-old, believes that experiencing an unnecessary and emotionally traumatic cesarean section is the reason she decided not to have more children. "I can still feel my voice get louder and angrier when I talk about it. The grief subsides, the disappointment does too, but the anger doesn't seem to go away. It's impossible to explain how cheated and sad I felt after having a cesarean forced on me because my labor was simply too long for the hospital's policy."

In one study, 72 percent of women who delivered vaginally felt that they had regained their normal energy by six weeks after birth, whereas only 34 percent of women delivered by cesarean had done so.[58] Cesarean mothers were more self-oriented and felt less confident about their ability to care for their babies than vaginally delivered mothers in another study.[59] Most differences resolved within a year after birth. C-sections can sometimes interfere with the initial maternal-infant bonding at birth, due to hospital policies separating cesarean infants from mothers. Fortunately, these policies have been eliminated in most hospitals. One small recent study failed to document disturbances of mother-infant interaction.[60]

Of course, normal delivery is also associated with complications, such as injury to the uterus, vagina, rectum, and surrounding tissues. Lacerations are common complications in women delivering vaginally. Postpartum infections after vaginal delivery, once widespread, are far less common nowadays. Many injuries can be avoided by careful obstetric management. Others are appropriately avoided when certain difficult deliveries are by cesarean section, rather than by spontaneous vaginal delivery or by forceps. In addition to lower frequency, the complications of vaginal delivery are generally less severe than those of cesareans, as evidenced by the more rapid recovery of women from vaginal birth.

Clearly, cesarean section is not the fast, painless, and convenient "Hollywood" delivery that some believe it to be. It is a painful major abdominal operation, associated with infection or other significant injury or complication in 5 to 40 percent or more of women. While the initial pain of labor may be avoided or shortened, it is often replaced with postoperative pain and complications, and even, on occasion, death. The risk of these significant side effects can only be justified in those defined situations where cesarean section has been well documented to offer a better outcome for mother or child.

THE MYTH OF THE PERFECT CESAREAN BABY

Another prevalent myth surrounding cesarean section is that of the "perfect baby." It goes something like this: because families are having fewer children, there is increasing pressure for the perfect baby. Consequently, doctors are performing cesareans to guarantee this perfect baby. This myth is truly pernicious, falsely leading women to believe that they are guaranteed a better outcome for the baby if they expose themselves to the risks of a surgical delivery. In fact, outside of certain well-defined situations, cesarean sections have no advantage for infants and may, indeed, cause harm.

The most common complication is the result of delivering a premature infant with immature lungs. In the 1970s, between three and four percent of infants with respiratory distress syndrome were babies delivered by elective cesarean section.[61] Some of this doctor-induced prematurity can be avoided by waiting for labor to begin, or by performing amniocentesis (which has its own risks), or other tests to check the maturity of the baby. Clearly the best way to avoid causing this kind of prematurity is not to do unnecessary cesareans. Since most prescheduled cesareans are repeats, this problem is largely avoidable.

Cesareans are generally thought to protect against birth trauma, however they are clearly not a panacea. While they may offer protection from trauma for extremely large infants (especially those larger than 10 pounds), small infants in breech position, or infants with other abnormal positions in the uterus, for most other groups no advantage has been demonstrated. Infants between 5.5 and 8.4 pounds in breech position can be delivered with near equal safety by either route, although this area is still controversial.

One study comparing infants delivered vaginally with infants delivered by elective repeat cesarean section at term showed that the normal-sized cesarean babies had more low Apgar scores (an index of the well-being of the baby assigned immediately after birth, in which low scores are a sign of abnormal function) than the babies delivered normally.[62]

In sum, when cesareans are performed unnecessarily—such as elective repeats—there is no evidence that the baby's outcome is better, and it may be worse, as measured by Apgar scores.

In certain well-defined situations, the baby will clearly benefit by cesarean delivery. Examples include real, confirmed fetal distress which does not respond to other efforts; some premature breech infants; true arrest of labor despite adequate medical support; placenta previa (where the placenta blocks the exit of the womb); hemorrhage; an abnormally positioned umbilical cord; and certain abnormally positioned twins or single babies. However, these and other legitimate indications account for fewer than half of all cesareans performed today. For the other 500,000 babies born by cesarean each year, surgery is more likely to make the infant and/or the mother ill rather than perfect and whole. The myth of the perfect cesarean baby should be laid to rest.

AT WHAT RATE SHOULD C-SECTIONS BE PERFORMED?

The cesarean rate is always composed of two main components. The first is the primary rate: first-time cesareans, performed allegedly for a medical reason. In 1987, 17.4 percent of all deliveries were primary cesarean sections. The second component is the repeat cesarean rate, which accounts for 35 percent of all cesareans, 8.6 percent of all deliveries in 1987. While dramatic lowering of the repeat cesarean rate is unquestionably safe and possible in the short-term, a long-term decrease in the abuse of this surgery will depend on eliminating unnecessary first-time cesareans as well.

The proper c-section rate is one that provides the most safety for infants without unnecessarily endangering the mothers. Most academicians have shied away from defining this point and its consequences for practice. One exception is Dr. E. J. Quilligan, Dean of the School of Medicine and former Director of Maternal-Fetal Medicine at the University of California, Irvine. Dr. Quilligan suggests that the proper range for c-section rates, if the operation were used only when medically indicated, is between 7.8 percent and 17.5 percent.[63] The low rate of 7.8 percent would be appropriate at a community hospital which sees very few complicated patients, a middle rate of 10 to 12 percent applies to the average hospital, and a high rate of 17.5 percent could be appropriate at a university medical center, such as one with a neonatal intensive care unit, which sees more complicated cases. He estimates that for the entire United States population an optimal c-section rate would be 12 to 14 percent.[64]

These estimates are not random, but are based on data from around the world and careful analysis of the details of the current cesarean rate. These include:

- Cesarean rates and perinatal mortality data from other countries

- Cesarean rates at United States hospitals which have sought to stop unnecessary surgery and monitor infant outcomes, or which have always had appropriately low c-section rates

- Well designed clinical trials examining the usefulness of cesarean section for women with previous cesareans, dystocia, fetal distress, and breech babies

Dr. Quilligan's estimates should be regarded as conservative, obtainable targets, since there are many documented cases of hospital services having c-section rates less than seven percent without increased perinatal mortality. Obviously, one is concerned about overall infant well-being and not just mortality. The lowest cesarean rate which will lead to optimal infant outcome with the least injury to the mother is not yet absolutely clear. What is clear is that our current rate is far too high, and that these suggested targets are a fair margin above the cesarean rates achieved in hospitals which have preserved good infant outcomes while stopping unnecessary surgery.

NUMBERS TALK: WHAT IS YOUR PHYSICIAN'S C-SECTION RATE?

One of the important things to know about your obstetrician is his or her c-section rate. Regardless of all the reassuring things you may hear from your doctor, if he or she is performing c-sections at a rate of 17 percent or more, that clearly says something you should know about that practice. Maybe that doctor has a great many high risk patients, in which case a rate no higher than 17 percent is justified. However, doctors with low or average risk patients should not be doing c-sections at a rate higher than 10 to 12 percent.

Availability of information on the practice of individual physicians has been a controversial issue, which medical societies have vigorously opposed.[65] In Maryland, for example, cesarean rates for individual named physicians were not available, although the information allowed the identification of hospitals where individual physicians have extraordinarily high rates. In that state, in 1987, cesarean rates for individual physicians ranged from 0 to 57 percent.[66]

Beth Shearer of C/Sec, an organization which is working to reduce the number of c-sections in this country, advises women to ask their doctors directly about their c-section rates. She says very often women seeking support for a vaginal birth after cesarean (VBAC) call her organization because they don't feel they have honest support from their physicians. "Doctors will say one thing, yes you can have a VBAC, and mean another. When there is no real support for a VBAC, women usually get that message."[67]

Linda experienced exactly that when she tried to make it clear to her physician that she wanted to have a vaginal delivery after her previous c-section. "My doctor said if I wanted a VBAC I could have one, but that if I were his wife, he wouldn't want me to try. I felt all along that he was treating me like a high-risk patient, instead of a woman having a normal pregnancy and expecting a normal delivery." Despite the clear evidence that ruptures and other complications for VBACs are rare, this woman and many like her are still given the long disproven message that attempting VBAC puts their lives at risk.

When choosing a doctor it is important to ask about his or her attitude concerning situations which may come up in your pregnancy, such as a breech baby or fetal distress. Also, potential mothers with uncomplicated pregnancies may wish to consider the option of using certified nurse-midwives, who generally have far lower rates of referring low-risk women for cesarean section. Most nurse-midwives today work in teams with obstetricians who can provide backup if complications arise.

HOSPITAL CESAREAN RATES

Throughout the country there is extraordinary variation in rates of cesarean section, from 63.6 percent of all deliveries (in Jellico Community Hospital in Tennessee) to none.[68] This variation bears little relation to the severity of the patients seen in a given hospital.

Based on an extensive survey published in 1989 based on 1987 data,[69] private, for-profit hospitals had the highest cesarean rates, averaging 24.6 percent, followed by voluntary and church-run hospitals at 23.3 percent, and state and local government hospitals at 20.9 percent. The fourteen hospitals run by the Federal Government for which we had information, including military and Public Health Service hospitals, had the lowest cesarean rates at 15 percent. Outside the hospital setting, freestanding birthing centers have by far the lowest cesarean section rate, according to a study published in 1989.[70] At these centers, which are usually staffed by midwives, the c-section rate averaged four percent in the years studied from 1985 to 1987.

Knowing the c-section rate at the hospital where you plan to deliver is important. For one thing, hospital policy affects how you will be handled by the nursing staff. They usually decide when to call in the doctor, so the way they monitor your labor is important. Once you are in the hospital, decisions can be made rapidly for you. If you know the kind of setting you are entering, you may be confronted with fewer surprises.

Betty, for example, had no idea that her baby would be taken away from her for 24 hours after delivery if she didn't give birth within a limited number of hours after her water broke. (The hospital had a rigid policy that required the newborn to be kept in isolation if delivered more than 24 hours after the mother's membranes broke. The policy was intended to decrease the elevated risk of infection for these newborns.) As her labor proceeded slowly, she was pressured to have a c-section to avoid giving up the baby immediately after birth. "It was horrible. I didn't feel ready to deliver and yet they said if I waited, the baby would be taken away. This hospital policy was completely new to me and I felt like a total victim."

WHAT'S A HOSPITAL TO DO?

It has been shown that voluntary initiatives within hospital obstetric departments can substantially reduce the c-section rate without jeopardizing the quality of care to either the mother or infant. At the Mount Sinai Hospital Medical Center in Chicago, a program establishing new, stricter guidelines for c-sections reduced the rate performed between 1985 and 1989 from 17.5 to 10.3 percent, far below the national average of 24.7 percent in 1988. The program included the following:

- A second opinion, by an obstetrician certified by a board, was required for all cesarean sections except in acute emergency situations.

- The department recognized that vaginal delivery was preferred after every previous cesarean, and that a patient's desire for repeat cesarean was not automatically acceptable as a reason to do one.

- The diagnosis of dystocia was changed to include stricter criteria, thus reducing the number of instances where this diagnosis was cited as a reason for terminating labor and resorting to a cesarean delivery.

- The diagnosis of fetal distress was accepted only after a confirming blood test (when technically possible).

- Most breech births were to be avoided by using external cephalic version at approximately 37 weeks whenever possible.

Obviously, a few clearly defined changes in clinical practice, which Mt. Sinai and an increasing number of other American hospitals are implementing, could dramatically lower the frequency of cesarean section in the United States without jeopardizing infant health. By following a consistent policy of encouraging vaginal birth after cesarean section, approximately 237,000 cesarean sections could have been avoided in 1987. Through the consistent use of external cephalic version, roughly another 65,000 cesareans for breech deliveries could be avoided. Both of these interventions involve virtually no added risk to mother or child, and indeed, would protect mothers from the hazards of cesarean surgery. These two policies alone would lower the United States cesarean rate to 16.5 percent from its current level of 24.7 percent.

The ideal rates of cesarean section for dystocia and fetal distress are less clear. However, the current rates are without question too high, as demonstrated by excellent outcomes at hospitals with far fewer cesareans for these indications. A 40 percent reduction in the rate of diagnosis of dystocia and fetal distress would lead to 142,000 fewer cesareans annually, and to a lowered national cesarean rate of 12 percent.

WHY DOCTORS IGNORE THE MEDICAL EVIDENCE ON UNNECESSARY C-SECTIONS

Several reasons have been suggested for the rising use of cesarean sections in the face of convincing evidence that they are only beneficial in certain situations. The threat of malpractice suits when a baby is born less than perfect, financial incentives for doctors and the hospital, and physician convenience have been the most plausible explanations.

An important factor to be considered in analyzing the rise in c-sections is the increased money that it brings to both physicians and hospitals. Physicians often receive as much as 20 to 40 percent more for doing a c-section, charging a median fee of $561 extra for a c-section in 1989. This is in addition to a doctor's charge for total maternity care which averaged $1,492 in 1989.[71]

The influence of financial incentives for c-sections was suggested in several studies which found that women with private physicians were more likely to receive a c-section than women receiving care in a public clinic or on a ward service.[72] One study of women in Los Angeles County found that women whose median household income was greater than $30,000 were nearly twice as likely to have first-time c-sections as women whose income was under $11,000.[73] This could occur either because physicians are being influenced by financial incentives to do more c-sections, or because their decision-making process is influenced by patients' social class, or both.

These influences are suggested when looking at c-section rates for women in relation to the source of payment for their care. In 1987, national c-section rates were the highest for patients covered by Blue Cross/Blue Shield and other private insurance companies and lowest for Medicaid beneficiaries and self-paying patients. While self-paying women are probably somewhat less poor than Medicaid enrollees, they have a lower cesarean rate. In short, patients with the best paying insurance plans have the highest c-section rate. A clear relation between cesarean rate and wealth has been seen in other countries such as Brazil, where the cesarean rate increases in direct proportion to family income.[74]

While physicians may or may not be deliberately or consciously performing c-sections for financial reasons, these findings, replicated in studies in the U.S. and other countries, clearly show a probability that financial factors are associated with a physician's decision to perform a c-section. The alternative explanation, that privately insured women have a different rate of legitimate medical indications for cesareans, seems unlikely to account for the wide variation. In fact, medically, one would expect poor women to need more cesareans, since they have a higher incidence of complications of pregnancy such as eclampsia, premature delivery, poor fetal growth, and other conditions which might lead to real fetal distress.

The other component of cost, perhaps more important than physician fees, is the issue of hospital charges. The bulk of the

Table 2. Cesarean Rate by Who Pays (Cesareans as % of All Deliveries)[75]

	Self Pay	Medicaid	HMO	BC/BS	Other Private Insurance
United States (1987)	19.3%	24.0%	n/a	26.5%	25.3%
California (1984)	17.2%	21.2%	20.3%	n/a	26.8%
Maryland (1987)	20.0%	23.0%	26.7%	28.5%	28.5%
New Jersey (1986)	21.9%	22.8%	28.4%	28.5%	28.1%

cost to society for unnecessary cesarean sections is from hospital costs. The extra two to three days spent in the hospital for a c-section roughly doubles the hospital revenues, bringing in as much as $2,000 to $2,500 extra revenue.

Rather than take responsibility for unnecessary surgery taking place within their walls, hospitals across the United States are more likely to be driven by opposite incentives. Hospitals have relatively low occupancy rates and are seeking to fill beds. They are competing with each other to attract patient referrals from obstetricians and other physicians, as demonstrated by the billboards of cherubic newborns which decorate the roads of many towns. Many hospitals have been unwilling to alienate private physicians, upon whom they depend, by interfering in their c-section glutted practices, no matter how outrageous those practices might be.

BAD MEDICINE OR THE SOLUTION TO MALPRACTICE LITIGATION?

It is commonly perceived that the threat of malpractice suits is a major cause of the increasing c-section rate. To be sure, physicians practicing obstetrics and gynecology are among the most

===== Questions to Ask a Hospital Administrator =====

1. What is the c-section rate for this hospital? If it is a community hospital, how close is it to seven percent? If it is a university hospital with a neonatal intensive care unit, which sees more difficult cases, lower than 17 percent may be okay.

2. Does this hospital offer a "trial of labor" to patients who have had a previous c-section? If so, what percentage of patients who have had a previous c-section do deliver vaginally? The percentage should ideally be greater than 60 percent. Real success rates with VBAC have been as high as 90 percent in some studies.

3. Is fetal blood sampled or a fetal stimulation test routinely done prior to doing a cesarean section if electronic fetal monitoring suggests fetal distress? At least one of these tests should ideally be performed unless a real emergency is noted.

4. Is a second opinion required before a nonemergency c-section is performed? A second opinion has been shown to lower c-section rates without affecting the quality or safety of care.

5. Do you have any other policies to help prevent unnecessary c-sections?

likely to be sued for malpractice. In a 1985 survey, the American College of Obstetricians and Gynecologists found that over 70 percent of its members have been sued once and that over 25 percent have been sued at least three times.[76] Obstetricians and gynecologists also have, by far, the highest number of successful suits—those where money is paid out to the patient—of any medical specialty in the country.[77]

While there has been a lot of talk about physicians performing more cesarean sections out of fear of malpractice suits, there is no real evidence of this. Cesarean rates in military and Public

Health Service hospitals have risen considerably (albeit more slowly than the national average), even though their physicians are not anywhere near as subject to malpractice liability. The explosion in cesarean surgery has occurred in other countries, such as Brazil, where there is no malpractice crisis, and Canada, where the cesarean section rate has trailed only slightly behind the U.S., again implying that other incentives are operating. More likely, in the United States the threat of malpractice litigation has served as one of several impediments to physicians heeding the results of research and the recommendations of their own professional leadership to reverse this trend.

Legal liability in relationship to c-sections can occur in four different categories: negligence in the failure to perform a c-section, negligence in delaying before performing a c-section, negligence in the performance of a c-section, or performance of an unnecessary c-section. Concern over liability in the first two areas might, theoretically, motivate a physician to do an unnecessary c-section. However, the 1980 National Institutes of Health consensus conference reviewed a number of successful lawsuits against doctors in these first two categories and found:

> In most of them, there was evidence of gross deviation from the appropriate standard of care, and not merely a situation in which a physician made an honest error in judgment in not performing or in delaying a cesarean.[78]

In other words, physicians rarely lose malpractice suits for not performing or delaying to perform c-sections in cases involving small or subtle errors in judgment. While some settlements do appear unjustified, gross negligence on the physician's part is the basis of most lost malpractice suits. Yet many physicians perceive that a c-section is easier and will result in less legal risk than a difficult labor, as demonstrated in the common saying among obstetricians and gynecologists, "I never regret having done a section, only not having done a section."

In fact, there is no empirical evidence that the performance of unnecessary cesarean sections lessens the legal risk for an obstetrician. A similar misperception is the widely held belief that poor people sue more, a myth which has been debunked by hard research. For example, a study in Maryland found that Medicaid beneficiaries had not initiated lawsuits with any greater frequency than the rest of the population.[79] The true solutions to the obstetric malpractice crisis lie in the improvement in quality of medical care, better communication between doctors and patients, and greater availability of desperately needed services and support for families of children with developmental disabilities.

It is clear that all hospitals and obstetricians with unnecessarily high c-section rates can lower those rates without any compromise in maternal or infant safety. This should demonstrate that unnecessary c-sections do not make the delivery process safer and, as a result, do not reduce legal risk. Concern for legal issues cannot be allowed to cover up for, or even cause, bad medical practice. As research data on infant outcomes accumulates, obstetricians should be increasingly able to defend a decision not to perform a cesarean in situations where the facts show that surgery does not significantly improve infant outcome.

HELP YOURSELF AVOID UNNECESSARY CESAREAN SURGERY

The most important force for stopping this epidemic is the concern and involvement of women, the targets of unnecessary cesarean surgery. There are a growing number of groups around the country trying to reduce the number of unnecessary cesarean sections. They also offer information and general support to pregnant women and their families. Two of the most active groups working on reducing the excessive number of c-sections are C/Sec Inc. (617-924-2681) and the National Cesarean Prevention Movement (315-424-1942.) Many childbirth educators have become interested in preventing unnecessary cesarean sections.

One indispensable component of involving consumers is providing access to information. For an expectant mother, the most important information needed to avoid unnecessary cesarean surgery is full knowledge of the cesarean "track record" of available doctors and hospitals, in addition to information about other aspects of their quality of care. It is clear that the factor which is most likely to decide how a woman delivers her baby is the practice style of her obstetrician, not the size of her pelvis or the health of her baby. While hospitals have tremendous variability in their overall rates, in many hospitals this variation can be accounted for by a few physicians who dramatically abuse cesarean surgery.

In 1985 Massachusetts passed a bill (Chapter 714) which obligates hospitals to provide women with their most recent cesarean rate and rate of vaginal birth after cesarean, as well as other data about common maternity practices. A similar bill passed in New York State. Several state government agencies are already publishing brochures with data on individual hospital cesarean rates. This is true in New York State, New Hampshire, and Nevada. These are important initiatives.

========= Questions to Ask an Obstetrician =========

1. What is your c-section rate? Doctors with high-risk practices should be less than about 17 percent. Doctors with low-risk practices should be under 10 percent.
2. Do you offer a "trial of labor" to women who have had a previous c-section? If so, what percentage of them deliver vaginally? The percentage should ideally be at least 60 percent to 70 percent.
3. Do you use fetal blood sampling or fetal stimulation techniques prior to performing a c-section if electronic fetal monitoring suggests fetal distress? Both of these tests should ideally be done.
4. Do you consider it good medical practice to seek an independent second opinion for elective c-sections?
5. When confronted with a baby in breech position, do you routinely perform external cephalic version (turning the baby) after 37 weeks?

Unfortunately, no state has yet made public the cesarean rates of individual physicians. This will be the most useful information for women. It is also important that all expectant mothers receive information on cesarean rates and other maternity practices, not just the small group who are informed enough to know that the data is available. The New York bill calls for information to be provided to all expectant mothers when they preregister with hospitals.

Over 30 states already have good publicly available data on cesarean sections by hospital, and many could easily calculate it for each physician. With the advent of the new standardized birth certificates in 1989, which include more information about delivery, virtually every state health agency will have excellent, detailed information on cesarean section rates by hospital, and, if they choose, by physician. It will also permit monitoring of repeat cesarean sections, dystocia, fetal distress, breech deliveries, and other obstetric procedures. This wealth of information should be made widely available to the general public as soon as possible. One way to do so is through the passage of legislation mandating that expectant mothers receive information on maternity practices. One model of such legislation is in Appendix B. State governments should make it a priority to tabulate and disseminate the data available on the new birth certificates beginning in 1989.

Insurers, employers, women's groups, and childbirth educators should consider promoting this type of maternity information legislation. In the absence of legislation, insurers, employers, and others can use publicly available data such as that included in this report to make this information widely available to families.

What can you do as an individual? Ask obstetricians about their cesarean rate. Some important questions include 1) their rate of c-section and vaginal birth after cesarean (if the woman has already had one), 2) their policy for fetal monitoring and whether they generally confirm suspected fetal distress using fetal stimulation or blood sampling, and 3) whether they are agreeable to obtaining a second opinion before performing any nonemergency cesarean. If you encounter a physician who is unwilling to answer or discuss these important questions, you should seriously consider seeking a different physician or a midwife. The impact on physician practice of hundreds of people like you asking questions may be greater than all the reports and articles of academia put together.

Cesareans are one of those issues where the interests of good health coincide with those of cost containment. On this particular issue, consumer groups seeking to stop unnecessary cesarean sections may find that they have common ground with those who pay for medical care.

1. Feldman GB, Freiman JA. Prophylactic cesarean section at term? New England Journal of Medicine 1985; 312:1264–7.

2. Jones OH. Cesarean section in present-day obstetrics. American Journal of Obstetrics and Gynecology 1976; 126:521–30.

3. Taffel SM, Placek PJ, and Liss T. Trends in the United States cesarean section rate and reasons for the 1980–85 rise. American Journal of Public Health 1987; 77:955–9.

4. Taffel SM, Placek PJ, Moien M. 1988 U.S. cesarean-section rate at 24.7 per 100 births—a plateau? New England Journal of Medicine 1990; 323:199–200; Myers SA, Gleicher N. 1988 U.S. cesarean-section rate; good news or bad. New England Journal of Medicine 1990; 323:200.

5. Placek PJ, Taffel SM, Liss TL. The cesarean future. American Demographics 1987; September.

6. O'Driscoll K, Foley M. Correlation of decrease in perinatal mortality and increase in cesarean section rates. Obstetrics and Gynecology 1983; 61:1–5; Taffel SM et al. Trends, op. cit.; Powell-Griner E. Perinatal mortality in the United States: 1981–1985. National Center for Health Statistics 1989; 37.

7. Notzon FC. International differences in the use of obstetric interventions. Journal of the American Medical Association 1990; 263:3286–91; Brazilian infant mortality data is from Magalhaes S. et al. Impacto da crise economica nos servicos de saude: o caso do Brasil. Unpublished paper, November 1987.

8. Notzon, op. cit.; The Health of America's Children. Children's Defense Fund, Washington, DC, 1988.

9. Taffel et al. Trends, op. cit.

10. Craigin E. Conservatism in obstetrics. New York State Medical Journal 1916; 104:1.

11. Taffel SM, Placek PJ. An overview of recent patterns in cesarean delivery and where we are today. Paper presented at the American Public Health Association annual meeting, Boston, November 13–17, 1988.

12. Taffel SM et al., Trends, op. cit.

13. Paul RH, Phelan JP, Yeh S. Trial of labor in the patient with a prior cesarean birth. American Journal of Obstetrics and Gynecology 1985; 151:297–304; Lavin JP, Stephens RJ, Miodovnik M, Barden TP. Vaginal delivery in patients with a prior cesarean section. Obstetrics and Gynecology 1982; 59:135–48; Gibbs CE. Planned vaginal delivery following cesarean section. Clinical Obstetrics and Gynecology 1980; 23:507–15.

14. Flamm BL. Vaginal birth after cesarean section: controversies old and new. Clinical Obstetrics and Gynecology 1985; 28:735–44.

15. Klein L. Cesarean birth and trial of labor. The Female Patient 1984; 9:106–17.

16. Pruett KM, Kirshon B, Cotton DB, Poindexter AN. Is vaginal birth after two or more cesareans safe? Obstetrics and Gynecology 1988; 72:163–5.

17. Pruett KM, Kirshon B, Cotton DB. Unknown uterine scar and trial of labor. American Journal of Obstetrics and Gynecology 1988; 159:807–10.

18. Endler GC, Mariona FG, Sokol RJ, Stevenson LB. Anesthesia-related maternal mortality in Michigan, 1972 to 1984. American Journal of Obstetrics and Gynecology 1988; 159:187–93.

19. Petitti DB. Maternal mortality and morbidity in cesarean section. Clinical Obstetrics and Gynecology 1985; 28:763–9.

20. Taffel SM and Placek P. Overview, op. cit.

21. Ibid.

22. Taffel et al., Trends, op. cit.

23. Ibid.

24. Placek PJ, Taffel SM. Recent patterns in cesarean delivery in the United States. Obstetrics and Gynecology Clinics of North America 1988; 15:607–27.

25. Ibid.

26. Neel J. Medicolegal pressure, MDs' lack of patience cited in cesarean 'epidemic'. OB/Gyn News May 15, 1987; 22:1 and 44.

27. Bottoms SF, Hirsch VJ, Sokol RJ. Medical management of arrest disorders of labor: a current overview. American Journal of Obstetrics and Gynecology 1987; 156:935–9.

28. Neel, op. cit.

29. Taffel SM, Trends, op. cit.

30. Freeman JM, Nelson KB. Intrapartum asphyxia and cerebral palsy. Pediatrics 1988; 82:240–9.

31. Friedman EA. The obstetrician's dilemma, how much fetal monitoring

and cesarean section is enough? New England Journal of Medicine 1986; 315:641–3.

32. Helfand M, Marton K, Ueland K. Factors involved in the interpretation of fetal monitor tracings. American Journal of Obstetrics and Gynecology 1985; 151:737–44

33. Schrock A. An assessment of the usefulness and predictive value of intrapartum monitoring. Wiener klinische Wochenschrift 1988; 100:145–53.

34. Zalar RW, Quilligan EJ. The influence of scalp sampling on the cesarean section rate for fetal distress. American Journal of Obstetrics and Gynecology 1979; 135:239–46.

35. Clark SL, Paul RH. Intrapartum fetal surveillance: the role of fetal scalp blood sampling. American Journal of Obstetrics and Gynecology 1985; 153:717–20.

36. Clark SL, Gimovsky ML, Miller FC. The scalp stimulation test: a clinical alternative to fetal scalp blood sampling. American Journal of Obstetrics and Gynecology 1984; 148:274–7; Smith CV, Nguyen HN, Phelan JP, Paul RH. Intrapartum assessment of fetal well-being: a comparison of fetal acoustic stimulation with acid-base determinations. American Journal of Obstetrics and Gynecology 1986; 155:726–8; Rice PE, Benedetti TJ. Fetal heart rate acceleration with fetal blood sampling. Obstetrics and Gynecology 1986; 68:469–72.

37. Pritchard J, MacDonald P, Gant N. Dystocia caused by abnormalities in presentation, position or development of the fetus. In Williams Obstetrics. Seventeenth Edition. Appleton-Century-Crofts, Norwalk: 1985, 651.

38. Taffel, Overview, op. cit.

39. Placek, Patterns, op. cit.

40. Pritchard et al., op. cit., 656.

41. Amon E, Sibai BH, Anderson GD. How perinatologists manage the problem of the presenting breech. American Journal of Perinatology 1988; 5:247–50.

42. Pritchard et al., op. cit., 656.

43. Amon et al., op. cit.

44. National Center for Health Statistics. Advance report of final mortality statistics, 1987. Monthly Vital Statistics Report, 1989; 38.

45. Petitti, op. cit.

46. Willson JR. The conquest of cesarean section-related infections: a progress report. Obstetrics and Gynecology 1988; 72:519–32.

47. Health Care Financing Administration. Medicare Hospital Mortality Information. U.S. Department of Health and Human Services, Washington, DC, 1987.

48. Sachs BP, Yeh J, Acker D, Driscoll S, Brown DAJ, Jewett JF. Cesarean section-related maternal mortality in Massachusetts, 1954–1985. Obstetrics and Gynecology 1988; 71:385–8.

49. Rubin GL, Peterson HB, Rochat RW, McCarthy BJ, Terry JS. Maternal

death after cesarean section in Georgia. American Journal of Obstetrics and Gynecology 1981; 139:681–5.

50. Sachs, op. cit; Rubin, op. cit.

51. Miller JM. Maternal and neonatal morbidity and mortality in cesarean section. Obstetrics and Gynecology Clinics of North America 1988; 15:629–38.

52. Petitti, op. cit.

53. Jeffcoate T, Miller J, Roos RF, Tindall VR. Puerperal thromboembolism in relation to the inhibition of lactation by estrogen therapy. British Medical Journal 1968; 4:19–25; Tindall VR. Factors influencing puerperal thromboembolism. Journal of Obstetrics and Gynecology of the British Commonwealth 1968; 75:1324–7.

54. Miller, op. cit.

55. Stedman CM, Kline RC. Intraoperative complications and unexpected pathology at the time of cesarean section. Obstetrics and Gynecology Clinics of North America 1988; 15:745–69.

56. LaSala AP, Berkeley AS. Primary cesarean section and subsequent fertility. American Journal of Obstetrics and Gynecology 1987; 157:379–83.

57. National Institutes of Health. Cesarean Childbirth. Publication 82–2067, 419–29, 1981.

58. Tulman L, Fawcett J. Return of functional ability after childbirth. Nursing Research 1988; 37:77–81.

59. Garel M, Lelong N, Kaminski M. Follow-up study of psychological consequences of cesarean childbirth. Early Human Development 1988; 16:271–82.

60. Kochanevich-Wallace PM, McCluskey-Fawcett KA, Meck NE. Method of delivery and parent-newborn interaction. Journal of Pediatric Psychology 1988; 13:213–21.

61. Miller, op. cit.

62. Burt RD, Vaughan TL, Daling JR. Evaluating the risks of cesarean section: low Apgar score in repeat cesarean section and vaginal deliveries. American Journal of Public Health 1988; 78:1312–4.

63. Quilligan EJ. Controlling the high cesarean section rate. Contemporary Obstetrics and Gynecology, January 1983: 221.

64. Quilligan, EJ. Personal communications with author, October 9, 1987.

65. Massachusetts Medical Society vs. Peter Hiam, et al. Suffolk, Massachusetts Superior Court, C.A. No. 54057, March 1982.

66. Silver L, Wolfe SM. Unnecessary c-sections: how to cure a national epidemic. Health Research Group 1989: 90A–94A.

67. Shearer B. Interview with author, January 1990.

68. Data gathered by Health Research Group. See Appendix A.

69. Silver L, op. cit. 10.

70. Rooks JP, Weatherby NL, Ernst EKM, Stapleton S, Rosen D, Rosenfield

A. Outcomes of care in birth centers. New England Journal of Medicine 1989; 321:1804–11.

71. Minor AF. The cost of maternity care and childbirth in the United States, 1989. Health Insurance Association of America, 1989.

72. De Regt RH, Minkoff HL, Feldman J, Schwarz RH. Relation of private or clinic care to the cesarean birth rate. New England Journal of Medicine 1986; 315:619–24.

73. Gould JB, Davey B, Stafford RS. Socioeconomic differences in rates of cesarean section. New England Journal of Medicine 1989; 321:233–9.

74. Dados, Oswaldo Cruz Foundation, October 1986, 14.

75. Silver, op. cit.

76. Needham, Porter, and Novelli. Professional liability insurance and its effects: report of a survey of ACOG's Membership, November 1985.

77. Government Accounting Office, "Medical Malpractice—Characteristics of Claims Closed in 1984," Human Resources Division GAO/HRD-87-55. Washington DC, 1987: 55.

78. National Institutes of Health, op. cit., 488.

79. Morlock LL. Impact of states reforms: the Maryland experience. In "Health Care Improvement and Medical Liability." Department of Health and Human Services, Washington DC, 1988.

PART II

Pills

Birth Control Pills, Tranquilizers and
Sleeping Pills, Lactation Suppressing Drugs,
Hormone Replacement Therapy, Accutane

BIRTH CONTROL PILLS

Serious Problems of Safety

In the United States, 13 million women between ages 15 and 44 use oral contraceptives. In this country the number of women relying on the Pill has risen since the early 1980s, reversing a steady decline in Pill use over the previous decade. Now an estimated 32 percent of women of childbearing age use the Pill. The increase in Pill use includes both married and unmarried women.

Risks

- Recent evidence shows that women who have used oral contraceptives for many years may be twice as likely to get breast cancer before age 45.

- Women who smoke more than 15 cigarettes a day and use oral contraceptives are 21 times more likely to suffer a heart attack than Pill users who don't smoke.

- As of 1988 between 100,000 and 200,000 women in the United States still used birth control pills with needlessly high doses of estrogen (over 35 μg) or progestins, thus increasing the risk of stroke, heart attack, and blood clots. (μg = one-millionth of a gram)

- Current product labeling on oral contraceptives is misleading and minimizes adverse effects of Pill use.

- Women having multiple sexual relationships who depend on oral contraceptives alone run a higher risk of contracting AIDS than women who rely on condoms.

Benefits

- Oral contraceptives are the most effective form of approved birth control if properly used.

- They are now proven—at least high-dose pills—to reduce the risk of ovarian and endometrial cancer.

Recommendations

- If you choose oral contraception, use only a Pill with the lowest dose of both estrogen and progestin, and don't smoke.

- We recommend against using any oral contraceptive that has more than 35 µg of estrogen. For example, do not use: Norlestrin 1/50(Parke-Davis), Ortho-Novum 1/50 (Ortho Pharmaceutical), Demulen 1/50-28 (Searle).

- If you smoke and are over 35, choose a different method of birth control. Even if you don't smoke, consider a different method of birth control after age 35.

- If you develop high blood pressure, switch to another form of birth control.

- Use barrier methods (condoms, diaphragms) with spermicide to reduce your risk of contracting sexually transmitted diseases.

*S*EVENTY years ago, Margaret Sanger preached to scandalized audiences that women must be able to control their own bodies. The mother of the birth control movement in this country, Sanger believed that sex without contraception led to generations of unwanted children and promoted repressed sexual behavior resulting in "the monotonous misery of millions who do not die nor end violently, but who are, nevertheless, devoid of the joys of natural love life."[1]

Her colleague, Robert L. Dickinson, envisioned an oral contraceptive that would solve all the problems of women unwilling to use diaphragms or condoms (which had been around since the nineteenth century). Years before the Pill was available, Dickinson dreamed of a physiological method that was completely removed from the act of intercourse. He wanted a device for those who would not use mechanical methods that required sacrifice of pleasure or attention to details. He anticipated the day when "sexual intercourse without procreation could become a completely spontaneous act requiring no forethought. Passion no longer would be dampened by messy fumbling. A method that saved physicians from the awkward chores of diaphragm fitting while increasing their incomes might end the last vestiges of medical hesitancy to prescribe contraception. The magic of science would make contraception easy and aesthetic for physician and patients alike."[2]

Other twentieth century visionaries were more concerned with the problem of worldwide overpopulation and saw birth control as the panacea for solving it. In fact, Aldous Huxley, when he revisited his "Brave New World" in 1958, may have inadvertently jettisoned the term "the Pill" into its present usage in the English language.

We are given two choices—famine, pestilence and war on the one hand, birth control on the other. Most of us choose birth control and immediately find ourselves confronted by a problem that is simultaneously a puzzle in physiology, pharmacology, sociology, psychology and even theology. "The Pill" has not yet been invented. When and if it is invented, how can it be distributed to the many hundreds of millions of potential mothers (or, if it is a pill that works upon the male, potential fathers) who will have to take it if the birth rate of the species is to be reduced?[3]

Huxley's brave new world was dawning. In a handful of years, the Pill would be released straight from animal laboratories onto the American market and there would be nothing less than a virtual stampede for it. By the middle of the 1960s, millions of women would be using birth control pills, and despite early evidence of acute cardiovascular side effects such as increased blood clotting, strokes, and heart attacks, all warnings would be drowned out by the exuberant applause of physicians, profit-hungry drug companies, and their media trumpeteers.

Today, highly effective and convenient contraceptive pills are available for a few dollars a month. Decades after Sanger and Dickinson first preached about a sexually healthier society, 60 million women worldwide are on the Pill. In the United States more than 13 million women use oral contraceptives.[4] Many will use oral contraceptives for the duration of their reproductive years. Just as the early birth controllers imagined, a vast number of women in the 1990s are literally married to the Pill.

THE PILL AND QUALITY OF LIFE IN THE 1990s

Why shouldn't women be married to the Pill? Women need to control their fertility. Family planning is basic to modern life and few rely on chastity, or "goodsex," as writer George Orwell planned in his novel *1984*. Orwell suggested the population could be controlled through the eradication of the sex instinct. "Procreation will be an annual formality like the renewal of a ration card. We shall abolish the orgasm."[5]

If anything, post-1984 is quite the opposite. Women seem to be more sexually active, not less. The percentage of women aged 18 to 44 who have never married and have had intercourse rose from 68 to 76 percent between 1982 and 1987.[6] Women are sexually active sooner and the Pill has been more successful at preventing teenage pregnancies than telling young people to abstain from sex. Especially for the youngest at risk of pregnancy, contraception that is private and partner-independent is important.

For many women, both married and unmarried, convenient birth control is virtually synonymous with a decent quality of life. For many Pill users, life without it is simply unthinkable. As of 1987, even as sexually transmitted diseases threatened the health of every sexually active person, condoms and other barrier methods made no significant gain against oral contraceptive use.[7] This situation may have improved but is still serious.

Furthermore, male involvement in responsibility for contraception has also not changed much throughout the history of birth control in this country. One avowed Pill user complains, "In the 15 years we've been together, he has never even asked what time of the month it is for me. He wouldn't consider a condom. I think if I had depended on him for protection, I would have been pregnant a dozen times." Since women ultimately bear the unwanted pregnancy resulting from any failure of birth control, women and not men most often decide what to use.

Gregory Pincus, creator of the birth control pill, put it quite simply. "I invented the Pill at the request of a woman."[8]

THE QUESTION OF RISKS

Why not use the Pill? The question of whether or not birth control pills are the safest option for you is the subject of this chapter. There are many issues to consider, and like every other decision concerning your health, this is a highly individual one. Unfortunately, you will not be able to base your decision on assurances of absolute safety. In fact, even after 30 years of studying the Pill, much about its long-term effect on human physiology is still unknown.

Although the convenience of the Pill is obvious from the start, soon its problems may also be evident. Many women suffer from headaches, bloating, nausea, irregular bleeding, breast tenderness, weight gain, or optical changes. Other unpleasant effects that can occur from a few months to a few years after starting oral contraceptive use include high blood pressure, gallbladder disease, liver tumors, depression, and metabolic disorders, such as diabetes. Temporary infertility has been associated with the period of time right after Pill use is stopped.

But the long-term risks—which you should also consider— are still not fully known to medical science. True, oral contraceptives have come a long way since the early days—the 1960s and 1970s—when women were first given hormone doses so potent that heart attacks and strokes were not unusual among Pill users. The quantities of hormones in the early pills were safe in test animals, but too often lethal in humans. With hormone levels in the Pill now much lower, the number of women suffering from heart attacks and strokes also appears to have dropped.

Today's Pill is clearly safer in many respects. When used properly it prevents pregnancy 98 percent of the time, and its unwanted clotting properties have been significantly reduced. But serious questions remain concerning the Pill's relationship to breast cancer. Recent persuasive evidence says that some women are more likely to get breast cancer before age 45 if they start taking the Pill in their teens or 20s and continue for many years. To what extent is oral contraceptive use contributing to the rise in breast cancer in this country? Unfortunately, the jury is still out.

THE PILL MAKES A COMEBACK

In the early days, the Pill enjoyed what one physician called "diplomatic immunity" from criticism. The 1960s were a time when everyone saw the need to press for solutions to the awesome problem of world population growth, so criticizing the Pill was considered counterproductive. Women who started using the Pill in the early days may remember how easy it was to feel confident of the safety of what they were doing. In his 1969 book *The Pill: A Shock Report from America,* journalist Morton

Mintz recalls the "avalanche of pro pill pressures exerted on women."

> If you picked up the Helen Gurley Brown book *Sex and the Office* . . . you would be advised in the chapter on management of an affair during the lunch hour: 'If you use pills, so much the easier.' If you picked up *McCall's* for May 1967 you would read that Jeanine Deckers, the former Singing Nun, had composed 'La Pilule d'Or' ('The Golden Pill'); in her fresh, beautiful voice 'she was singing a hymn of praise to God for inspiring mankind to invent the birth-control pill.' If you went to the movies you might see *Prudence and the Pill,* a 20th Century-Fox production described by a *New York Times* reviewer as a 'nauseating little sex comedy in which somebody is always substituting a vitamin or an aspirin for somebody else's oral contraceptive until everyone gets confused or pregnant.' If you read [the July 3, 1964 issue of] *Life* to find out what Dr. Joseph F. Sadusk, Jr., the top doctor in the Food and Drug Administration, had to say, you would be given reassurance: 'We are not taking a dogmatic attitude that oral contraceptives are absolutely safe—and we do intend to review the evidence immediately. But the indications so far are that they are safe, when given under the supervision of a doctor . . . we are not worried. But we're going to watch it.'[9]

Women's confidence didn't shatter until the mid-1970s, when the immunity barrier crumbled and the public finally realized that oral contraceptives were causing women to suffer strokes, blood clots, and heart attacks. Paul Rheingold, a New York litigation attorney who represented many women in Pill-related lawsuits, vividly remembers the days when he was getting many calls about women who were suffering from strokes related to Pill use. Rheingold said it was hard to keep up with for a while. "An entire litigation industry was spawned over the Pill and how it was killing women."[10]

With the news of its harmful effects reaching women in the mid-1970s, Pill use temporarily plummeted. After lower dose pills proved to be just as effective and safer in at least some ways than high dose Pills, women returned to using the Pill. By the early 1980s Pill use began to revive, and according to a 1987 study, it hasn't stopped making a comeback.[11] It is now by far the most widely used form of contraception among unmarried women, used by almost half of those who are exposed to the risk of unintended pregnancy. Next to sterilization, it's the preferred choice of married women too.[12] In all, 32 percent of women at risk of pregnancy ages 18 to 44 use oral contraceptives, an increase since 1982, when 27 percent of this group were users.[13] In a 1987 survey of women's attitudes about contraception, the Pill received by far the most favorable rating of all birth control methods from both married and unmarried women. Three quarters of all women said they had a favorable opinion of the Pill and 95 percent of Pill users were satisfied with it.[14] The Pill is back.

ARE LOW DOSE PILLS THE ANSWER?

In the last 15 years, researchers have learned much more about the potentially lethal properties of the Pill. That information has not come easily, because the Pill itself has changed so much over the years. Now women generally take "low dose" Pills, but what does that mean? Usually, doses of estrogen and, to a lesser extent, progestin are reduced from the levels that were more harmful to women. A dose reduction, however, must not be interpreted as a blanket assurance of safety, as many would have you believe.

It took many years for scientists to figure out the role estrogen plays in changing the properties of blood to speed up clotting, the source of many of the Pill's dangerous side effects. The precise mechanisms for this are still unclear. As currently understood, changes in the coagulability of the blood occur at both high and low doses of estrogen and the risk posed to women depends on individual factors. The likelihood of developing blood clots is higher in women with a family history of stroke, heart attack, or blood clotting. It is also higher in women

> Comparison of pregnancy rates for birth control methods when used **exactly as directed** under conditions of perfect use:[15]
>
> - IUD: 96–99% effective (considered 100 percent effective if used with contraceptive cream, jelly, or foam)
> - Diaphragm: 90–98% effective
> - Condom: 90–97% effective (but close to 100 percent effective if used with spermicidal cream or jelly)
> - Sterilization: 100% effective
> - Combination (estrogen and progestin) Pills: 99% effective

who smoke, probably because tobacco proteins increase blood clotting on their own by making blood platelets stick together.

So even with doses of estrogen much reduced, thromboembolic disease is still the most important risk factor for taking the Pill for some women, especially those who smoke. But also important is the fact that research, much of it published in the 1980s, has linked oral contraceptives to breast cancer.

While no one knows for certain exactly what property of the Pill is responsible, it is thought that estrogen speeds up the growth of breast tumor cells in some women. Several studies have shown the risk of getting breast cancer is increased in women who use the Pill, but not all women are affected, and the most susceptible group of users is still unidentified. The real missing link in understanding the long-term risks of the Pill is older women, the very first Pill users, who are now approaching age 60, the age when increased amounts of cancer would be expected to show up. A big question also looms over those women in their mid-thirties, who were the first to take the Pill as teenagers. (The first Pill users were older, married women who used it to space births. It wasn't until the early 1970s that single teenagers started using the Pill. This is important because the young breast may be more susceptible to carcinogens.)

Over the next 15 years, the changes in the incidence of

breast cancer and other disease among these two groups of women will teach us a lot about the real safety of long-term Pill use. For women on lifetime low doses (less than 50 μg—first available in the mid-1970s) the breast cancer incidence won't be available for at least ten years.

Low dose Pills do not necessarily contain comparably lower doses of the other hormone, progestin (synthetic form of the naturally occurring progesterone). While there are basically only two types of estrogen used in the Pill, there are 19 different progestins that can be used. Some commonly used forms of progestins are as much as five times more potent than others. Progestins are known to increase blood pressure and to raise the level of unwanted cholesterol (low density lipoprotein, LDL) in the blood. The implication is that over many years of use, progestins may contribute to hardening of the arteries. The manifestations of this cardiovascular disease do not develop in most women until midlife or beyond, but the pathologic changes in the arterial vessels are known to begin at a young age.

Furthermore, there is growing scientific evidence of some association between progestins and an increased risk of blood clotting, which suggests that some property in progestins acts the way estrogen does, increasing the risk of diseases related to clotting problems, including strokes and heart attacks.

Years of engineering different forms of synthetic progestins have complicated scientific understanding of the role of the potential hazards of that element of the Pill. Progestins have been heralded as protection against endometrial cancer, and they also serve to maintain regular periods for Pill users. But their side effects are still largely unknown.

In addition to the above effects, progestins in birth control pills have been thought to contribute to breast cancer in younger women.[16] There is also recent evidence that progestins used in hormone replacement therapy for postmenopausal women may be linked to breast cancer.[17] These findings are preliminary. Research on Pill use is like peeling an onion: there are always new layers of understanding beneath what is known. Unfortunately, users are generally the last to be told.

HEART DISEASE AND ORAL CONTRACEPTIVES

The problems with heart disease have not vanished since low dose formulations of the Pill have become more widely prescribed. Women are not getting heart attacks, strokes, or other manifestations of thromboembolic disease at the rate they were when the Pill was much more potent (over 50 μg of estrogen), but the threat of cardiovascular disease remains. Today physicians are being warned to keep women off oral contraceptives for the same reasons given 15 years ago. You should not use the Pill if you have a personal history of:

- blood clots
- strokes
- high blood pressure
- heart disease

The Pill has been implicated in serious or fatal cardiovascular disease in two ways. Most of the evidence points to a mechanism called thrombogenesis, which has to do with the way that blood platelets stick together and coagulate blood. Estrogen accelerates this process, thus increasing the risk of unwanted blood clots. When these clots plug a blood vessel, the result can be fatal. The most common plug is a "venous thrombus," which can lodge in a deep vein of the lower body or break loose and travel to the lung. When the latter happens it is called a pulmonary embolism and can be fatal. Other plugs can form on the arterial side of the circulatory system. When these occur, heart attacks and strokes may result.

Most, but not all, research has demonstrated that the increased risk of thromboembolic disease goes away rapidly once Pill use is stopped.[18] In other words, blood coagulation returns to normal after women go off oral contraceptives.

However, this is not true in women who smoke. Smoking is highly thrombogenic, causing clots on the arterial (more dangerous) side of the circulatory system. A recently published study showed that cigarette smoking was by far the most important independent risk factor for heart attack in young women. The same study showed that women who smoked heavily (defined as 15 or more cigarettes per day) and who were also current users of oral contraceptives, had a whopping 21-fold increased risk of heart attack.[19] Clearly, any woman considering oral contraception should definitely not smoke. Any woman who smokes—at any age—should not use the Pill.

The other cardiovascular problem that can be lethal results from the slow deposition of fat in the arteries (atheromas). The eventual outcome is atherosclerosis, or hardened arteries which eventually choke off the blood supply to the heart, leading to heart attacks. This is a highly unusual condition in women under the age of menopause. It is suspected that naturally occurring estrogen levels during reproductive years have a protective effect, increasing levels of the desirable cholesterol (high density lipoproteins, HDLs) and reducing the unwanted cholesterol (low density lipoproteins, LDLs).

However, researchers have wondered whether the use of oral contraceptives throughout the reproductive years could have any other effect on lipid levels that would increase the risk of heart attacks induced by atherosclerosis. The most recent evidence suggests that oral contraceptives do not accelerate atherosclerosis and that there are no long-term accumulated effects leading to higher incidences of heart attack from this type of cardiovascular disease.[20]

While it doesn't appear that estrogens in birth control pills create problems with lipid levels, some controversy remains about the role of progestins, the other hormones found in the majority of birth control pills. Recent studies indicate that they may counteract the positive cardiovascular effects of estrogens on lipid levels.[21] It may be that progestins increase unwanted cholesterol (LDL). This effect may be particularly dangerous to older women because atherosclerosis is vascular wall damage that takes time to develop and is known to start at an early age.

Dr. Bruce Stadel, Director of Epidemiology in the drug division of the FDA, believes that tailoring contraceptive dose to individual chemistry is ultimately the new frontier. This would theoretically fully address the complicated scenario surrounding cardiovascular risks.

With sex hormones it's clear that too much is bad for you, and too little is bad for you. Too little estrogen (after menopause) and your vascular lining may harden up (atherosclerosis). Too much estrogen and you may get thromboembolic effects.

Sixty million women worldwide take oral contraceptives and we have no way of knowing how much individually each woman needs to suppress ovulation but not disturb lipid levels. The science is relatively undeveloped. Women generally take what they get. They get the Pill.[22]

TAKING THE PILL AFTER 40

Even without any history or present use of oral contraceptives, the risk of heart attack goes up as women age. The reason is simple enough. The incidence of all cardiovascular disease goes up as the vascular system ages and becomes less responsive. Therefore, women have been advised for years not to take birth control pills after age 35 if they smoked, or after 40 if they didn't smoke. According to the FDA's Dr. Stadel, "Especially if women smoked, if they were over 35, add high dose pills and boom, you've really got matches to gasoline."[23]

However, that thinking changed recently in some people's minds. In a surprising decision in October 1989, an advisory panel to the FDA recommended the age limit for using oral contraceptives be lifted from the present age limit of 40. Since the FDA has taken the advice of this panel, it has the effect of giving physicians "permission" to prescribe the Pill to women until they reach menopause.

In general, the reasoning beind the move was that age alone should not rule out Pill use. If a woman doesn't smoke, or doesn't have other vascular problems, there is little reason why she shouldn't be using a low dose Pill rather than other less effective methods of birth control, the panel said.[24]

That was the reasoning after a day of testimony by medical experts who showed evidence that women over 40 are very sexually active, have a high rate of abortions for their number of pregnancies, run higher risks of maternal death, and have children with higher incidences of congenital problems. "We are talking about a total of more than 10 million women (between ages 40 and 54) in the United States who need to control their fertility," said Judith A. Fortney of Family Health International.

Unfortunately, the recommendation was made in the absence of any data to support the safety of continued use of birth control pills beyond age 40. By making this recommendation, the panel added new meaning to the practice of "long-term use." Now women in so-called low risk groups could be on the Pill for another 15 or so years. "I was shocked," said Dr. Robert Hoover, a leading government cancer researcher. "They did it in a vacuum."[25]

This was confirmed by the comments of an invited guest speaker before the FDA panel. "We really do not have epidemiologic studies relating to current prescribing practice in which the majority of women use pills containing less than 50 μg. We probably will not have these studies for another 5–10 years because of the necessity to derive data and analyze them."[26]

In his independent review of the evidence, leading researcher Paul D. Stolley of the University of Pennsylvania School of Medicine confirmed that the new recommendation to raise the age limit was ill-advised. "The earlier advice to physicians still seems prudent . . . try to avoid prescribing oral contraceptives for women over 35 years of age."[27]

BREAST CANCER AND THE PILL

Since the Pill first came on the market 30 years ago, researchers have tried to determine if its manipulation of the body's hormone profile contributes to cancers of the reproductive system. The evidence shows that oral contraceptives protect against endometrial and ovarian cancers.[28] We will discuss those benefits later. The area that is not quite as crystal clear is how the Pill relates to breast cancer, a deadly disease which takes years or even decades to develop and that strikes thousands of women, usually at older ages.

During their lifetime, about one out of eleven American women develops breast cancer.[29] At 30 years old, 28 in every 100,000 women in the United States are diagnosed. At age 50 the incidence is 195 in every 100,000. At age 70 the number rises to 362 women in every 100,000.[30] Despite the fact that cancer has always been considered an old age disease, the incidence of breast cancer in women under age 45 is increasing very rapidly at a rate of 1.5 to 2 percent a year.[31]

Breast tissue has receptors for both estrogen and progesterone, and high levels of either have been implicated as a cause of breast cancer in both animals and humans.[32] Although increasing exposure of breast tissue to estrogens and perhaps progestins is thought to enhance the risk of malignancies, no one is sure how or why. In addition, some studies suggest that estrogen exposure at certain times in life, such as under age 25 or before having a first child, may be more likely to stimulate breast cancer than exposure years later.[33] But that remains controversial.

In his summary of a decade of research on the impact of oral contraceptives on breast cancer, researcher Dr. James J. Schlesselman wrote:

> If one understood the hormonal events that determine whether or not a breast cancer will develop, one could better infer the likely effects of oral contraception. In the absence of such knowledge, one may either speculate about what ought to occur, or turn to studies that report what in fact does happen. Regrettably, many of the "facts" are presently in dispute. The picture that currently emerges might well be described as kaleidoscopic.[34]

Before we look at this kaleidoscope of research and consider the speculation, let's look at what are considered basic risk factors for breast cancer aside from oral contraceptive use. Most studies categorize individual risk based on reproductive and family histories. Having an immediate relative, a sister, mother, aunt, or grandmother who has suffered from the disease increases your personal risk. Other factors for increased risk are age (older women have increased risk) and nationality (women in the United States are at greater risk than, for example, Japanese women).[35] Reproductive risk factors relate to the amount of time a woman is exposed to cyclical hormonal fluctuations. So other increased risk factors include early age at start of menstruation (before age 15),[36] a late age at menopause, childlessness, and a late age at first pregnancy. Obesity after menopause may also increase your risk.[37]

Ever since breast cancer was discovered it has been known that ovarian hormones play a role in its development, which partially explains why women whose ovaries are active longer (early menstruation, late menopause) statistically show an increased incidence of breast cancer. For example, women who go into menopause at age 55 have about twice the risk of breast cancer as women who become menopausal at 45. So about 10 additional years of cyclic ovarian activity at that time of life tends to double a woman's risk of breast cancer.[38]

Conversely, halting ovarian activity reduces the risks of breast cancer. That is why women whose ovaries are surgically removed before menopause have a reduced risk of breast cancer. Pregnancy also halts cyclic ovarian action, so women with children and women who get pregnant early in life have less breast cancer.

One theory on why childbearing reduces breast cancer risks relates to the breast tissue itself. During the last part of pregnancy, breast tissue cells mature, or "differentiate," dramatically. It is thought that once the previously immature cells go through this change, they are less vulnerable to carcinogens. If this is true, it may partially explain some studies which suggest that early Pill use (before first pregnancy) is linked to breast cancer. Theoretically, estrogen from the Pill is "hitting" immature breast tissue.

Given these many reproductive factors, breast cancer studies look for groups of women who might be more susceptible to the cancer-causing properties of the Pill than others. They want to know how and if the following affect the breast cancer risk associated with Pill use:

- age of first menstruation
- age of first Pill use relative to first pregnancy
- number of pregnancies, if any
- age of menopause (if menopause has occurred)

Also, any adverse effect of oral contraception ought to show a dose response by duration of use. In other words, a woman's risk of developing breast cancer should increase as the amount of exposure to contraceptive hormones adds up. Unfortunately, dose and duration variables are extremely difficult to nail down because the Pill has changed so much over the 30 years it's been around. For example, it is nearly impossible to study a group of Pill users who all used the same dose. No study has been able to sort out the combinations and types of products that have been available over the years.

Furthermore, women tend to change Pills and forget what they used and for how long. By necessity researchers have had to lump research participants together using terms like "ever-users" versus "never-users." These factors make any analysis of long-term Pill safety extremely difficult.

There are other intrinsic limitations to oral contraceptive research when long-term effects are under scrutiny. For one thing, breast cancer may have a very long latency period, up to 20 years or more. Since oral contraceptives did not come on the market until 1960, relatively few women now older than 60 would have ever used the Pill, and women in their 50s could not have taken it early in their reproductive years. Consequently, most studies of the relationship between the Pill and breast cancer have been confined to younger women who make up only a fraction of women who get breast cancer.

Since 1977, six studies have reported an elevated risk of breast cancer in some women who used oral contraceptives before their first delivery.[39] In four of these studies the authors noted that duration of use before the first birth played a role in the cancer outcome.[40]

■ In a study from San Francisco of women under the age of 50 (who had not reached menopause) researchers reported that women who used oral contraceptives before their first delivery were 2.7 times more likely to get breast cancer.[41]

■ In Los Angeles, increased breast cancer risk was identified among women who were diagnosed with it before age 33 and had used oral contraceptives before their first pregnancy. These women showed a risk of breast cancer 3.5 times that of nonusers after eight years. When this study was updated in 1983, results seemed to indicate that having taken the Pill before age 25 was the critical risk factor.[42]

■ In 1982 a study showed that women aged 35 to 54 who had ever used oral contraceptives before their first delivery had a threefold risk of developing breast cancer. In that study the risk seemed to increase with duration of use.[43]

■ In a 1986 study from Sweden, women under age 45 who had used the Pill for longer than eight years before having a child were twice as likely to develop breast cancer.[44]

■ In 1987 researchers reported a more than twofold increase in the risk of developing breast cancer under age 45 in women who used oral contraceptives for more than four years before their first delivery.[45]

These and other studies over the past 10 years have linked the Pill to breast cancer. However, they seem not to have jolted some of the nation's leading researchers. "The cumulative risk of breast cancer through 59 years of age appears to bear no relationship to oral contraceptive (OC) use, whatsoever," wrote Dr. James Schlesselman, in a recent analysis of studies over the past decade. "Studies restricted to women [with breast cancer diagnosed] under age 45, however, raise concern about a possible adverse effect from OC use before a first-term pregnancy."[46] While claiming not to be worried, Schlesselman and others acknowledge that recent evidence is also not particularly reassuring.

Dr. Bruce Stadel, leading author of the Cancer and Steroid Hormone Study (CASH), found that "oral contraceptive use in the 1960s and 1970s may have promoted earlier onset of breast cancer in susceptible women." In this study, women of ages 20 to 54 whose breast cancer was diagnosed between December 1980 and December 1982 were personally interviewed at home about their reproductive history. The study found that women who had never given birth, who had used the Pill for more than eight years, and who had started menstruating before age 13, showed an increased risk of developing breast cancer before age 45, and a decreased risk after that age.[47]

Why? "Our studies indicate that oral contraceptives may speed up the rate of growth of [breast] cancer in susceptible women." Stadel emphasized that the CASH study pointed to earlier onset of breast cancer but did not show increased risk to the general population of Pill users. "This is consistent with laboratory evidence that high doses of hormones—especially estrogen—may promote the growth of existing tumors."[48]

Does it follow, in this expert's opinion, that lower doses are safer, that women who have children are protected, or that only women who have existing tumors will get breast cancer from the Pill? "I won't go any further," says Stadel. "I can't go any further. People who do are stretching what we really do and do not know. We have a lot of reason to think that in general lower doses are probably safer, but that's a pretty general statement."[49]

Like the CASH investigators, researchers from Britain's Royal College of General Practitioners found that the Pill probably accelerates latent cancer rather than initiates it. A study from the College began enrolling oral contraceptive users and an equal number of nonusers in 1968. The data analyzed in 1985 showed an increased risk of breast cancer among women of ages 30 to 34 who had "ever-used" oral contraceptives and had only one child at the time their cancer was diagnosed.[50]

Clifford Kay, director of the Royal College study, speculated that the Pill might negate the otherwise protective effect against breast cancer that first pregnancies normally provide.[51]

Further evidence on the promotional effects of the Pill on breast cancer development are more recent and perhaps even more compelling. A hospital-based study conducted between 1983 and 1986 in 16 hospitals on the East Coast showed that among women diagnosed with breast cancer under age 45, the relative risk of the disease rose to four times that of nonusers after 10 years of contraceptive use.[52] The authors of the study said: "[Our] results suggest that oral contraceptive users, particularly those with very long duration of use, may be at increased risk of breast cancer." They also noted that "this study provides new evidence to suggest that the risk of breast cancer is increased among women below the age of 45 years who have used oral contraceptives. The risk appeared to be approximately doubled for use of less than 10 years duration, and quadrupled for 10 or more years of use."

Other respected researchers in foreign studies reached similar conclusions. A study of Swedish and Norwegian women found: "Our data for long-term use of OC (oral contraceptives) beyond 7 years and particularly for 12 years or more are suggestive of an association with an increased risk of premenopausal breast cancer."[53] Another study in Sweden concluded: Our "findings indicated that early OC [oral contraceptive] use was associated with a high risk of breast cancer development among premenopausal women."[54] Finally, another recent study from Great Britain showed once again that young women who use the Pill for long periods are at an increased risk for early breast cancer. The United Kingdom Case-Control Study Group demonstrated that women diagnosed with breast cancer under age 36, who had used the Pill for between four and eight years, were 1.43 times more at risk for the disease. The risk crept higher for women who had used it longer.[55]

On the other hand, there have also been 20 reports on 13 independent studies published since 1980 that show no association between Pill use and breast cancer. However, this evidence is neither conclusive nor reassuring:

- Most studies were conducted on women who had little early, long-term Pill use, because they were older when Pill use became widespread.[56]

- Three previously "negative" studies have since yielded positive findings when updated or refocused on a younger age group.[57]

- Six of eight "negative" reports on women with extensive early Pill use are based on data collected from just one population of women. Under reanalysis the data revealed an elevated risk of breast cancer with Pill use for some women.

- The most widely cited persuasive evidence refuting any link between oral contraceptives and breast cancer comes from a study conducted in New Zealand. However, even this study raises concern that women who use the Pill may be at an elevated risk of developing breast cancer under age 36.[58]

The argument that is repeatedly used to refute a connection between Pill use and breast cancer is that low doses are safer than high doses. By necessity, most of the research thus far has used data on higher doses of the Pill than are prescribed today. According to this argument, evidence on high doses may be questionable, but lower doses are undoubtedly safer.

In fact, no one can safely speculate that far. If low doses allow women to use the Pill for a longer period of time, perhaps the accumulated effect by age 60 is worse. Without data, no one can be sure whether low doses are safer or not. For epidemiologic evidence on the association between low dose Pills and breast cancer, we will have to wait quite a while, maybe 20 years, until the young women now taking lower doses of the Pill reach the age at which they may or may not develop breast cancer.

Dr. Robert Hoover, leading cancer researcher at the National Institutes of Health, explained the present state of cancer research and oral contraceptives. "If we knew what it is about the

Pill that increases the risk of breast cancer, then we might be able to rest easier with lower doses. But since we don't, saying that lower doses will be safer is more than a little speculative."[59]

BENEFITS OF THE PILL

The Pill has some lesser known beneficial effects on such diseases as acne and iron deficiency anemia due to menstrual bleeding, but its most important beneficial side effect is that it reduces the risk of two cancers—cancer of the ovary, which is often fatal, and cancer of the uterine lining, the endometrium, which is less serious and more easily treated.

Approximately two percent of American women develop endometrial cancer.[60] Women at greatest risk are white, obese, childless and have a late age of menopause.[61] In the United States, 95 percent of endometrial cancers are diagnosed in women over age 45.[62]

Studies published since 1980 showed that women who used combined oral contraceptives (estrogen and progestins in a cyclic regimen) for at least one year have a significantly reduced risk of endometrial cancer. The combined data of six studies show that one year of using the Pill reduces the risk by about 20 percent, two years doubles that reduction, and four years or more provides about a 60 percent reduction in risk.[63] It is still unclear whether this protection lasts after Pill use ceases.

Ovarian cancer is a much more deadly form of cancer and afflicts approximately one percent of American women. It is harder to detect than other cancers, and 60 percent of the time it has spread to other body locations before it is found. Consequently, survival rate is poor. Only about 40 percent of all women diagnosed with ovarian cancer are alive five years later.[64]

Every study of this issue has found that the Pill offers protection against ovarian cancer after three or more years of use.[65] Studies also suggest the reduced risk of ovarian cancer remains in effect long after oral contraception is stopped.[66]

These positive findings, however, for both ovarian and endometrial cancers, should be looked at with a balanced view.

Most studies showing a reduction of ovarian and uterine cancer were done on women using Pills containing 50 μg or more of estrogen. It has not yet been established whether this protective effect will still be present in women on the lower dose 35 μg Pills. Since the benefits, like the risks, appear to derive from the dosage of estrogen and progestins, it is possible that a lower dose pill will have less of these benefits as well.

DECIDING ON SAFE CONTRACEPTION: DON'T TRUST THE PILL LABELS

Obviously, what you don't know about the Pill can hurt you. Unfortunately, you can't look at the product labels for guidance. They tell you about the "current conflict in research," but generally don't mention which groups of women may be more susceptible to Pill effects.

One of the most blatantly inaccurate labels comes out of Parke-Davis, the maker of Loestrin and Norlestrin. It states in the warning section: "The overwhelming evidence in the literature suggests that use of oral contraceptives is not associated with an increase in the risk of developing breast cancer, regardless of the age and parity of first use."[67]

Most warning labels do not include the most recent findings, which suggest elevated risk of developing breast cancer under age 45 in long-term users, women who use the Pill before their first delivery, and those with a long history of Pill use under age 25.

The pack of new studies showing an association between the Pill and breast cancer did prompt the FDA to rethink the accuracy of labels on oral contraceptives, but they were urged by their outside advisory committee, made up largely of obstetrician/gynecologists, not to change current labeling. Their argument was that if women were informed of this new evidence (even though it was "balanced" by mentioning that there were also negative studies) they might change their contraceptive practices. So despite the newest reports, the FDA committee concluded, "The existing data do not support a change in prescribing practices by physicians or in the use of oral contraceptives by women."[68]

COMPARING THE PILL TO OTHER ALTERNATIVES

The most recent survey of contraceptive failure rates published in 1989 showed, as expected, that the Pill remains the most effective means of birth control. However, the report indicated a higher than expected failure rate of six percent for all Pill users, including married and unmarried women, and young users under 20. The data showed that young (under 20), unmarried, nonwhite women experienced as much as an 18 percent failure rate with the Pill, while the oldest group, over 35, white, and married, became pregnant at a rate of less than two percent a year.[69]

Overall, use of the Pill as directed prevents pregnancy over 99 percent of the time. Most of the failure rate can be attributed to skipping Pills, which in the case of low dose formulations greatly increases the chances of ovulation. Perfect use makes a considerable difference, and with low dose pills that can be tricky. They have to be taken every 24 hours without skipping a pill. This kind of strict requirement obviously reduces its effectiveness for some women. "While in theory oral contraceptives offer almost complete protection against pregnancy, failures occur fairly often in practice because women do not always exactly follow the regimen for taking the pill," concluded the study's authors.[70]

Failure rates for IUDs were not included in the study, but currently two IUDs are available in the United States: the only copper-containing IUD on the market, the Copper T 380A (ParaGard), and the progesterone-releasing IUD (Progestasert). A report published in 1989 suggests that the progesterone-releasing IUD, which must be changed every 12 months, is effective 94 percent of the time, and the copper IUD, inserted for four years, is effective 97 percent of the time.[71] However, the same report emphasized that these IUDs are not recommended for every woman. "The IUD is an acceptable method of contraception, especially for those women who are in the middle to older reproductive years, unable to take oral contraceptives, in a stable monogamous relationship and not at risk for sexually transmitted diseases."[72]

Pelvic inflammatory disease (PID) is one serious complication of IUDs. There is an increased relative risk of PID from 1.5 to 2.6 in women using IUDs compared with women using no form of contraception.[73] Other complications include uterine perforation, expulsion, pregnancy, ectopic pregnancy, pain, and bleeding.

Because of side effects and complications associated with both IUDs, they are not recommended in women with multiple sexual partners or a history of pelvic infections, bleeding disorders, or previous ectopic pregnancies. Due to the increased risk of PID they are not recommended for women who have never had children.

Failure rates for surgical sterilization were not included in the study because accidental pregnancy from that method of contraception is so rare. For older women who are finished with childbearing, sterilization via tubal ligation is an excellent method of birth control. It entails only a one-time surgical risk, which makes it, overall, safer for many older women. One disadvantage is its cost, which can be up to $2,000, including anesthesia.

The diaphragm provides up to 98 percent effectiveness when combined with spermicidal jelly and otherwise used correctly.[74] The two percent failure rate for the diaphragm (when used perfectly) may be due to the fact that it moves around some during intercourse. It may also be related to improper fitting.

Obviously, the success of "barrier methods" has a lot to do with how well you are instructed to use them and how well you follow the directions. Diaphragms and condoms are excellent forms of birth control, not only because they are highly successful at preventing pregnancies, but also because they help protect against sexually transmitted disease, including AIDS. However, the diaphragm does not afford as much protection against any sexually transmitted disease as the condom does. Your own ability to use these methods will depend somewhat on the type of sexual relationships you have, your attitudes about pregnancy, your feelings about the method, and whether you know how to use them.

IF YOU CHOOSE THE PILL, HOW CAN YOU DECREASE YOUR RISK?

A woman's decision on contraception must take into account both the risks and benefits. Certainly, if the Pill is the only contraceptive that a women feels she is able to use consistently, the risk of unplanned pregnancy may outweigh potential side effects. However, there are safer contraceptives, such as a diaphragm with spermicide, that if used properly are quite effective without the potential side effects of the Pill. Further, unless you are having sex with someone with whom you have had a long-term monogamous relationship, if you use the Pill you must also get your partner to use a condom. AIDS kills and a condom can probably protect you.

If you decide to use the Pill, you should take one with the lowest amount of estrogen and progestin. If you are on a Pill containing 50 μg of estrogen, discuss with your doctor the desirability of switching to a lower dose, such as 35 μg. Since this higher dose (50 μg) Pill provides little if any additional benefits, only risks, most women should never take them. One frequently voiced reason for prescribing it is bleeding between periods, but this can usually be controlled somewhat with lower dose Pills.

Higher estrogen Pills are a relic from the past, an historic attempt at an effective oral contraceptive whose unique usefulness has worn out but whose danger remains. Although Pills with greater than 50 μg of estrogen are now finally off the market, between 100,000 and 200,000 women in the U.S. were still taking pills with 50 μg as late as 1988.[75]

1. Reed J. From Private Vice to Public Virtue, The Birth Control Movement and American Society Since 1830. Basic Books, New York: 1978, 138.

2. Ibid., 311.

3. Huxley A. Brave New World Revisited. Harper & Row, New York: 1958, 111–2.

4. Forrest JD, Fordyce RR. U.S. women's contraceptive attitudes and practice: how have they changed in the 1980s? Family Planning Perspectives 1988; 20:3, 112–118.

5. Orwell, G. 1984. Harcourt Brace Jovanovich, Inc. Signet Edition, New York: 1949, 220.

6. Forrest, op. cit.

7. Ibid.

8. Pincus G. Interview in Candide, 1966. As quoted in Reed, op. cit., 309.

9. Mintz M. The Pill: A Shock Report from America. Fawcett Publications Inc., New York: 1969.

10. Rheingold P. Interview with author, November 1989.

11. Forrest, op. cit.

12. Ibid.

13. Ibid.

14. Ibid.

15. Tatum HJ, Connell-Tatum EB. Barrier contraception: a comprehensive review. Fertility and Sterility 1981; 36:10; Hatcher RA, Stewart GK, Guest F, Finkelstein R, Godwin C. Contraceptive Technology 1976–1977. Eighth edition. Irvington Publishers, New York: 1976.

16. Henderson BE, Pike MC, Ross RK. Epidemiology and risk factors. In Bonadonna G, ed. Breast Cancer: Diagnosis and Management. John Wiley & Sons, New York: 1984, 15–33.

17. Bergkvist L, Adami HO, Persson I, Hoover R, Schairer C. The risk of breast cancer after estrogen and estrogen-progestin replacement. New England Journal of Medicine 1989; 321:293–7.

18. von Kaulla E, Droegemueller W, Aoki N, von Kaulla KN. Antithrombin III depression and thrombin generation acceleration in women taking oral contraceptives. American Journal of Obstetrics and Gynecology 1971; 109:868–73.

19. Croft P, Hannaford PC. Risk factors for acute myocardial infarction in women: evidence from the Royal College of General Practitioners oral contraception study. British Medical Journal 1989; 298:165–8.

20. Stampfer MJ, Willett WC, Colditz GA, Speizer FE, Hennekens CH. A prospective study of past use of oral contraceptive agents and risk of cardiovascular diseases. New England Journal of Medicine 1988; 319:1313–7.

21. Knopp RH. Arteriosclerosis risk: The roles of oral contraceptives and postmenopausal estrogens. Journal of Reproductive Medicine 1986; 31:913–21.

22. Stadel B. Interview with author, November 1989.

23. Ibid.

24. Fertility and Maternal Health Drugs Advisory Committee, FDA, summary minutes, October 26–27, 1989.

25. Hoover R. Interview with author, November 1989.

26. Testimony of Dr. Daniel R. Mishell before Fertility and Maternal Health Drugs Advisory Committee, FDA, October 26–27, 1989.

27. Stolley PD, Strom BL, Sartwell PE. Oral contraceptives and vascular disease. Epidemiologic Reviews 1989; 11:241–3.

28. Schlesselman JJ. Cancer of the breast and reproductive tract in relation to use of oral contraceptives. Contraception 1989; 40:1.

29. Willis J. Progress against breast cancer. FDA Consumer, May 1986, 6–11.

30. Cancer Statistics Review 1973–1987. National Cancer Institute, 1990.

31. Hoover, op. cit.

32. Henderson, op. cit.; Petrakis NL, Ernster VL, King MC. Breast. In Schottenfeld D, Fraumeni JF, eds. Cancer Epidemiology and Prevention. Philadelphia: WB Sanders Co, 1982; 855–70

33. Schlesselman, op. cit.

34. Ibid.

35. Henderson, op. cit.

36. Helmrich SP, Shapiro S, Rosenberg L, Kaufman DW, Slone D, Bain C, Miettinen OS, Stolley PD, Rosenshein NB, Knapp RC, Leavitt T, Schottenfeld D, Engle RL, Levy M. Risk factors for breast cancer. American Journal of Epidemiology, 1983; 117:35–45.

37. Drife JO. Evolution, menstruation and breast cancer. In Bulbrook RD, Taylor DJ, eds. Commentaries on Research in Breast Disease. Vol 1. Alan R. Liss, New York: 1979; 1–23; Henderson, op. cit.; Sattin RW, Rubin GL, Webster LA, Huezo CM, Wingo PA, Ory HW, Layde PM. Family history and the risk of breast cancer. Journal of the American Medical Association 1985; 253:1908–13.

38. Hoover, op. cit.

39. Paffenbarger RS, Fasal E, Simmons ME, Kampert JB. Cancer risk as related to the use of oral contraceptives during fertile years. Cancer 1977; 39:1887–91; Pike MC, Henderson BE, Casagrande JT, Rosario I, Gray GE. Oral contraceptive use and early abortion as risk factors for breast cancer in young women. British Journal of Cancer 1981; 43:72–6; Harris NV, Weiss NS, Francis AM, Polissar L. Breast cancer in relation to patterns of oral contraceptive use. American Journal of Epidemiology 1982; 116:643–51; Meirik O, Lund E, Adami H, Bergstrom R, Christofferson T, Bergsjo P. Oral contraceptive use and breast cancer in young women. A joint national case-control study in Sweden and Norway. Lancet 1986; ii: 650–4; McPherson K, Vessey MP, Neil A, Doll R, Jones

L, Roberts M. Early oral contraceptive use and breast cancer: results of another case control study. British Journal of Cancer 1987; 56:653–60; Olsson H, Moller TR, Ranstam J. Early oral contraceptive use and breast cancer among premenopausal women: final report from a study in southern Sweden. Journal of the National Cancer Institute 1989; 81:1000–4.

40. Pike, op. cit.; Harris, op. cit.; Meirik, op. cit.; McPherson, op. cit.

41. Paffenbarger, op. cit.

42. Pike, op. cit.; Pike MC, Henderson BE, Krailo MD, Duke A. Breast cancer in young women and use of oral contraceptives: possible modifying effect of formulation and age at use. Lancet 1983; 2:926–30.

43. Harris, op. cit.

44. Meirik, op. cit.

45. McPherson, op. cit.

46. Schlesselman, op. cit.

47. Stadel BV. Oral contraceptives and premenopausal breast cancer in nulliparous women. Contraception 1988; 38:287–99.

48. Stadel, interview, op. cit.

49. Ibid.

50. Kay CR, Hannaford PC. Breast cancer and the pill: a further report from The Royal College of General Practitioners' oral contraception study. British Journal of Cancer 1988; 58:675–80.

51. Johnson JH. Weighing the evidence on the pill and breast cancer. Family Planning Perspectives 1989; 21:89–92.

52. Miller DR, Rosenberg L, Kaufman DW, Stolley P, Warshauer ME, Shapiro S. Breast cancer before age 45 and oral contraceptive use: new findings. American Journal of Epidemiology 1989; 129:269–80.

53. Meirik, op. cit.

54. Olsson, op. cit.

55. UK National Case-Control Study Group. Oral contraceptive use and breast cancer risk in young women. Lancet 1989; 1:974–82.

56. Kelsey JL, Fischer DB, Holford TR, LiVoisi VA, Mostow ED, Goldenberg IS, White C. Exogenous estrogens and other factors in the epidemiology of breast cancer. Journal of the National Cancer Institute 1981; 67:327–33; Trapido EJ. A prospective cohort study of oral contraceptives and breast cancer. Journal of the National Cancer Institute, 1981; 67:1011–5; Brinton LA, Hoover R, Szklo M, Fraumeni JF. Oral contraceptives and breast cancer. International Journal of Epidemiology 1982; 11:316–22; Vessey MP, McPherson K, Yeates D, Doll R. Oral contraceptive use and abortion before first term pregnancy in relation to breast cancer risk. British Journal of Cancer 1982; 45:327–31; Centers for Disease Control Cancer and Steroid Hormone Study. Long-term oral contraceptive use and the risk of breast cancer. Journal of the American Medical Association 1983; 249:1591–5; Vessey MP, Baron J, Doll R, McPherson K, Yeates D. Oral contraceptives and breast cancer; final report of an epidemiological study. British

Journal of Cancer 1983; 47:455–62; Hennekens CH, Speizer FE, Lipnick RJ, Rosner B, Bain C, Belanger C, Stampfer MJ, Willett W, Peto R. A case-control study of oral contraceptive use and breast cancer. Journal of the National Cancer Institute 1984; 72:39–42; Talamini R, LaVecchia C, Franceschi S, Colombo F, Decarli A, Grattoni E, Grigoletto E, Tognoni G. Reproductive and hormonal factors and breast cancer in a northern Italian population. International Journal of Epidemiology 1985; 14:70–4; Ellery C, MacLennan R, Berry G, Shearman RP. A case control study of breast cancer in relation to the use of steroid contraceptive agents. Medical Journal of Australia 1986; 144:173–6; Lipnick RJ, Buring JE, Hennekens CH, Rosner B, Willet W, Bain C, Stampfer MJ, Colditz GA, Peto R, Speizer FE. Oral contraceptives and breast cancer: a prospective cohort study. Journal of the American Medical Association 1986; 255:58–61; La Vecchia C, Decarli A, Fasoli M, Franceschi S, Gentile A, Negri E, Parazzini F, Tognoni G. Oral contraceptives and cancers of the breast and of the female genital tract. British Journal of Cancer 1986; 54:311–17; Vessey MP, McPherson K, Villard-MacKintosh L, Yeates D. Oral contraceptives and breast cancer: latest findings in a large cohort study. British Journal of Cancer 1989; 59:613–7.

57. McPherson, op. cit.; Stadel, op. cit.; Miller, op. cit.

58. Paul C, Skegg DCG, Spears GFS, Kaldor JM. Oral contraceptives and breast cancer: a national study. British Medical Journal 1986; 293:723–6.

59. Hoover, op. cit.

60. Schlesselman, op. cit.

61. Kelsey JL, Hildreth NG. Breast and Gynecologic Cancer Epidemiology. CRC Press, Boca Raton: 1983 as cited in Schlesselman, op. cit.; Henderson BE, Casagrande JT, Pike MC, Mack T, Rosario I, Duke A. The epidemiology of endometrial cancer in young women. British Journal of Cancer 1983; 47:749–56.

62. Young JL, Percey CL, Asire AJ, eds. Surveillance Epidemiology End Results. Incidence and Mortality Data: 1973–1977. Bethesda: National Institutes of Health, 1981 as cited in Schlesselman, op. cit.

63. Schlesselman, op. cit., 13.

64. National Cancer Institute, Cancer Statistics Review, op. cit.

65. Schlesselman, op. cit., 17

66. Ibid.

67. Physician's Desk Reference 1990. 4th Edition. Oradell NJ: Medical Economics Company, 1619–38.

68. Food and Drug Administration, Fertility and Maternal Health Drugs Advisory Committee. Summary minutes. Rockville, Md.; January 5–6, 1989.

69. Jones EF, Forrest JD. Contraceptive failure in the United States: revised estimates from the 1982 national survey of family growth. Family Planning Perspectives 1989; 21:103–9.

70. Ibid.

71. Questions and Answers: Diagnostic and Therapeutic Technology As-

sessment (DATTA), Intrauterine Devices. Journal of the American Medical Association 1989; 261:2127–30.

72. Ibid.

73. Grimes DA. Intrauterine devices and pelvic inflammatory disease: recent developments. Contraception 1987; 36:97–109.

74. Lane ME, Arceo R, Sobrero AJ. Successful use of the diaphragm and jelly by a young population: report of a clinical study. Family Planning Perspectives 1976; 8:81–6.

75. Estimate of high-dose pill users based on data from National Prescription Audit. IMS, Ambler PA, 1988.

TRANQUILIZERS AND SLEEPING PILLS

Two Groups of Dangerously Overprescribed Drugs

Each year, there are approximately 100 million prescriptions filled for tranquilizers and sleeping pills in the United States. But according to data from a nationwide survey of doctors' offices, two-thirds of these prescriptions are for women, only one-third for men. In other words, women get twice as many prescriptions for these drugs as men, about 66 million to 33 million, and women are therefore the principal targets of the gross overprescribing of these too-often dangerous drugs. (The survey was done by IMS, Inc., Ambler, PA.)

- Even at the recommended doses tranquilizers such as Valium, Librium, Xanax or Tranxene, or sleeping pills such as Dalmane, Restoril, or Halcion can cause unwanted and often debilitating mental, physical, and emotional changes. Daytime sedation, confusion, memory loss, poor coordination causing falls and hip fractures, impaired learning ability, slurred speech, even death are possible side effects of these drugs.

- Drowsiness, fatigue, dizziness, lightheadedness and slowed reaction times are all common problems of tranquilizer users. At least one in five people taking tranquilizers will be disturbed by unwanted drowsiness.

- Although tranquilizers are supposed to calm you down, some people feel more aggressive and hostile after taking them. These paradoxical reactions include rage, excitement, and violence.

- A large proportion of people who use tranquilizers or sleeping pills at the recommended doses for more than one or two months will become addicted. Over two million American women are taking a sleeping pill or tranquilizer every day for a year or more, longer than any evidence shows they are effective.

- Older women are at particular risk for dangerous effects because they have more difficulty clearing the drug from their systems, resulting in increased toxicity. Furthermore, older women are more likely to use them for extended periods of time.

- Using tranquilizers during pregnancy or while pregnancy or while you are nursing poses serious health threats to your infant.

Recommendations

- Many people with anxiety, panic attacks, posttraumatic stress disorder, and depression-based insomnia would benefit from a mental health specialist.

- Absolutely avoid the "jet lag" sleeping pill Halcion (triazolam), a drug with many serious side effects.

- Avoid tranquilizers if you drink alcohol, drive, or do anything that requires coordination, or if you are pregnant or nursing. Those with a history of problem drinking or drug dependence should especially avoid these drugs.

> - The only prescription tranquilizer or sleeping pill that we advise for use, albeit limited use (one week or less), is oxazepam, available generically, and under the brand name of Serax.
>
> - Before using any tranquilizer, make sure that your doctor knows whether you are taking other drugs with a sedative or "downer" effect, such as antidepressants, antipsychotics, antihistamines, narcotic painkillers, epilepsy medications, barbiturates, or other sleeping medications. Oxazepam taken with other drugs with sedative effects dangerously increases the risks of both.

*W*E all suffer from stress and anxiety, and the urge to take a pill to get some relief, relax, and get a good night's sleep may be very tempting. But too often, physicians comply with their patients' pleas for relief by prescribing mild tranquilizers or sleeping pills. Unfortunately, physicians who prescribe them may dismiss the risks with the assertion that, in general, these drugs are remarkably safe.

Tranquilizers can be safe, but they can also be very dangerous. Certainly they are grossly overprescribed, especially to older women, for periods five to ten times longer than the drugs have been proven to be effective. Long-term use increases your risk of addiction and mental, physical, and emotional impairment. Also, underlying problems may go ignored when they are masked by the effects of the drugs. In short, when you take pills to ease your anxiety or help you sleep, you have brought new reasons to worry into your life.

Tranquilizers (minor tranquilizers or antianxiety pills) and sleeping pills are discussed together because the most commonly used drugs in both classes belong to the same family of chemicals, called benzodiazepines. The vast majority of prescriptions filled in retail drugstores for minor tranquilizers or antianxiety pills include: Valium (diazepam), Librium (chlordiazepoxide), Xanax (alprazolam), and Tranxene (clorazepate).

Similarly, most sleeping medication prescriptions are benzodiazepine hypnotics (or sleep-inducing benzodiazepines) such as Dalmane (flurazepam), Restoril (temazepam), or Halcion (triazolam).

In the last few years, Halcion has led the pack of sleeping pills in popularity and as we will discuss later, it has proven to be extremely dangerous. In addition, many of the tranquilizers, such as Valium, are used as sleeping pills.

Other commonly used tranquilizers or sleeping pills include the following:

- Barbiturates
- Meprobamate (Miltown, Equanil)
- Hydroxyzine (Atarax, Vistaril) as a sleeping pill or tranquilizer
- Glutethimide (Doriden)
- Chloral hydrate
- Methyprylon (Noludar)
- Diphenhydramine (Benadryl)
- Buspar (Buspirone)

THE RISKS OF TRANQUILIZERS AND SLEEPING PILLS

After you pay for your prescription for tranquilizers, you continue to pay for the calming effect when you experience their unwelcome side effects. If you take tranquilizers, you may experience unwanted mental, physical, and emotional changes, some subtle, others profound. Daytime sedation, confusion, memory loss, poor coordination causing falls and hip fractures, impaired learning ability, or slurred speech are all well documented adverse effects of benzodiazepine tranquilizers and sleeping pills.

Furthermore, the longer you take these drugs, the greater your chances of becoming addicted. According to national prescribing data, more than two million American women are taking a sleeping pill or tranquilizer daily for a year or more even though there is no evidence that tranquilizers work for longer than four months or sleeping pills for more than two to four weeks. You will find that breaking your addiction will be much harder than addressing the reasons for your anxiety and sleeplessness without pills.

The problems described in this chapter can happen to anyone on tranquilizers, but they can worsen with higher doses and longer periods of taking the pills.

Mental Impairment

Many cognitive abilities decline measurably with tranquilizer and sleeping pill use. Memory and learning ability become predictably worse. Concentration is often affected.[1] While you may not even notice the subtle differences in your ability to grasp new information or remember a name or an address, the changes in your ability to think clearly may hamper you outright.

According to Johns Hopkins researcher Dr. Nathan Hendler, "I would say that 75 to 80 percent of the patients taking Librium or Valium, or similar drugs, have impaired intellectual functioning and this occurs at normal, if you will, prescribing ranges— between 5 and 40 milligrams a day [for Valium]."[2]

For the Librium user described below, taking sleeping pills resulted in a trade-off: she got nighttime relief (improved sleep) in exchange for daytime problems (impaired mental functioning).

> The patient was sleeping well, but had noticed loss of ability to concentrate. She no longer could read a book, although previously she had habitually read five or six weekly. Minor lapses of memory had been noted; she would start to look for something in the house and then forget what she was looking for.
>
> —description of an anonymous Librium user

This patient was taking higher than recommended doses of tranquilizers, but even at the usual dose these drugs have been shown to diminish alertness, learning, and memory.

Physical Deficits

Drowsiness, decreased coordination, fatigue, dizziness, light-headedness, slowed reaction times are all common problems of tranquilizer and sleeping pill use. At least one in five people taking tranquilizers will be disturbed by drowsiness. In one study, the majority of users experienced this side effect.[3]

Obviously, impaired driving is one very dangerous consequence. Driving skills such as braking ability and reaction time become significantly worse after taking tranquilizers. In an actual driving test people took Librium and then drove a car at low speeds. Their driving performance deteriorated visibly—and they did not realize it.[4]

Tranquilizer use has been studied among people involved in repeated traffic accidents. The risk of having a traffic accident was increased almost five times in people who had used a tranquilizer in the previous three months.[5]

Tranquilizers decrease attention and concentration, slow reaction time, and impair eye/hand coordination. It is not surprising, then, that taking them results in poor driving performance, both in laboratory studies and in real-life situations.

Adding alcohol to tranquilizers and sleeping pills results in even greater danger. The combined damage from taking both these drugs at once seriously impairs the physical and mental skills you need to drive safely.

Emotional Changes

Though less common, the other mental reactions to tranquilizers or sleeping pills may be severe or even life-threatening. They include:

■ Hostility and rage: Although tranquilizers and sleeping pills are supposed to relax you, some people feel more aggressive and hostile after taking them. These paradoxical reactions include rage, excitement, and violence. This seems to happen especially often with Halcion (see pages 166–168).

- Confusion: Some people become extremely confused when they take tranquilizers and sleeping pills. Older people who are branded as senile or depressed may turn out instead to be victims of confusion induced by the drugs.[6]

- Suicide: Some people taking tranquilizers may become very depressed. Reports have linked suicides to tranquilizer use, especially in combination with alcohol. It is thought that these drugs can exacerbate depression and promote or worsen suicidal thoughts.[7]

- Nightmares: Both sleep disturbances and nightmares may be side effects of tranquilizers.[8]

ADDICTION

What is addiction and who gets addicted?

By addiction we mean the regular use of a substance for such a long period of time that upon stopping, especially stopping suddenly, the person develops physical signs and symptoms of withdrawal. These include sweating, nervousness, or when more severe, hallucinations or seizures. Psychological addiction often accompanies the physical problems.

The myth used to be that only people who were prone to addiction, as judged by a prior history of alcoholism or other drug problems, would possibly become addicted to benzodiazepine tranquilizers or sleeping pills. According to this lore, only if you have a drug-prone history and use very large doses of these drugs for a long period of time do you risk addiction.

This attitude, intended to cover up a major national problem, was pushed by the president of Hoffmann-LaRoche, the world's biggest benzodiazepine maker (Valium, Librium, and Dalmane). Testifying before U.S. Senate hearings on the abuse of these drugs in 1979, President Robert Clark said that "true addiction is probably exceedingly unusual and, when it occurs, is probably confined to those individuals with 'abuse-prone' personalities who ingest very large amounts."[9]

But even then it was quite clear and is now even clearer that a large fraction, probably the majority, of people who use any of the benzodiazepines at the recommended dose for more than one or two months will become addicted.[10]

In fact, many people experience an unpleasant withdrawal syndrome when they suddenly stop taking the drug (as opposed to gradually tapering the dose to reduce, if not eliminate, the withdrawal symptoms). The only difference between addiction to the longer acting drugs such as Valium, Tranxene, and Dalmane, and the shorter acting drugs such as Halcion, Xanax, and Ativan is the time, after the drug is suddenly stopped, that it takes before withdrawal symptoms occur.

The myth that tranquilizers are not addictive has been slow to die in medical circles. In spite of over 20 years of published reports showing addiction to tranquilizers, some doctors continue to believe that tranquilizers are not—or hardly ever—addictive.

The evidence from medical studies has shown just the opposite:

- Every drug in the tranquilizer and sleeping pill family can cause physical addiction. People who stop taking these drugs suddenly, after taking them for months, develop serious withdrawal symptoms, including hallucinations and seizures.

- Even low doses of tranquilizers can cause both physical and psychological addiction. People who take prescribed doses for several months can become physically addicted.

- Anyone can become addicted to tranquilizers and sleeping pills. Even if you have no mental or emotional problems, you can still become addicted.

- Thousands of people are or have been addicted to tranquilizers and sleeping pills, and over three million Americans have taken tranquilizers or sleeping pills long enough that they are in danger of becoming addicted.

Danger with Continuing Use

Many of the people who have become addicted to tranquilizers have been taking them for a long time, often for several years. But addiction may develop over a few months, even at low doses. For example, people taking as little as 15 mg of Valium per day for a few months may develop typical withdrawal symptoms when they quit.

However, no studies have proven a therapeutic benefit to long term use (more than four months for tranquilizers, four weeks for sleeping pills). It therefore makes no sense at all to keep taking these drugs in the face of their proven addictive risk.

How Can I Tell if I'm Getting Addicted?

You can be addicted to tranquilizers or sleeping pills and not know it. If you have taken them for months, your body may have become dependent on them. If you have taken tranquilizers daily for four months or more, addiction is a serious possibility. Some of the warning signs of addiction are:

- Relying on the drug: If you feel you need tranquilizers or sleeping pills to function, you may be addicted. You may feel you can't cope without your daily pill. Or you may just think that you're not at your best without it. Either way, the drugs have become a crutch for you. This is a danger sign.

- Needing more to have the same effect: Addicting drugs lose their effectiveness when taken every day. You may be tempted to keep taking more so the drugs will work as well as they did before. You are in particular danger if you are taking higher doses of tranquilizers or sleeping pills than your doctor has prescribed.

- Not being able to quit: When you are physically dependent on tranquilizers or sleeping pills, quitting suddenly can make you downright sick. You feel tense and can't sleep, and you may go on to develop a full-blown withdrawal reaction—shakiness, headache, nausea, vomiting, changes in sensation, and at times hallucinations or seizures. When you resume taking tranquilizers, the symptoms usually go away quickly.

Withdrawal symptoms are a very serious danger sign. If you are physically addicted to tranquilizers, you should be under a doctor's care to withdraw from the drug safely.

If you have any of these warning signs, you may be addicted to tranquilizers. Even if you don't, you are at risk if you have taken tranquilizers for several months. Either way, it's time to find help and get to work on stopping tranquilizers.

Withdrawal

Withdrawal symptoms from tranquilizers may start as early as a few hours or as late as several days after you stop taking them. Some of the members of the tranquilizer family of drugs (Ativan, Xanax, Halcion) disappear from the body more rapidly and may produce withdrawal symptoms within a day.

The symptoms almost always include anxiety, restlessness, and trouble sleeping. Headache, muscle twitching and pain, shaking, and changes in vision are also common.

Many people going through tranquilizer withdrawal have various changes in sensation, including unpleasant feelings, tastes, and smell. They may become nauseated and vomit; they may also lose their appetite and lose weight. They often feel listless, depressed, and miserable.

More dangerous reactions also occur. Withdrawal from tranquilizers can cause full-blown seizures. It also can cause temporary psychosis, with paranoia, hallucinations, and loss of touch with reality. One former tranquilizer user had this experience:

> I stopped, and for the first couple of weeks it was terror; multiple muscle contractions. I think one of the best descriptions I have heard is if somebody pours kerosene over your skin and then every so often they touch a torch to it or set it to fire; this is one of the feelings I had.

I became very paranoid; everybody was out to get me and nobody was a friend any longer. These kinds of things began to happen, and I became so uptight that I could not sleep; I could not eat. In the darkness of the night, I do not know whether I was actually hallucinating or I was having delusions, but they were a very frightening experience.

If a person having withdrawal symptoms starts taking tranquilizers again, the symptoms rapidly disappear. (This is a typical feature of withdrawal reactions.) Otherwise, without resuming drug use, the symptoms begin to get better after a week to 10 days. They may take weeks or longer to disappear entirely.

TRANQUILIZERS AND SLEEPING PILLS AND YOUR BABY: PREGNANCY AND NURSING

If you are or might be pregnant, tranquilizers and sleeping pills are particularly dangerous. Risks include:

- Birth defects: Several studies have found that taking tranquilizers early in pregnancy (in the first trimester, especially for the first six weeks) may increase the danger of birth defects. Studies have found increases in cleft lip and cleft palate and an increased risk of severe malformations, such as mental retardation.[11] The evidence of birth defects is strong enough that the FDA-approved doctor labeling warns that using tranquilizers in pregnancy "should almost always be avoided."

- Floppy baby: Using tranquilizers late in pregnancy (near delivery) has other dangers. The newborn infant may be weak and floppy, may suck poorly and be unable to get enough milk, and may even have serious breathing problems.[12]

- Withdrawal symptoms: Several doctors have reported withdrawal symptoms in newborn infants when the babies' mothers took tranquilizers continuously during late pregnancy. Dr. Loretta Finnegan described these babies: "They arch their back[s], they have a large difficulty with feeding, and are much more difficult to treat than the infants undergoing heroin withdrawal."[13]

■ Nursing mothers: tranquilizers get into mother's milk. A nursing infant whose mother is taking tranquilizers will get a hefty dose of the drug. This will make the baby groggy. Over time the baby may eat poorly and lose weight.[14]

During pregnancy and nursing, you should take no drugs unless they are absolutely essential. Tranquilizers or sleeping pills are rarely if ever essential, and their hazards are considerable. Do not take them while pregnant or nursing.

SPECIAL HAZARDS IN OLDER WOMEN

In older people, tranquilizers and sleeping pills are especially dangerous. Because older adults have a much more difficult time clearing benzodiazepines and similar drugs from their bodies and are more sensitive to the effects of many of these drugs than younger adults, there are significantly increased risks of adverse drug effects. These include serious ones such as unsteady gait; dizziness; falling, causing an increased risk of hip fractures; drug-induced or drug-worsened impairment of thinking; memory loss; and addiction.[15]

Despite these significantly increased risks to older adults, sleeping pills and minor tranquilizers are prescribed much more often than they are for younger adults, for much longer periods of time, and usually not at the reduced dose that could decrease the risks. In comparison with younger people, older adults, especially women, are more likely to be given a prescription for tranquilizers or sleeping pills, are not usually given the reduced dose that would at least diminish the odds of serious adverse effects, and are prescribed these drugs for longer periods of time than are younger people. Therefore, it is not surprising that older adults are at much greater risk of suffering adverse effects, and, when they occur, they are much more serious.

One of the biggest impediments to discovering and eliminating these drug-induced problems is their frequent attribution to the aging process instead of to the drugs. The onset of impaired intelligence with memory loss, confusion, or impaired learning, or the onset of loss of coordination in a younger person will more likely prompt an inquiry leading to identification of the drug as culprit. But the same symptoms in an older person, especially if they develop more slowly, are often dismissed with a familiar remark, "Well, she is just growing old; what do you expect?" This lack of suspicion allows the drug to keep doing damage because the doctor keeps up the prescription.

Hip Fractures

A recent study of 1,021 older adults with hip fractures found that 14 percent of these life-threatening injuries are attributable to the use of mind-affecting drugs, including sleeping pills and minor tranquilizers, antipsychotics, and antidepressants.[16] Since there are approximately 227,000 hip fractures each year in the United States, virtually all in older adults,[17] this means that if the results of the study are projected nationally, approximately 32,000 hip fractures a year in older adults are caused by the use of mind-affecting drugs. Of these, about 30 percent, or almost 10,000 hip fractures a year, are caused by sleeping pills and minor tranquilizers, particularly the long acting drugs such as Valium, Librium, and Dalmane.

Another recent study on fractures in older adults found that the increased occurrence of falls resulting in such fractures could often be reduced by removing the offending drug.[18]

Drug-induced or Drug-worsened Senility (Decreased Mental Functioning)

Drug-induced impairment of thinking is one of the most reversible, or treatable, forms of dementia. It is a by-product of the increased use of drugs during the past few decades. Among the 28,500,000 people 65 and over in the United States, approximately 5 out of every 100 have dementia, with an estimated one of these five due to "reversible" conditions such as treatable diseases (thyroid disease, for example) or adverse effects of drugs.[19]

A recent study of 308 older adults with significant intellectual impairment found that in 11.4 percent of these people the problem was caused or worsened by a drug.[20] This study, the first ever to analyze this problem systematically, revealed that after stopping the use of the dementia-causing drugs, all persons had long-term improvement of their mental function. The most common class of drugs to cause the impairment of mental function was the sleeping pill/tranquilizer group. It accounted for 46 percent of the dementia induced or worsened by drugs.

Serious Breathing Problems in Older Women

Another serious adverse effect of the benzodiazepines is their effect on respiration, which occurs in two different ways. The first has to do with sleep apnea, a common condition in older adults in which breathing stops for varying periods of time while asleep. Dr. William Dement, an expert in sleep research, has found that older people with sleep apnea who use sleeping medications can stop breathing for much longer—dangerously longer—periods of time as a result of the respiration-suppressing effects of the drugs. He told a government task force on sleeping problems that people over 65 should not use Dalmane because of the risk of worsening sleep apnea.[21]

A second problem in this category is in people with severe lung disease. Such persons should be extremely cautious if they use benzodiazepines because they decrease the urge to breathe, which can be life-threatening.[22]

Other Adverse Effects in Older Women

The following problems have been linked to tranquilizer use. They are not common, but they can be serious.

- Jaundice and liver problems: tranquilizers may cause liver abnormalities and jaundice. People taking tranquilizers for more than a few weeks should have periodic tests of liver function.

- Low blood counts: Some people develop low blood counts while taking tranquilizers. Since this can lower one's resistance to infection, people taking tranquilizers for more than a few weeks should have blood counts done periodically.[23]

- Allergy: tranquilizers and sleeping pills may cause rash, hives, sudden shortness of breath, or other allergic reactions.[24]

- Glaucoma: tranquilizers and sleeping pills may cause an attack of glaucoma in people who have narrow-angle glaucoma. People with this condition should not use these drugs.[25]

- Abnormal facial movements: Doctors have described uncontrolled abnormal facial movements caused by tranquilizers.

Since older people are more likely to be taking several drugs, they are particularly prone to develop dangerous drug interactions. Many tranquilizers also stay in the body for a much longer time in the elderly. As a result, the drugs can accumulate to hazardous levels. If an older person "must" have tranquilizers, the dose should be no more than half the usual dose.

ALTERNATIVES TO TRANQUILIZERS

What if you are not elderly, are not pregnant, are not using alcohol, other mind-altering drugs, or other drugs which interfere with tranquilizers, but are anxious or having difficulty coping? Aren't tranquilizers worth considering?

First, consider other solutions. Do you have somebody to talk to: a friend, a spouse, a family member, a professional counselor? Many people with anxiety, panic attacks, posttraumatic stress syndrome, and depression-based insomnia would benefit from a mental health counselor.

Have you tried some form of regular exercise? Have you thought about getting a new job, if that is possible? Sometimes when people think that there is a relatively easy pill "solution" rather than the more difficult solutions that involve coping with causes rather than symptoms, they tend not to put as much energy into solving their problems.

What about the benefits or effectiveness of tranquilizers?

On a very short-term basis, there is no question that tranquilizers may help some people to relieve anxiety and can also help people through an occasional sleepless night. However, there is no evidence that tranquilizers continue having their tranquilizing effect for more than several months, or their sedative effect for more than a week or two, and there is significant risk of addiction.

In a recent discussion about the use of tranquilizers and sleeping pills the World Health Organization (WHO) experts said:

> Anxiety is a normal response to stress and only when it is severe and disabling should it lead to drug treatment. Long-term treatment . . . is rarely effective and should be avoided. . . . short-term use (less than two weeks) will minimize the risk of dependence.[26]

They concluded that "discussion of the problems of sleeplessness and anxiety and the drawbacks of drug therapy will often help the patient to come to terms with his or her problem without the need to resort to drugs."

Two studies on alternatives to the use of minor tranquilizers highlight how much of the present use is unnecessary. Ninety patients, mainly suffering from anxiety, were randomly divided into two groups when they went to see their family doctors. The first group was given the usual dose of one of the benzodiazepine tranquilizers.[27] The other group was given a small dose of a much safer treatment consisting solely of "listening, explanation, advice, and reassurance." The two treatments were equally effective in relieving the anxiety, but those receiving the informal counselling were more satisfied with their treatment than those given minor tranquilizers.

In a second study, patients with anxiety were either given one of three different tranquilizers or a placebo (sugar pill).[28] At the end of a month, with weekly evaluations of their anxiety levels being made by the patients themselves and by professional

evaluators, the results showed "all four treatments to be effica-
cious in their therapeutic effects on relieving anxiety." That is,
placebos worked as well as tranquilizers.

Talking to nonmedical people—a friend, a spouse, a relative,
a member of the clergy—may help to identify causes of anxiety
and potential solutions, as well as allow for sharing of feelings
and reassurance. Gathering the courage to talk about difficult
concerns will generally be a better solution than taking pills.
Getting regular exercise can also help relieve anxiety.

In addition, the use of foods, beverages, and over-the-
counter (nonprescription) or prescription drugs that have significant stimulant effects can also cause a chemically-induced
anxiety that can be remedied. (See the list of such substances
below.)

Try These Alternatives to Drugs for Your Sleeping Problems

If the cause of the sleeping problem is depression, this condition
should be addressed directly instead of using sleeping medication to treat its symptoms. In fact, using benzodiazepines can
worsen depression. A mental health specialist may be helpful for
insomnia which is caused by depression. If the cause is a medical
condition with pain as one of the components, the pain has to
be treated rather than turning to a sleeping pill to induce sleep
despite the pain.

Other causes of sleeping problems that can also be treated
without drugs include the following:

- Daytime napping or going to bed too early;
- Inaccurate idea of how much sleep you require each night. If
  you do not feel tired during the day, you had enough sleep
  the night before;
- Environmental factors such as light and noise. A quieter, darker
  room may promote a more restful sleep;
- Drinking stimulants—coffee, tea, or cola beverages—or eating
  chocolate within eight hours of when you want to sleep. Some

sensitive people cannot use these stimulants even in the morning.

- Lack of a nighttime routine. A warm bath, a pleasant book, a light but bland snack, no working just before going to bed or while in bed are ways to encourage sleep.
- Over-the-counter (nonprescription) drugs: sleeplessness can be caused by caffeine, found in Anacin and other drugs; PPA (phenylpropanolamine), the decongestant found in Contac, other decongestant products, and most over-the-counter diet pills; the ingredients in many asthma drugs;
- Prescription drugs—asthma drugs containing theophylline or aminophylline; amphetamines such as Benzidrine and diet pills; thyroid drugs; and the withdrawal from the use of sleeping pills, tranquilizers, and antidepressants.

If you have a sleeping problem and use one of these drugs, or if the problem began when you started using another drug, talk to your doctor. Tell him or her all the drugs (over-the-counter and prescription) you are taking. It might be possible to change the drug or lower the dosage to help you sleep. Returning to sleeping pills to get past withdrawal effects will only place you in a vicious cycle. Do not use L-tryptophan, an amino acid which has recently been found to cause serious debilitating disease.

WHICH TRANQUILIZERS OR SLEEPING PILLS SHOULD YOU USE, IF ANY?

Although we strongly discourage the use of these drugs in most situations, especially for older adults, there are some perfectly competent physicians who, in very well-defined circumstances and for very short periods of time, will prescribe them. They can be helpful for short-term use (seven days or less) for people with severe anxiety disorders, panic attacks, alcohol withdrawal syndrome, and severe situational stress (severe grief, marital separation, etc.). But even the labeling approved by the Food and Drug Administration for all of the tranquilizers has to state, "Anxiety or tension associated with the stress of everyday life usually does not require treatment with an anxiolytic [tranquilizer]."[29]

Consequently, the only prescription tranquilizer or sleeping pill that we advise for use, albeit limited use, is oxazepam, available generically, and under the brand name of Serax.

Rules for Safer Use of Oxazepam:

1. For older women, the dose should be no more than 7.5 milligrams, one to three times a day, if used as a tranquilizer, or 7.5 milligrams at bedtime, if used as a sleeping pill. (This is 1/2 of a 15 milligram, generically available, tablet.) Younger women might be prescribed 10-milligram pills.[30]

2. Ask your doctor to limit the size of the prescription to seven days' worth of pills.

3. Ask your doctor to write NO REFILL on the prescription so that you will not be inclined (because of the "good chemical feelings" these pills may provide) to refill the prescription without seeing the doctor again. The dangerously lax refill policy (allowing up to five refills without seeing the doctor) is legal because oxazepam and other similar drugs are not carefully controlled by the government. By urging your doctor to write NO REFILL you are making sure that he or she will reevaluate your condition after you use oxazepam for a short time. You want to discuss how you are doing with your anxiety or sleeping problem, rather than continuing to take the drug without a reevaluation. Continuing to take oxazepam without talking to your doctor could be the first step to addiction or other drug-induced problems.

4. At the end of the first day, and every day you use oxazepam, evaluate what you have done, on your own or by talking to others, to find out what is making you anxious. This includes evaluation of what you have done to alter the internal or external circumstances causing your anxiety. Keep a record of these evaluations. As soon as possible try reducing the dose, in consultation with your doctor. Since you only have enough medication for one week, it is unlikely that you will have become addicted this quickly.

5. Do not drive a car or operate dangerous machinery while using oxazepam.

6. Do not drink alcohol. The combination of this drug with alcohol dangerously increases the effects of both. An overdose of oxazepam in combination with alcohol can be fatal.

7. Before using oxazepam, make sure that your doctor knows if you are taking other drugs with a sedative or "downer" effect, such as antidepressants, antipsychotics, antihistamines, narcotic painkillers, epilepsy medications, barbiturates, or other sleeping medications. Oxazepam taken with other drugs with sedative effects dangerously increases the risks of both.

8. If you are elderly, pregnant, or nursing or have narrow angle glaucoma or serious lung disease, you should not use tranquilizers.

The following drugs should also not be used with tranquilizers:

■ **Tagamet:** This ulcer drug keeps most of the tranquilizers from leaving the body. Because of this, a larger amount of the drug builds up in the body; drowsiness and other problems will result. Ativan and Serax do not appear to show this effect.

■ **Antabuse:** Like Tagamet, Antabuse keeps those drugs from leaving the body so they can build up to dangerous levels. Again, this interaction probably does not occur with Ativan or Serax.

- **Larodopa, Levodopa, Sinemet:** Tranquilizers may make these drugs (which treat Parkinson's disease) less effective.

THE HALCION STORY: WHAT YOU NEED TO KNOW (BUT THE FDA WON'T TELL YOU)

Since its introduction in late 1982, Halcion has become the most widely prescribed sleeping medication in the United States, with over 11 million prescriptions in 1988. It is in a class of drugs known as benzodiazepine hypnotics (or sleep-inducing benzodiazepines) along with Restoril and Dalmane, but chemically it is a fairly drastic modification on the established chemical structure of a benzodiazepine. The chief selling point of Halcion, compared to its competitors, has been its very short half life in the body, under three hours,[31] which reduces the daytime "hangover" the drug produces.

However, Halcion's short half life appears to be a mixed blessing, since it is reported to cause insomnia in the early morning and to actually increase a person's feeling of anxiety during the day. In addition, there may be an intense "rebound" of insomnia and anxiety after the drug is stopped.

In fact, since this popular sleeping pill was put on the United States market in December 1982, the FDA has received nearly 2,000 reports of dangerous reactions to the drug, over five times as many per prescription as have been reported for a similar sleeping medication, Restoril, since its introduction in 1981.[32] Reported harmful reactions to Halcion have included:

- anterograde amnesia (amnesia to events which occur after the drug was taken)
- anxiety
- anorexia
- agitation
- bizarre and aggressive behavior
- confusion and delirium
- depression
- paranoia

Extreme reactions include:

- seizures
- hallucinations
- suicidal thinking

Some, but not all, of these adverse effects occurred in people who had taken a high dose (.5 mg or more) of this potent drug. These undesirable effects appear to be more prevalent in the elderly, and may occur even at the lowest recommended dose (.125 mg). This is serious, since people over 60 make up over half (51 percent) of the market for sleeping medications. Also, rebound insomnia and anxiety may foster a sense of dependence on the drug, causing people to take it for long periods when, in fact, tolerance to the drug's benefits develops quickly, within two to three weeks of continuous use.

In response to accumulating evidence of dangerous side effects and international pressure (the Netherlands banned the sale of the drug entirely in 1979 after one year on the Dutch market; France, Italy and West Germany suspended the sale of the .5 mg dose between 1987 and 1988), Upjohn voluntarily suspended the sale of the .5 mg tablet in the United States market in June 1988. The company began recommending that lower doses be prescribed: .125 mg for the elderly, .25 mg for most others, .5 mg only for "those patients who do not respond adequately to a lower dose." The company expanded its warning label to warn of the risk of anterograde amnesia and "paradoxical" reactions (agitation, insomnia, hallucinations, sleepwalking, and inappropriate behavior) following even low doses of Halcion.

However, reports of side effects from Halcion continued to pour into the FDA, and four different studies concluded that the number of reported adverse reactions to Halcion, especially psychological and behavioral reactions, was far higher than for other drugs in its class. The Food and Drug Administration (FDA) convened a special meeting of its Psychopharmacological Drugs Advisory Committee on September 22, 1989, to discuss the issue.

Partly as a concession to the consumers' right to more

information, the committee recommended that the label warn more strongly of the risk of anterograde amnesia to travelers who take Halcion for "jet lag," and urged the development of a patient package insert (an information sheet that patients receive with their medicine) for all three drugs in Halcion's class, the benzodiazepine hypnotics. But they stopped short of announcing that, based on their own data, Halcion appears to produce more psychological and behavioral side effects (amnesia, agitation, confusion, delirium, hallucinations, seizures, hostility, and aggression) than other benzodiazepine sleeping pills on the United States market.

Despite its popularity as a fast acting sleep-inducing drug, Halcion's chemical structure, its relative potency, and its rapid elimination contribute to an incredible array of unwanted and dangerous side effects. We do not recommend the use of this very dangerous drug.

FIND A HELPFUL, SUPPORTIVE DOCTOR

If you think you may be addicted to tranquilizers or sleeping pills and would like to do something about it, the first thing to do is to have a talk with your doctor. Depending on what kind of doctor you have, you will get a receptive or not so receptive response. What follows are scenarios, each representing a type of doctor or situation you may encounter.

Scenario A: Doctor Knows Best?

Edith has had a rocky year. Her divorce became final after years of bitter wrangling with her now ex-husband. Required to work for the first time in her life, she started out as a salesperson in a boutique. Soon her natural fashion sense landed her the job of buyer and assistant manager.

The divorce, her job, her relationship with two lively children now entering adolescence, and her reentry into the "singles" scene have all been sources of anxiety as Edith attempted to cope with the many changes in her life.

About two years ago, when it was clear that her marriage

was breaking up, Edith went to see her doctor about a backache brought on by strenuous household work. During the conversation she told her doctor about the tension at home. Her doctor gave her a prescription for tranquilizers for both problems. At first her prescription was for 5 mg three times a day, and it made her feel more in control of her life; but mounting tension at home, protracted legal proceedings, and entry into the job scene all increased her anxiety until her doctor suggested that more tranquilizers might be in order. Now she is taking one 10 mg pill four times a day, as her doctor has prescribed.

On a recent buying trip for the boutique, Edith picked up a book at the airport: *I'm Dancing as Fast as I Can,* an autobiography of a professional woman who had become addicted to tranquilizers. She noticed the parallels between her life and the author's, and when she returned from the trip she made an appointment with her doctor.

Edith: Doctor, I am worried about the tranquilizers I'm taking. I have been taking tranquilizers for over two years now, and I wonder if I could be getting addicted.

Doctor: Well now Edith, I guess you've been reading some of those scare stories in the popular press.

Edith: Yes, I have, Doctor. I read a book about a woman a lot like me who began taking tranquilizers because of the stress in her life, and wound up in terrible shape when she tried to quit. Ann Landers wrote a warning about tranquilizers, too, and now I'm worried.

Doctor: Well, I can assure you, that I keep right up to date with professional literature, not the headline-making stuff you've been reading, and there really isn't any danger.

Edith: But, Doctor, I asked the druggist about this, and he showed me the *Physicians' Desk Reference,* and it said that I was taking the maximum dosage permitted, and that even the manufacturer doesn't know very much about the long-term effects of the drug. The book also said I shouldn't be taking it with alcohol. I had two glasses of wine with dinner just a few days ago.

Doctor: And did anything bad happen?

Edith: Well, no, not really, but . . .

Doctor: So you see, it's perfectly safe!

Edith: The book the druggist showed me also said I should be careful driving. I do a lot of driving as part of my job.

Doctor: And have you had an accident?

Edith: Well, no, but maybe I've been lucky.

Doctor: I don't see why you are complaining. These pills are doing you good and I don't see why you are taking up my time with these questions.

Edith: I'm worried about taking these pills. I think they are bad for me to be taking for such a long time. My life is on a pretty even keel now and I don't think I need a crutch; in fact, I wonder if I ever really did. I know now I could have used a counsellor during the time of my divorce, but no one ever suggested it and I didn't think of it myself. I really don't like the idea of using chemicals like this, and I think it would be best if I stopped using tranquilizers.

Doctor: You do, eh? Now where did you get your medical degree? Don't you think I know what's best for you? Of course I do.

Edith: Oh, Doctor, I don't want to have a fight over this, but I would like your help; I know I still have some personal problems, but my back feels fine now, and perhaps with counseling . . .

Doctor: I can see you are not interested in my advice. Well then, do whatever you want to do. If you don't want to take the pills, just don't take them. I don't care. It's your problem. Now, I think the appointment is over.

Edith: But Doctor, is it safe to just stop all of a sudden like that? Couldn't I get withdrawal symptoms?

Doctor: If you really wanted my advice you would have taken it, and taken your pills just as I prescribed. I'm really very busy now; good day.

Edith left the doctor's office. She still had one refill of her tranquilizer prescription, so she continued using it as directed.

However, she went directly to a drug information hotline for a referral to a physician who would help her get off tranquilizers safely. She was lucky, for if she had followed her doctor's advice and quit cold turkey she might have experienced severe withdrawal symptoms.

Scenario B: Working With The Doctor

Ann is a housewife and mother of three. Two years ago, her doctor prescribed tranquilizers for her after one of her children was seriously injured in an accident. The child is now fine, but keeping a home and raising three children has brought many new stresses, and Ann is always expected to be friendly and responsible. Tranquilizers seemed to help, so her doctor has kept giving her prescriptions for tranquilizers and she has kept taking them. She takes tranquilizers only as directed: a 10 mg pill two to three times a day. Ann also has had several attacks of lower back pain since she hurt her back a few years ago. Her doctor has told her that tranquilizers will help her back pain, too.

Recently, Ann has read articles warning that tranquilizers can be addicting. Although she is taking it only as prescribed, she is worried. After some thought, Ann writes down a list of questions and decides to talk to her doctor about tranquilizers.

Ann: Doctor, I recently read that taking tranquilizers can be addicting. I've been taking the tranquilizers you prescribed for me for two years, now, and I'm a little worried. Could I be getting addicted to tranquilizers?

Doctor: You certainly shouldn't take more tranquilizers than you need, Ann, but tranquilizers are actually quite safe. Very few people get addicted to tranquilizers. And people who do get addicted are usually those who take very high doses of tranquilizers.

Ann: I understand that. But I've read that even doses of tranquilizers prescribed by doctors can be dangerous if I take them for a long time. Isn't two years getting to be a long time?

Doctor: Well, yes, it's a pretty long time. You certainly don't want to take it if you don't need it. But if you do need a drug for tension, it's really a pretty safe drug.

Ann: Is it really safe? I've read that tranquilizers can affect my mind—that it could make my memory worse, or make it harder for me to think clearly. I do seem to forget things more than I did. Could that be the tranquilizers?

Doctor: Well, many things can make you forgetful, and I wouldn't just blame the drug. Tranquilizers do seem to have some effects on a few people's mental functions. But so does anxiety! It's very hard to think well when you're upset.

Ann: That's true, but I do worry about muddling up my mind even more. And I'm also worried about drowsiness. I do feel a little slow sometimes after taking tranquilizers. Is it safe for me to drive?

Doctor: It is pretty common for tranquilizers to slow you down. Some studies even suggest that it slows your reactions down and may affect your coordination. You certainly don't want to drive when you're at all drowsy, or to take anything else that could make you drowsy when you're taking tranquilizers.

Ann: You mean things like sleeping pills?

Doctor: Yes, sleeping pills. And also alcohol, and other tranquilizers. And antihistamines, too.

Ann: I'm glad you told me that. But it does worry me; I often have my children in the car with me, and I'd hate to drive if I'm not quite alert. I'm still a little worried about addiction, too. Wouldn't taking a tranquilizer for this long change my system somehow? Ten milligrams of tranquilizers used to knock me out, and now I take it and hardly notice the difference.

Doctor: It's true, you do seem to get used to a drug when you take it a long time.

Ann: Then is it really worth the risk? If it can slow me down, and if there's even a small chance I could get addicted, should I be taking a drug like this?

Doctor: That depends on whether you need it.

Ann: Does it even work when you take it for this long? It really knocked me out at first, but is it doing anything now?

Doctor: It's hard to say. The label does say that it hasn't been studied well for periods over four months.

Ann: Do you have a copy of the label that I can see? My bottle just says, "Take one pill two or three times a day as needed."

Doctor: You can get the label from your pharmacist. But it's written for doctors, and you may find it hard to read.

Ann: Can I call you if I have any questions?

Doctor: Of course.

Ann: But if you're not sure the tranquilizers are doing anything, and if they can be dangerous, wouldn't I be better off trying to do without them?

Doctor: Well, if you'd like to try, it might be a good idea to try to cut down.

Ann: How about trying to do without them entirely?

Doctor: You could try that too, if you want.

Ann: Can I just quit "cold turkey"?

Doctor: Well, it might not be a good idea. If you stop taking tranquilizers suddenly after two years, you can have bad reactions. You get nervous or shaky, or you may have trouble sleeping.

Ann: It sounds like I could be a little addicted, then.

Doctor: Well, you're used to the drug. Or it could just be your old anxiety coming back.

Ann: But I wasn't that anxious before my son was hurt. And since then, I've been taking tranquilizers all the time.

Doctor: You are used to taking tranquilizers, too. So it is better if you cut back gradually.

Ann: How should I take them when I'm cutting back? I'm taking two to three pills a day.

Doctor: You want to lower your dose over about four weeks. So take two pills a day for a week. Then take 1 1/2 pills a day for the next week. Then take one pill a day or half a pill twice a day for a week. Then cut down to half a pill a day for a week, and then stop.

Ann: Will I have problems right away if I quit suddenly?

Doctor: No. If you stop taking tranquilizers after taking them a long time, they stay in your body in some form for over a week. So it takes a few days before you develop symptoms.

Ann: But I've heard that you can still get withdrawal symptoms.

Doctor: Well, if you were addicted, you could get severe symptoms. They start a few days after you stop.

Ann: What about my back pain? Will that get worse if I don't use tranquilizers?

Doctor: Tranquilizers are only one of the treatments for back pain, and they shouldn't be used alone. Aspirin, rest, and heating pads are very helpful, and they probably will be all you need. You should also be doing back exercises to keep your back from acting up. I can give you a sheet describing some back exercises, if you'd like.

Ann: That would be nice. What about tension? What can I do for tension besides take pills?

Doctor: It depends on what causes it. If you have serious problems, you may want to get counselling. If someone upsets you, try talking to that person. When you can do it, changing situations that upset you is the best thing to do to help tension.

Ann: That makes sense to me. I think I could really use a week's vacation. I haven't had a vacation in years!

Doctor: It sounds like a good idea.

Ann: It sounds much better to me than taking pills. I really like the idea of getting off these tranquilizers. I've felt sort of guilty about them, like they're a crutch. I'd feel a lot more free if I could do without them. I do want to quit, even though it's a little scary.

Doctor: You seem to have thought about it a lot. And I'll be happy to try to help you through the rough spots, if you find you have trouble quitting.

Ann: Good. I need your help.

Doctor: Let me write down a schedule for cutting down, and I'll see you in a month. Give me a call if you have any problems while you're cutting down your dose.

Ann: Thanks. I will.

Doctor: You may find that you need to cut down your dose more slowly. Don't feel that you need to keep to this schedule. Some people take months to stop entirely.

Ann: I'll see how I do.

Doctor: I'll see you in a month, but call me sooner if you have any problems.

Ann: See you then. Hey! I'm leaving here without any prescriptions at all! I feel better already.

1. Wittenborn JR. Effects of benzodiazepines on psychomotor performance. British Journal of Clinical Pharmacology 1979; 7:61S–7S; McKay AC, Dundee JW. Effect of oral benzodiazepines on memory. British Journal of Anaesthesiology 1980; 52:1247–56.

2. Hendler N. Use and Misuse of Benzodiazepines. Testimony at Hearings before the Senate Subcommittee on Health and Scientific Research. September 10, 1979, 33.

3. Davies DM. Textbook of Adverse Drug Reactions. Oxford University Press, Oxford: 1977, 337.

4. Betts TA, Clayton AB, MacKay GM. Effects of four commonly-used tranquillizers on low-speed driving performance tests. British Medical Journal 1972; 4:580–4.

5. Skegg DCG, Richards SM, Doll R. Minor tranquillisers and road accidents. British Medical Journal 1979; 1:917–9.

6. Choice of benzodiazepines. The Medical Letter 1981; 23:41–3.

7. Drugs that cause psychiatric symptoms. The Medical Letter 1981; 23:9–12.

8. Greenblatt DJ, Shader RI. Benzodiazepines. New England Journal of Medicine 1974; 291:1239–43.

9. Clark RB. Hearings, op. cit., 309.

10. Busto U, Sellers EM, Naranjo CA, Cappell H, Sanchez-Craig M, Sykora K. Withdrawal reaction after long-term therapeutic use of benzodiazepines. New England Journal of Medicine 1986; 315:854–9; Murphy SM, Owen RT, Tyrer PJ. Withdrawal symptoms after six weeks treatment with diazepam. Lancet 1984; 2:1389.

11. Milkovich L, van den Berg BJ. Effects of prenatal meprobamate and chlordiazepoxide hydrochloride on human embryonic and fetal development. New England Journal of Medicine 1974; 291:1268–71; Saxen I. Associations

between oral clefts and drugs taken during pregnancy. International Journal of Epidemiology 1975; 4:37–44.; Safra MJ, Oakley GP. Association between cleft lip with or without cleft palate and prenatal exposure to diazepam. Lancet 1975; 2:478–80.

12. Speight ANP. Floppy-infant syndrome and maternal diazepam and/or nitrazepam. Lancet 1977; 2:878; Rowlatt RJ. Effect of maternal diazepam on the newborn. British Medical Journal 1978; 1:985.

13. Finnegan L. Testimony before the House Narcotics Committee, Feb. 6, 1980. Quoted in FDC Reports, Feb. 11 1980, T&G-14.

14. Rowlatt, op. cit.

15. Boston Collaborative Drug Surveillance Program. Clinical depression of the central nervous system due to diazepam and chlordiazepoxide in relation to cigarette smoking and age. New England Journal of Medicine 1973; 288:277–80; Committee on the Review of Medicines. Systematic review of the benzo-diazepines. British Medical Journal 1980; 1:910–12; Ramsay LE. Tucker GT. Clinical pharmacology: drugs and the elderly. British Journal of Medicine 1981; 282:125–7.

16. Ray WA, Griffin MR, Schaffner W, Baugh DK, Melton LJ. Psychotropic drug use and the risk of hip fracture. New England Journal of Medicine 1987; 316:363–9.

17. Riggs BL, Melton LJ. Involutional osteoporosis. New England Journal of Medicine 1986; 314:1676–86.

18. Buchner DM, Larson EB. Falls and fractures in patients with Alzheimer-type dementia. Journal of the American Medical Association 1987; 257:1492–5.

19. Beck JC, Benson DF, Scheibel AB, Spar JE, Rubenstein LZ. Dementia in the elderly: the silent epidemic. Annals of Internal Medicine 1982; 97:231–41.

20. Larson EB, Kukull WA, Buchner D, Reifler BV. Adverse drug reactions associated with global cognitive impairment in elderly persons. Annals of Internal Medicine 1987; 107:169–73.

21. Dement W. Presentation before the HEW Joint Coordinating Council for Project Sleep. July 28, 1980.

22. Lakshminarayan S, Sahn SA, Hudson LD, Weil JV. Effect of diazepam on ventilatory response. Clinical Pharmacology and Therapeutics 1976; 20:178–83.

23. Hoffmann-LaRoche. Prescribing information for Valium, Aug. 1, 1981.

24. Ghosh JS. Allergy to diazepam and other benzodiazepines. British Medical Journal 1977: 1:902–3.

25. Hyams SW, Keroub C. Glaucoma due to diazepam. American Journal of Psychiatry 1977; 134:447–8.

26. Drugs for the Elderly. World Health Organization, Denmark: 1985; 121.

27. Catalan J, Gath D, Edmonds G, Ennis L. The effects of non-prescribing of anxiolytics in general practice—I: controlled evaluation of psychiatric private practices. British Journal of Clinical Psychiatry 1984; 144:593–602.

28. Zung WK, Daniel JT, King RE, Moore DT. A comparison of prazepam,

diazepam, lorazepam and placebo in anxious outpatients in non-psychiatric private practices. Journal of Clinical Psychiatry 1981; 42:280–4.

29. Physicians' Desk Reference. 41st ed. Oradell, N.J.: Medical Economics Company, 1987, 1697. The FDA-approved labeling for all benzodiazepine tranquilizers states that there is no evidence of effectiveness for more than four months.

30. Vestal RE, ed. Drug Treatment in the Elderly. ADIS Health Science Press, Sydney, Australia: 1984: 317–37.

31. Dukes MNG, Side Effects of Drugs Annual 3, Amsterdam: Excerpta Medica, 1979.

32. Testimony by Dr. Charles Anello presented to the Psychopharmacological Drugs Advisory Committee meeting on September 22, 1989.

LACTATION SUPPRESSING DRUGS

Parlodel and Others: Do Not Use

Lactation suppressants are potent drugs with potentially dangerous side effects. They are prescribed to nearly 20 percent of postpartum women in this country (over a third of women who do not want to breast feed) with the hope that they will prevent short-lived breast discomfort, a condition in nonnursing mothers that typically resolves itself in fewer than 10 days without any drugs.

- Repeated studies have shown that 95 percent of non-nursing postpartum women consider their breast discomfort mild and don't want any drugs.

- Despite the clear lack of need, up to 800,000 women a year receive potent drugs to suppress lactation. These include bromocriptine (brand name Parlodel), TACE, diethylstilbestrol (DES), Testosterone, Delestrogen, and Deladumone.

Risks

- Mild reactions to lactation suppressants include nausea, dizziness, headaches, vomiting, abdominal cramps, diarrhea, or lightheadedness.

- Serious reactions include dramatic changes in blood pressure, seizures, strokes, heart attacks, blood clots, and psychosis.

- Up to 75 percent of women taking these drugs lactate once their pill supply is used up. Lactation suppressants postpone rather than prevent breast pain.
- In late 1989, most of the manufacturers of drugs used for lactation suppression withdrew them from the market for that use. The only exception was Sandoz Ltd., the makers of Parlodel, which is by far the most widely used lactation suppressant. The company has refused to withdraw this popular drug and now the FDA is pursuing legal action against them.

Benefits

- The benefit of these drugs is short-term relief—actually, in most cases merely postponement—of breast discomfort and inconvenience from the buildup of unused milk in nonnursing mothers.

Recommendations

- Before you have your baby, if you know you don't want to nurse, tell your doctor you don't want any Parlodel (bromocriptine), estrogens, or any other pills to help dry up your milk supply. To suppress milk production, wear a snug wrap or bra for several days after you deliver. The pressure will hasten the process of shutting down your milk supply. Ice packs and cool compresses also help. If you still experience pain, you may want to take low doses of acetaminophen.
- According to Dr. Ruth Lawrence, a pediatrician from the University of Rochester School of Medicine quoted in the magazine *FDA Consumer* April 1990, the risks of letting lactation end naturally "seem to be close to zero. I think that in some respects we've assumed that women would rather be medicated than experience any discomfort at all, and that is probably not true."

*B*REASTFEEDING is a perfect system of supply and demand. After a woman gives birth, the suckling of an infant, the sound of its cry, even touching its body will initiate a powerful physiological response from the new mother, and milk production begins within hours. When a baby is stillborn or a mother doesn't want to nurse, milk soon dries up. Either way, nature accommodates.

Despite this exquisite mechanism which has worked well in all mammals since the beginning of time, modern medicine has found an opportunity to interfere and try to improve things. Today up to half of all new mothers don't nurse, and for these women there are two choices—one medically safe, one not. They can let their breasts fill up with milk and then wait about 10 days for their milk to dry up. Or they can take drugs to temporarily suppress the body's process for making milk (lactation suppressants). Over the last decade lactation suppressants have been so well received by the medical community that they have been prescribed for up to 20 percent of women giving birth each year. According to the Food and Drug Administration, 800,000 women yearly take drugs to suppress lactation.[1]

The first option—no drugs—is virtually free of risk. It may be unpleasant to have temporarily sensitive, enlarged breasts, and sometimes the unwanted milk will inconveniently leak out. But there are no health hazards involved in simply waiting for nature to take its course.

Not surprisingly, taking drugs to prevent milk production or to reduce the pain when breasts become swollen with unwanted milk is not free of risk. Not only do these drugs introduce health risks, often they don't even work. In up to 40 percent of medicated new mothers, milk production is merely postponed and returns anyway, immediately after the drug regimen is over. This means that many mothers may take a potent and potentially dangerous drug for two weeks, only to find they eventually have all the problems with unwanted milk anyway.

Furthermore, there is plenty of evidence that most women don't feel the need for these drugs to begin with, despite the fact that many doctors routinely prescribe them. Repeated studies show that only a small percentage of postpartum women who don't nurse experience serious pain from breast engorgement. For the vast majority, the soreness can be easily treated for the few days of discomfort without using drugs of any sort. The oldest and best remedies still work today, as they have for centuries. Using cold compresses and wrapping breasts securely against the chest for as little as 12 hours still provides the safest and most efficient mechanism for stopping milk supply and reducing swelling. But many nurses and doctors today are not trained to take time with such measures. Offering a pill is much quicker.

RISKY DRUGS YOU DON'T NEED

The drugs used to curtail milk flow are either injected or given orally soon after delivery and before breasts become engorged. By far the most popular is bromocriptine, brand name Parlodel. More than half a million women receive this drug each year as a lactation suppressant. It works by affecting hormonal activity in the brain to suppress milk production. But it is also known to trigger dramatic, sometimes lethal changes in blood pressure. Bromocriptine accounts for an estimated 83 percent of the lactation suppressant market in this country.[2]

The other popular lactation suppressants prescribed by doctors are sex hormones, used to treat breast engorgement (called postpartum breast engorgement or PPBE) at their target site, the breast tissue itself. High doses of estrogens (female hormones) and androgens (male hormones) are given to relieve breast swelling and soreness. These include the long lasting synthetic estrogen TACE (chlorotrianisene), and DES (diethylstilbestrol) which account for 13 percent and 3 percent of the lactation market respectively.[3] Another medication consists of an injectable combination of estrogens and androgens, most commonly administered as a drug called Deladumone. Androgens are also used alone.

The drugs used to curtail lactation and reduce pain have well documented side effects, both serious and mild. They appear to speed up nature's process, but of course they do much more. Unwittingly and without their informed consent, many healthy postpartum women exchange initial short-lived breast discomfort for nausea, dizziness, headaches, vomiting, abdominal cramps, diarrhea, or lightheadedness. These reactions have been acknowledged by the manufacturers themselves and are predictable in view of the drugs' known dangers:

- dramatic changes in blood pressure
- seizures
- strokes
- heart attacks
- blood clots
- psychosis[4]

While these severe reactions are rare, they do occur; the Food and Drug Administration has been gathering reports about them for years. One of the agency's own physicians recently characterized these drugs this way:

> In my view, there is no way to predict ahead of time who may be susceptible to strokes, hypertension, and MIs [heart attacks] that have been reported so far and could represent young women who react idiosyncratically to this drug. The above findings again reemphasize the clinical risks taken with giving a potent drug for a trivial indication.[5]

Needless to say, new mothers are not typically told they could have life-threatening reactions to these drugs. And physicians, in their efforts to ward off possible complaints of swelling and discomfort from their patients who decide not to nurse, relay only half the truth.

WHO NEEDS THEM?

That question has interested researchers since the use of these drugs first became widespread. One way to approach the question has been to look at the natural course of lactation in women who didn't get drugs. Was it terribly painful in most cases? Did most women suffer fevers, soreness, and other symptoms that provoked them to ask for medication? When the FDA looked into the need for lactation suppressants, they were repeatedly shown that most women are satisfied with nature's mechanism when it is given a chance to work.

One of the best studies on this subject was done in 1979 by Dr. Jennifer Niebyl.[6] She found that by the third day following childbirth, only seven percent of the nonnursing women in her study who had taken no lactation suppressants required an analgesic painkiller, and only four percent had a mild fever. Furthermore, according to Niebyl, 89 percent didn't complain of severe or even moderate breast engorgement. By the eighth day, the number of new mothers who had even mild problems with breast engorgement had dropped to five percent. That means that according to Niebyl's study, 90 percent of women had no further problem with postpartum breast engorgement by just over a week after delivery without using lactation suppressant drugs.

Another study looked at the natural resolution of breast discomfort and showed that for most women the painful period lasted only about 12 hours.[7] So why use drugs which, on average, must be taken two weeks or more, days longer than even the natural process?

Five years ago at the University of Rochester Medical Center, hundreds of new mothers were interviewed about postpartum breast pain and only a handful reported being uncomfortable. Follow-up studies there showed that after patients went home, even fewer women reported discomfort, leading one researcher to comment, "women are going home sooner, moving around earlier. They just aren't sitting around thinking about their breasts. Being more active in the postpartum period has changed the whole experience for non-lactating women."[8]

Dr. Ruth Lawrence of the University of Rochester Medical Center said that after research there, physicians at that institution virtually stopped prescribing drugs to suppress lactation. "We were suspicious that they were being overprescribed and we were right."[9]

Apparently other major university hospital-based practices have also independently decided the same thing. In a survey conducted by Public Citizen Health Research Group, the following institutions use no lactation suppressants at all: Johns Hopkins, the University of North Carolina (Chapel Hill), Yale, Iowa, U.C.L.A, and The Brigham and Women's Hospital. Other institutions such as University of Texas-Southwestern, Mount Sinai (New York), and the University of Pittsburgh, use Parlodel occasionally, but not routinely, and TACE and Deladumone are never used. Androgens are never used at any of these institutions.

REBOUND LACTATION

Lactation suppressant drugs may be the classic example of adding insult to injury. According to the FDA's own analysis, between 18 and 40 percent of the women receiving Parlodel and an even larger percentage of women taking estrogens will develop breast soreness or fullness and will leak new milk (rebound lactation) after finishing a 14 day course of treatment.[10] In one of the early studies on rebound lactation from estrogen use, 75 percent of those treated with it required further treatment for breast pain days after they had gone home.[11] These studies demonstrate that for many women these drugs don't prevent problems, they just postpone them.

POSTPARTUM WOMEN RECEIVING HORMONES TAKE RISKS

There are many physiologic changes going on in women right after delivery which make it a time of instability even without the introduction of drugs. Postpartum fluctuations in body fluids can lead to changes in blood pressure under perfectly normal circumstances. Research has shown that during and after delivery, natural changes in the blood have the effect of boosting a woman's clotting tendencies.[12] This is a normal part of the postpartum healing process, but it also slightly increases the risk of developing unwanted blood clots.

Some of the most serious problems now associated with hormonal lactation suppressants have never been demonstrated in large scale, well-designed epidemiologic studies. However many experts have been concerned for years over reports of perfectly healthy new mothers suddenly developing blood clots or dying of heart attacks a few days after taking them. Estrogens such as TACE or DES have been linked to the formation of blood clots in the large veins of the legs (venous thromboembolism) and pelvis. These can travel to the lungs (pulmonary embolism) and cause death. A study from Great Britain in the 1960s showed a fourfold increase in the risk of blood clots for women with fewer than three children taking postpartum estrogens, and a tenfold increase if the women were over 25.[13] Other research showed that women over 35 having "assisted" deliveries (cesarean section, for example) had 10 times the risk of thromboembolism if they received estrogen to suppress lactation.[14] Since the number of older mothers having cesarean sections is increasing,[15] there is a growing population of women who might use these drugs who have at least one other risk factor for thromboembolism.

In 1978 the FDA found these negative reports about estrogen-containing hormonal lactation suppressants so compelling that the agency issued a notice proposing to withdraw a so-called "New Drug Application" for their use in treating postpartum breast engorgement.[16] Basically the agency was poised to withdraw its approval for use of these hormones as lactation suppressants.

The notice listed many estrogens, including TACE as well as Deladumone-OB, an estrogen and testosterone combination. Withdrawing approval was not the same as a ban on all of these drugs, some of which could remain on hospital and neighborhood pharmacy shelves for other uses. However, it would have vastly increased the liability physicians faced if they used the drug for unapproved treatments. When a specific use for any drug is withdrawn, the manufacturer must also change its drug labeling, eliminating any recommendation for the unapproved use. In 1978 the FDA was set to ask companies to stop marketing estrogens for use as lactation suppressants.

Incredibly, the FDA never formally followed through until 1988, and the message to stop using hormonal lactation suppressants didn't get out to practitioners for more than a decade after FDA investigators and other researchers initially questioned the drugs. For a variety of reasons, including the introduction of a new drug, bromocriptine, the regulatory process simply petered out. The result is that hormones are still being used today.[17]

BROMOCRIPTINE

Bromocriptine (Parlodel) is not a hormone; it acts as a neurotransmitter, relaying messages within the brain and central nervous system. It belongs to a family of drugs known as ergot alkaloids, which also affect the tone of blood vessels and are used to treat conditions such as migraine headaches. To stop milk flow, bromocriptine mimics a chemical transmitter in the brain called dopamine that stops the body's production of prolactin. When prolactin is turned off, so is milk production. Bromocriptine is thus somewhat effective in temporarily slowing down milk production.

But of course this drug does more, because it copies the

other properties of naturally occurring dopamine. Operating within the central nervous system, dopamine has significant effects on blood pressure. When massive amounts of bromocriptine are introduced into the central nervous system, blood pressure can plummet. This effect is well-known.[18] Thus, during the postpartum period, when blood pressure may be unstable, the addition of bromocriptine can initiate a life-threatening change in blood pressure.

Bromocriptine was first approved in 1978 for the treatment of Parkinson's disease and pituitary tumors. In 1980 the approval was amended to include suppression of lactation, and by 1987 between 480,000 and 939,000 women were given bromocriptine postpartum.[19] However, from the beginning, the FDA had been receiving reports of young women on bromocriptine who had suffered strokes in the first few days after delivery.

The FDA has a system for receiving reports about any adverse reaction found with any medication approved by the government. These spontaneous reports reach the FDA in one of two ways: either directly from a health care professional or consumer, or through the pharmaceutical manufacturer. By law, pharmaceutical manufacturers must report all adverse reactions to the FDA at specified time periods. This is, of course, a very imperfect system. However, it does shed light on some side effects that do not show up in clinical studies.

It was clear from correspondence between the FDA and Parlodel's manufacturer, Sandoz Ltd., that by February 1983 the number and severity of these side effects concerned the FDA medical officers. In August 1983 a letter from the FDA stated that there was a "concern about the safety of Parlodel in the treatment of physiological lactation. This may be a problem only for individuals who have toxemia, hypertension or who have received ergots or other drugs which can alter blood pressure. While many of the individual cases are inconclusive, in the aggregate they are compelling."

At the time, Sandoz was instructed to change the labeling and was reminded that, under FDA regulations, they were to "include a warning as soon as there is reasonable evidence of an association of a serious hazard with a drug; a causal relationship need not have been proved."[20] These warnings were not included until nearly two years later.

Reports documenting episodes of high blood pressure, seizures, strokes, and even heart attacks have steadily continued since then, as bromocriptine sales have grown into a multimillion dollar a year business for Sandoz.

The FDA received reports of cases in which bromocriptine was the only explanation.[21] Some collected in 1988 include:

- A 38-year-old woman had a completely normal delivery and was discharged in good health with normal blood pressure. She was started on bromocriptine one day after delivery. Nine days later she came to the emergency room with a severe headache and a very high blood pressure. She had a stroke and died six weeks later.

- A 31-year-old healthy new mother without any history of seizures delivered a child by an uncomplicated cesarean section in May 1987. She was put on bromocriptine after delivery. She developed headaches two weeks later while still on the drug, and had a prolonged grand mal convulsion at home. She was resuscitated but remained in a coma for two months. She now has severe brain damage from oxygen deprivation during the seizure and is paralyzed.

- A healthy 22-year-old woman was started on bromocriptine after a cesarean section for fetal distress. She returned home three days after delivery. On the fifth day she died at home from a severe heart attack due to closing of one of the coronary arteries.

Bromocriptine has also been associated with postpartum psychosis, both in well individuals and in women with a history of psychiatric illness.[22] Postpartum depression, manic depressive disorder, and schizophrenia are common conditions in females of childbearing age (up to 10 percent may be affected),[23] and the use of a drug known to exacerbate or induce psychosis adds unnecessary risk. This is especially true because the postpartum period is a time when women are subject to the additional stress and responsibility of a newborn infant.

THE FDA ACTS ON KNOWN DANGERS

In February 1987, after reviewing reports of adverse reactions from bromocriptine, the FDA requested that the drug's manufacturer, Sandoz Pharmaceuticals Corp., change the label. They were instructed to add warnings of problems such as uncontrolled hypertension that had emerged since the last time the company was asked to add warnings in 1984. They were also requested to send a so-called "Dear Doctor" letter alerting all obstetricians and gynecologists to the health risks of postpartum use of the drug.[24]

It is critically important to notify practicing physicians of such risks, as history has demonstrated. Even after companies acknowledge the risks and add appropriate warnings, such information can go tragically unnoticed if physicians and the public remain uninformed. For example, the Eli Lilly Company voluntarily withdrew its promotion of DES for use in nonnursing postpartum women in 1981. Amazingly, DES still accounted for three percent of all prescriptions written for lactation suppression seven years later, according to the National Disease and Therapeutics Index. This implies that about 25,000 women a year are still receiving DES years after the company withdrew its use for breast engorgement. This figure also includes a large number of prescriptions for generic diethylstilbestrol (DES).[25]

In 1987 the FDA merely asked that doctors who use Parlodel be appraised of the findings by the company that manufactures the drug. A year later the FDA had to ask again.

PUTTING AN END TO LACTATION SUPPRESSANTS

In September 1989 the FDA finally asked drug makers to voluntarily stop marketing both hormonal drugs and bromocriptine for lactation suppression. Announcing the decision, former FDA commissioner Frank Young acknowledged years of accumulated evidence adding up to too much risk and too little benefit. "We estimate that, if 100 women are given these drugs, at best 10 may benefit, which means that at least 90 percent of the women who receive the drugs are exposed to possible side effects from these agents but are not benefited."[26]

Squibb Corp., which sells Deladumone, and Merrill Dow Co., which sells TACE, are among the manufacturers to have complied with the FDA's request. Those two drugs, however, make up only a fraction of the market for lactation suppressants. Sandoz, with its 83 percent market share, stands to lose much more money if Parlodel is yanked from the market, and has balked at the request. If history repeats itself, it may require more than merely asking them to voluntarily withdraw lactation suppression from the list of uses of this drug. As one commentator put it, "If voluntary compliance worked, Moses would have come down from Mount Sinai with ten guidelines."

Dr. David Winter, vice president of Sandoz, in his response to the FDA request, stated that to deny patients the freedom of choice would do a disservice to the U. S. medical community, "which has prescribed the drug safely and effectively for many years."[27] Fortunately, the FDA doesn't agree. But Sandoz has decided not to join other companies in taking voluntary action. Therefore, the next step involves legal proceedings, which could take years.

Doctors can, of course, use whatever is on the pharmacy shelf for whatever purpose. Since Parlodel is useful for treating other conditions, physicians may be willing to take the risk of prescribing it for lactation suppression, even if labeling changes occur. More likely, they may simply remain uninformed of its dangers. Adequate notification through the FDA Drug Bulletins, "Dear Doctor" letters, and physicians' associations must reach tens of thousands of family doctors, as well as obstetrician/gynecologists who treat postpartum women.

At the time this book is being written, the FDA is in the

process of initiating legal action to force the company to stop marketing their dangerous drug, Parlodel, for use in lactation suppression.

1. Extrapolation from Dianne Kennedy, June 1, 1989 Testimony.

2. Kennedy DL, R.Ph., M.P.H., National Disease and Therapeutic Index analysis, Testimony before Fertility and Maternal Health Drugs Advisory Committee, Food and Drug Administration, June 1, 1989.

3. Ibid.

4. Testimony of Dr. Wendy Nelson, Food and Drug Administration, Fertility and Maternal Health Drugs Advisory Committee Hearing, June 2, 1988, and additional updates obtained from the FDA September 22, 1988; Katz M, Kroll D, Pak I, Osimoni A, Hirsch M. Puerperal hypertension, stroke and seizures after suppression of lactation with bromocriptine. Obstetrics and Gynecology 1985; 66:822–4; Iffy L, TenHove W, Frisoli G. Acute myocardial infarction in the puerperium in patients receiving bromocriptine. American Journal of Obstetrics and Gynecology 1986; 155:371–2; Testimony of Sandoz Pharmaceutical staff, Fertility and Maternal Health Drugs Advisory Committee hearing, Food and Drug Administration, June 2, 1988; Watson DL, Bhatia R, Norman G, Brindley B, Sokol RJ. Parlodel (Bromocriptine mesylate) in pregnancy-induced hypertension; a risk factor for postpartum hypertension. Presentation, Meetings of the American College of Obstetricians and Gynecologists 1988.

5. Testimony of Vanaja V. Ragavan, M.D., Fertility and Maternal Health Drugs Advisory Committee, Food and Drug Administration, June 2, 1988.

6. Niebyl JR, Bell WR, Schaaf ME, Blake DA, Dubin NH, King TM. The effect of chlorotrianisene as postpartum lactation suppression on blood coagulation factors. American Journal of Obstetrics and Gynecology 1979; 134:518–22.

7. Turnbull AC. Puerperal thrombo-embolism and suppression of lactation. Journal of Obstetrics and Gynaecology of the British Commonwealth 1968; 75:1321–3.

8. Lawrence R, University of Rochester Medical Center, Interview with author, November 1989.

9. Ibid.

10. Turnbull, op. cit.; Summary basis for approval for bromocriptine mesylate to Food and Drug Administration, October 27, 1978.

11. Turnbull, op. cit.

12. Niebyl, op. cit.

13. Daniel DG, Campbell H, Turnbull AC. Puerperal thromboembolism and suppression of lactation. Lancet 1967; 2:287–9.

14. Jeffcoate TNA, Miller J, Roos RF, Tindall VR. Puerperal thromboembolism in relation to the inhibition of lactation of oestrogen therapy. British Medical Journal 1968; 4:19–25.

15. Silver L, Wolfe S. Unnecessary Cesarean Sections: A Rapidly Growing National Epidemic, Public Citizen Health Research Group, Washington, DC, January 1989.

16. Federal Register, October 24, 1978.

17. Kennedy, op. cit., June 1, 1989.

18. Mehta AE, Tolis G. Pharmacology of bromocriptine in health and disease. Drugs 1979; 17:313–25.

19. Testimony of Dr. Dianne Kennedy, Fertility and Maternal Health Drugs Advisory Committee, Food and Drug Administration, June 2, 1988.

20. Letter from Solomon Sobel, MD, Office of New Drug Evaluation, FDA, to Kalmar Magyar, Sandoz Inc.; August 10, 1983.

21. Adverse Drug Reactions reported to FDA, 1988.

22. Canterbury RJ, Haskins B, Kahn N, Saathoff G, Yazell JJ. Postpartum psychosis induced by bromocriptine. Southern Medical Journal 1987; 80:1463–4; Pearson KC. Mental disorders from low-dose bromocriptine. New England Journal of Medicine 1978; 305:173; Vlissides DN, Gill D, Castelow J. Bromocriptine-induced mania? British Medical Journal 1978; 1:510; Brook NM, Cookson IB. Bromocriptine-induced mania? British Medical Journal 1978:1:790.

23. Robins LN, Helzer JE, Weissman MM, Orvaschel H, Gruenberg E, Burke JD, Regier DA. Lifetime prevalence of specific psychiatric disorders in three sites. Archives of General Psychiatry 1984; 41:949–58.

24. Letter from Solomon Sobel, Office of Biologics Research and Review, to Eileen Ryan, Sandoz, February 11, 1987.

25. Testimony of Dianne Kennedy, June 1, 1989, op. cit.

26. Letter from Frank Young to Dr. Sidney M. Wolfe, August 23, 1989.

27. US FDA committee criticizes lactation products. Scrip 1989; 1420:32.

HORMONE REPLACEMENT THERAPY

The Most Abused "Wonder Drugs" of the Century

Millions of women today take, or plan to take, replacement hormones (primarily Premarin) from the onset of their menopause through age 70 to 80 or older—despite evidence that long-term use of these powerful drugs doubles their risk of breast cancer.

- In the 1990s estrogen is fast becoming the most popular cholesterol lowering drug for women, despite the lack of evidence from properly controlled studies that mass prescriptions of the drug are lowering the rate at which women die of heart disease.

- There has been a striking decrease in heart disease deaths in American women over the last 35 years but this has also occurred in a large number of other countries, in very few of which is there significant use of menopausal estrogens.

- Many women who take estrogen replacement therapy to prevent osteoporosis may be at little or no risk of developing the disease, and thus are needlessly exposing themselves to the dangers of these potent drugs.

- While estrogen lowers the rate at which bone loss occurs in postmenopausal women, lifelong moderate exercise and adequate calcium intake, neither of which pose any health risks, can also prevent bone loss, although not as well as estrogens.

- Today, the trend is to add progestins to estrogens, which may reduce your risk of uterine cancer, but may increase your risk of heart disease and, possibly, breast cancer.

Recommendations

- If you suffer from severe menopausal symptoms such as hot flashes and vaginal dryness, low dose menopausal estrogen replacement therapy (.625 mg) for several months will alleviate your symptoms. These drugs should not be taken for longer than a year. Once you discontinue therapy, the dryness will return (and can be treated with topical creams) but your hot flashes probably will not.

- Do not automatically refill your prescription for menopausal hormones. After a few months, try going without them and see if your hot flashes come back.

- Do not take menopausal estrogens as a hedge against osteoporosis or heart disease unless you are in a very high risk group. Diet and exercise in younger years are your best means of preventing these diseases in later life. But even if you did not do this previously, now is a good time to start.

*F*EMALE replacement hormones may someday be remembered as the most recklessly prescribed and dangerous drugs of this century. Since the 1940s when estrogens were first manufactured cheaply and made available by mouth, the story of their widespread use in treating women's "problems" is one of false promises, disregard for scientific evidence, and the wishful thinking of women and their doctors that all female health problems might vanish with the magic of pills. It is a story of well-meaning doctors eager to please, and of women too easily sold the wonders of pharmaceutical cures. Unfortunately, years after women have been routinely consuming hormones, many of these otherwise healthy people have slowly been getting sick from estrogens.

In 1989 over 3.5 million women were given estrogens for the symptoms of menopause: hot flashes, heavy sweating, and vaginal discomfort.[1] These women *began* hormone replacement therapy for the short-term problems associated with menopause. However, while the symptoms of menopause usually subside in less than two years, a large proportion of these women will take estrogen, and probably progestins (a synthetic form of the naturally occurring hormone progesterone) indefinitely.

By today's questionable medical reasoning, these potent drugs should be given to perfectly healthy women, not to treat any disease, but to decrease the potential of disease, specifically osteoporosis and heart disease.

Replacement hormones were the "feminine forever" drugs of the 1960s and 1970s, guaranteed to keep wrinkles away, hair glossy, and depression to a minimum. In the 1980s these drugs were advertised as the cure for osteoporosis, the long sought after answer to brittle bones. Now in the 1990s, estrogens are being touted as the solution to female heart disease. Whatever their mission, these recycled wonder drugs have securely found a permanent spot in the medicine cabinets of millions of healthy women over 45. But the dangers of hormone replacement therapy have been tragically underplayed by American doctors, the press, and of course the drug companies, who make hundreds of millions more dollars every time a new use for these drugs is found. Throughout the history of their application in American medicine, estrogens have proven to be as dangerous as they are helpful. As with so many medical products sold to American consumers, taking them has become a risk/benefit game; the difference here is that women are not making choices based on all the facts.

Ovarian hormones, especially estrogens, have been linked to breast cancer in animal studies since the 1930s. But if you ask your doctor if they cause human breast cancer, you will probably be told the evidence is still "inconclusive" and "inconsistent," or that women are not the same as rats or mice.

You may have heard or read that if you take menopausal hormones you increase your risk of endometrial (uterine) cancer, heart disease, stroke, gallbladder disease, uterine fibroids, liver disease, and migraine headaches. If you combine estrogens with progestins, you will reduce your risk of uterine cancer, but may simultaneously increase your risk of heart disease and breast cancer. Progestins may also cause abdominal bloating, headaches, depression, or acne. And you may begin to menstruate again.

Many women do not realize that menopausal hormones are grossly overprescribed for extraordinary lengths of time, now longer than ever before, longer than anyone can scientifically justify. Unless you are considered at high risk for potential problems associated with the treatment, physicians today are more likely to downplay any harm and persuade you that without them you will expire prematurely of a heart attack or snap under the weight of old age related osteoporosis.

Prescription practices for these potent drugs have subtly but dramatically shifted over time. Today it is not up to women to prove they need hormone replacement after menopause; the burden is on women to prove they don't. So widespread is the use that many women may not be completely sure why they are still taking estrogens at age 60.

These two grandmothers are examples:

> I have been taking estrogens since I can remember. I don't know whether I'd still get hot flashes, but I don't want to find out.

I started taking estrogens 12 years ago when my surgeon prescribed them following my hysterectomy. I was having terrible hot flashes then, and Premarin (the most widely prescribed estrogen) completely got rid of them. I'm still taking it, because somewhere along the line, I don't remember when, my doctor told me they would protect me against osteoporosis. I feel great and don't see a reason in the world I should stop taking that pill along with my vitamin every day.

HORMONES: NOT HARMLESS LITTLE TABLETS

Pills that deliver hormones to your body are not simply vitamins or candy coated aspirin. They are manufactured duplicates of substances that play amazingly diverse roles in women's bodies. Besides their role in maintaining reproductive cycles, estrogens alter lipid (fat) levels, metabolize carbohydrates, affect how blood coagulates, adjust blood pressure, and assist in calcium absorption, all of which are complex biologic events.

When the natural supply of estrogen slowly diminishes after menopause, can its functions all be "replaced" by a pill? Obviously not. The enormous and complicated functions of hormones are not completely understood by science. Experts are still exploring the effects—both good and bad—of replacement hormones. There is still a lot to know about their long-term risks, since long-term use is relatively new. In fact, it is still impossible to identify which women will ultimately benefit from these drugs, which is why their use is so general and widespread. There is an excellent probability that the vast majority of women receiving hormone replacement therapy will obtain no benefit at all while subjecting themselves to all the potential risks and side effects.

Since ovarian hormones have been known to promote cancer, the trend toward grossly overprescribing them can't be taken lightly. As Allan S. Brett, a researcher from the New England Deaconess Medical Center wrote in a 1989 editorial in the *New England Journal of Medicine,* "Pharmacologic interventions are powerful symbols of the triumph of medical technology. Patients are likely to believe implicitly that the benefits of drugs clearly outweigh the risks."[2]

This can be a very dangerous assumption.

CANCER AND HORMONE REPLACEMENT THERAPY

In the United States in 1990, an estimated 150,000 new cases of breast cancer will be diagnosed in women and 44,000 women will die of the disease.[3] In fact, one in every 11 women will eventually get breast cancer, which leads the list along with lung cancer in female cancer fatalities.[4] Because women of the "baby boom generation" are now reaching age 40, the number of breast cancer cases and deaths will increase substantially over the next 40 years. For this reason, even a small increase in the risk of breast cancer caused by menopausal estrogens will translate into a lot of lost lives.

That increased breast cancer risk is being further investigated now, while hundreds of thousands of women in menopause are being given replacement hormones. But accumulated evidence over the past decade shows that if you use menopausal estrogens for a long time, you roughly double your chance of getting breast cancer by the time you are 75.

What constitutes a long time? Let's take a brief look at the scientific studies. While they go back earlier than this, the first reliable studies of women taking menopausal estrogens for longer than five years were published between 1977 and 1983. These were strikingly consistent in their findings and, overall, showed that women using the most commonly prescribed dose of estrogen (1.25 mg tablets at the time) for five or more years double their chance of developing breast cancer.

Four of the five studies found that the risk of breast cancer was highest in women who used higher doses of the drug, women who used the drug for a long period of time, or both.[5]

In the first of these studies, researchers found that women

using doses higher than .625 mg per day (the dose most commonly prescribed today) were 2.7 times as likely to develop breast cancer 10 years after starting drug treatment as women who did not use the drug.[6]

In the second study, researchers found that women who received any dose of menopausal estrogens for at least seven years had an 80 percent increase in breast cancer.[7]

The 1981 study[8] found that women who had surgical removal of the ovaries and estrogen replacement therapy increased their risk of breast cancer dramatically the longer they were on estrogens. The risk worked out like this: in less than five years of estrogen replacement therapy these women had a 38 percent increased risk of breast cancer, at nine years their risk had increased to 55 percent, and after ten years it reached 70 percent.

In 1986, an expanded study of menopausal estrogen use showed that 20 years after first using estrogens, women had increased their risk by 50 percent.[9]

But all these findings have been called "inconclusive" because other studies have shown little or no connection between breast cancer and menopausal hormones.[10] Proponents of menopausal hormones are reluctant to implicate this wonder drug as a contributor to breast cancer, an admittedly complicated disease caused by many factors.

In 1990 at a meeting of the Food and Drug Administration Fertility and Maternal Health Drugs Advisory Committee in Washington D.C., leading researchers met to decide if the evidence over the last decade did indeed point to an increased risk of breast cancer in postmenopausal women.

At this meeting, Janet Daling from the Fred Hutchinson Cancer Research Center in Seattle called the question of risk "very tricky" to answer: " My conclusion would be that estrogen replacement therapy may have a modest effect on breast cancer risk, something in the range of 1.5 or 1.3 to 2.0 [times increased risk] in women who have used estrogens for long periods of time."[11]

The committee was also asked to review all the evidence

and they found that: "The committee's unanimous response is, while the evidence is not conclusive, some studies have reported an increased risk of breast cancer in long term use of estrogen replacement therapy. Other studies have not shown this relationship."[12]

Today, instead of getting only a prescription for estrogens, you will probably also get another little bottle, this one with progestins. You will take these for seven to ten days at the end of your cycle of estrogen pills. Progestins are added because in the mid-1970s three striking studies found that taking estrogen by itself increases your risk of endometrial or uterine cancer from five- to fourteen-fold.[13] This news sent shock waves through the medical community, but in 1989 it was shown that by adding progestins, the problem of endometrial cancer was largely ameliorated.

Good news and bad news. It was hoped by some doctors that progestin would also somehow offer women some protection from breast cancer, despite the known differences between how each organ responds to hormones. However, in the summer of 1989 a new study from Sweden suggested that progestins in combination with estrogen may cause more harm than good.[14] The study confirmed that women using estrogens alone for an extended period double their risk of breast cancer, but it also showed that when progestin was added there was no protection against breast cancer. Instead, the few women who used the two hormones together for more than six years had a higher risk of breast cancer than those taking estrogen alone.

The study has been criticized because the Swedish women who participated in it were given hormones manufactured differently and administered at different doses than women typically get in the United States. But one of the study's authors, Dr. Robert Hoover, Chief of the Environmental Epidemiology Branch of the National Cancer Institute, says the results shouldn't make any hormone proponent feel vindicated. "It looks as though the cancer risk may be an estrogenic effect and not some nuance of the chemical structure of different estrogen compounds."

The results of the Swedish study, says Hoover, are not surprising.

The fact that ovarian hormones might relate to increased risk of breast cancer is not on the bizarre fringe of biological reasoning. The biological plausibility was established 100 years ago, so new data which shows that women on replacement therapy have an increased risk is exactly what you would predict. You can argue about what level of risk there is, but the reasonableness of the observation is firmly steeped in biology.[15]

"Arguing about the level of risk" is what researchers are doing these days, which may be the reason that practicing physicians are told, and will tell you, that studies are inconsistent and inconclusive, so basically there is nothing to worry about. But, in fact, if these drugs increase your risk of breast cancer, that obviously *is* something to worry about.

GETTING STARTED ON REPLACEMENT THERAPY

Why have women adopted the notion that menopause is a cruel consequence of being female, "one of nature's mistakes,"[16] an illness that needs to be cured? Menopause is not a disease. No one has ever died from it. It is a natural event that results in some temporary and some permanent changes for all women. Physiologically it's the time when a woman's ovaries stop functioning, a process that can take several years. The cessation of periods and the thinning and drying of the vaginal tissues are among the two most obvious permanent changes associated with menopause. Hot flashes are temporary changes most women encounter.[17] However, many other psychological conditions have been described as "symptoms" of menopause. Irritability, depression, anxiety, loss of sexual feelings, and an almost limitless list of other states are all attributed to it, but not proven to be caused by it.

Menopause is not the first time most women experience

these symptoms, but they may be worsened at age 45 or 50 in a society that discriminates against aging women, promotes superficial notions of exclusively youth-related sex appeal, and encourages everyone to answer all problems with a pill. Menopausal estrogens will not eliminate wrinkles, increase your libido, or ameliorate all the psychological conditions that come with growing older. Those hoped for effects don't happen, plain and simple.

A small number of the disruptive and annoying symptoms of menopause may be alleviated by reintroducing estrogen as the body's own production is slowly reduced. Menopausal estrogens in low doses over short periods can eliminate hot flashes and night sweating associated with menopause. They can also reduce vaginal dryness. While useful for both problems, treatment seldom needs to continue for longer than several months. Most women are free of hot flashes in under two years[18] and vaginal dryness can be treated with topical creams.

While some women do experience hot flashes that are incapacitating, more frequent is the experience of Dorothy, a fifty-year-old psychologist:

> The first time I felt one I thought I had forgotten to turn on the air conditioner. Now I can feel one coming and I know it's going to last a minute or so. Occasionally I have to take off a sweater, or wipe my brow but it never gets in my way. It's simply not a big problem.

OSTEOPOROSIS: WHO'S AT RISK?

In the early 1980s, osteoporosis turned into one of the most well publicized health threats to women. The media attention it received ushered in a new era of hormone use in this country. Hormone replacement therapy thus became a powerful pharmacologic intervention for millions of women with and without menopausal problems.

If you are female, white, and thin you are, by today's standards, automatically at risk for getting osteoporosis in old age.

That's a lot of women. Whether or not you have symptoms related to menopause, your gynecologist may recommend you start taking replacement hormones, because despite your good health at 45, you qualify in 20 to 25 years as a prime candidate for osteoporosis. Very typically, it's as simple as that.

Of course physicians vary in their prescription practices. Some will only put those at highest risk for osteoporosis on replacement hormones. This would include women:

- whose ovaries have been removed before age 40
- who have a family history of osteoporosis
- who have been on long-term adrenal steroid therapy
- who have such conditions as hyperthyroidism, kidney disease, or gastrectomy (operation to remove part or all of the stomach)

But much of the time even if you are not in one of these high risk groups, if you are going through menopause, have a sedentary lifestyle, are thin, smoke, or drink, those factors alone may persuade your doctor to prescribe estrogens for the rest of your life.

What is osteoporosis? It's bone thinning to the point where the skeleton cannot support normal loads. The term literally means that the bones are porous, but the diagnosis simply means that the bones are fragile. What's important is that they break too easily. Hip fractures, spinal compression fractures, and broken vertebrae are the hallmarks of osteoporosis. Most of the time these breaks occur as the result of a fall. The effects of osteoporosis should not be underestimated: they can cost older people their independence, lots of money, and sometimes their lives.

Why Estrogen?

It has been recognized for several decades that estrogen plays an important role in the process of manufacturing bone in women. Bone is living tissue which is constantly being remodeled, broken down, and reformed throughout life. Until we reach our mid-30s, bone is usually added faster than it is removed.

However at around age 35 the balance begins to shift and slowly more bone is lost than is formed.

Bone loss happens in both men and women, but in women the loss is greater and the effects more severe. While it isn't clear how this happens, until menopause estrogen suppresses the rate at which calcium is broken down from bones and reabsorbed back into the body. After menopause when ovarian function stops and estrogens are no longer available, bone turn-over increases, but the loss occurs faster than formation.[19] The net result is accelerated bone loss for several years after the onset of menopause.

Estrogen replacement has gotten a lot of attention because studies have shown that daily doses above .625 mg conjugated estrogen (today the most common prescription in the U.S.) seem to retard bone loss for as long as the drug is taken.[20] Some studies also show that women on menopausal estrogens suffer fewer debilitating fractures.[21]

So the medical rule of thumb today is to prescribe estrogens as soon after the onset of menopause as possible, because 50 percent of bone loss in women occurs in the first seven years after menopause.[22] The therapy continues, uninterrupted, for 25 years or so, until bone loss slows down naturally around age 70. But if there is any interruption in the estrogen regimen women appear to return to their pretreatment bone loss rate.[23]

Questions about Estrogen and Bones

If estrogen deprivation were the entire reason older women get hip fractures, broken arms, and crushed vertebrae, then the mystery of osteoporosis would have been solved. However, although all women eventually live without estrogen, only some get debilitating osteoporotic fractures. There remain many questions about this potentially crippling disease. Why are some women so-called "fast bone losers" and others not? Why are there significant differences in the bone mass among all women? While blanket prescriptions for menopausal estrogens are being passed out by many doctors, these differences are not being taken into account. Most women on menopausal estrogens get the same dose, for an indefinite period of time, even though this medication has clear health risks of its own.

Furthermore, studies have not clarified the following questions about estrogen therapy itself:

- Do women started on estrogen several years after menopause receive any protection?
- What is the optimal dose for maximum benefit and minimal side effects?
- Does the cyclical addition of progestins to the estrogens provide more benefit than estrogens alone? (This also frequently reintroduces monthly periods.)
- Is the benefit of replacement therapy to reduce hip and forearm fractures lost within a few years after cessation of use?[24]

By definition, all postmenopausal women have estrogen deficiency, yet only a few develop osteoporosis within the 15 to 20 year period after menopause. Only 5 to 10 percent of those who ultimately get spinal (vertebral) fractures do so during this time.[25] Many women live with varying degrees of osteoporosis and don't even know they have it. As will be discussed below, you can effectively reduce your risk of having delicate bones at age 65 through lifelong attention to diet and exercise. Reducing your risk of suffering from fractures has a lot to do with safe habits which, unlike taking drugs, pose no new health risks to you.

The most common osteoporotic fractures—vertebral compression fractures—are not life-threatening, and their incidence in older women can be curtailed. As demonstrated by the comments of this 70-year-old woman, her life is active despite a diagnosis of osteoporosis and a vertebral fracture following a day of strenuous gardening:

I learned I have some degree of osteoporosis after I gardened too much. I lifted a load that was too heavy in the wheelbarrow and the next day my back was in real pain. It took a couple of weeks to get better and now I'm much more careful not to overdo.

What Doctors Fear Most: Hip Fractures

Preventing life-threatening fractures, primarily hip fractures, is one of the big reasons physicians are hooked on using menopausal estrogens. Hip fractures are, indeed, one tragic consequence of osteoporosis. They can lead to death, because the long recuperation increases vulnerability to such problems as blood clotting and pneumonia.

Furthermore, about 25 percent of those who suffer hip fractures after age 55 do not heal well enough to be able to walk again without help, and 15 to 20 percent are in long-term institutions one year after the injury.[26]

One physician who puts virtually all his postmenopausal patients on hormone therapy expresses fears typical of many physicians: "It's very traumatic seeing the life of an elderly person after hip fracture. They may be in painful rehabilitation for months. Their whole life has changed. It may be more devastating than a heart attack or cancer."[27]

Bone Mass Not the Only Culprit in Hip Fractures

Your bone mass is only one factor that predicts how likely you are to break your hip someday. It may, in fact, be a very crude predictor. Several studies show even bone density itself may not be the protection against fractures that estrogen replacement therapy supporters claim. Studies show patients with fractures have similar bone densities at various sites as those without fractures.[28] Other researchers have argued that bone mass in the hips of patients with hip fractures was similar to that in the general population.[29]

So what besides low bone mass accounts for fractures? Age, falling, and the way you live.

More than 90 percent of all hip fractures occur in individuals over age 70,[30] and about 90 percent of fractures of the hip, forearm, and pelvis result from a fall.[31] Clearly, the way you live in older age—especially avoiding falls—decides your fate as much as the density of your bones.

What about modifying the risk of falling? These problems cause falls:

- diminished vision
- cognitive losses
- balance problems
- disability in the legs
- the side-effects of psychotropic (mind-affecting) medications
- environmental hazards (tangled electric cords, stairs, slippery carpets)

Preventing Falls

As we age, our bones will thin, our muscle tone soften, our agility diminish. Whether or not you have osteoporosis, in older age you should take the following steps to decrease your risk of falling:

- Have your vision and hearing tested regularly
- Limit alcohol intake
- Consult a physician or pharmacist about possible side effects of any medicines that may cause dizziness or lightheadedness
- Use a cane or walking stick when needed, particularly if walking outdoors on wet or icy pavement
- Wear supportive, rubber soled, low heeled shoes
- Reduce home hazards that might cause falls; for example, install thick carpeting, bathroom safety bars, and bright stairway lighting

Over a lifetime bones react not just to hormonal influences but to mechanical use, good nutrition, and especially in old age, environmental factors. Sadly, in our rush to treat bodies medically we overlook the other well documented factors that combine to provide the most protection against osteoporosis. These include a diet adequate in calcium at all ages; consistent weight-bearing exercise to maintain balance, strength, and agility; reducing the environmental hazards of daily life; and careful attention to other drugs being consumed which could increase chances of falling.

What Improves Bone Mass in All Women?

Our bones are not simply the rigid structures around which the rest of us is assembled. Actually, the most important function of our bones is as a reservoir for the calcium needed by the rest of the body. Every cell requires calcium, and nature sees to it that cellular needs are taken care of first. In a sense, our bones are constantly tapped to serve the physiological need for calcium elsewhere in our bodies.

The demands for calcium are constant, but our supply is obviously not. It's important, therefore, that we keep our bodies supplied with adequate calcium and that we begin early in life.

Many experts agree that 60 percent of the human skeleton is laid down by the time bones fuse and growth stops, at around age 20. That means that during the adolescent growth spurt, most bone mass has been established. The National Research Council, recognizing the importance of early accumulation of calcium stores in young bones, increased its recommendation for daily calcium for ages 11 to 18 to 1,200 mg a day, up from 800. That is as much as the recommended amount for pregnant and nursing women. Unfortunately, teens on average consume less than half that amount of calcium.

The three things that potentially interfere with bone mass development are dietary insufficiency (mainly calcium), interruption of reproductive endocrine status (loss of menstrual period), and absence of adequate weight bearing or mechanical loading onto the skeleton. These three factors can set the stage for osteoporosis decades before old age.

The process of bone formation and reformation throughout life continues to be significantly impacted by diet and exercise. By age 35 a woman has the largest bone mass she is likely to get. While there is no evidence that even very high calcium diets started then will increase the amount of bone she has amassed or make up for early life calcium deficits, it remains important as a way of protecting what there is.[32]

Daily Calcium Requirements

	Mg calcium per day
Children	
Birth—less than a year	360
1–10	540
11–18	1,200
Premenopausal women	1,000
Estrogen-treated women	1,000
Postmenopausal women	1,500
Pregnant or nursing women under age 19	2,000
Pregnant or nursing women over age 19	1,400

Sources of Calcium

Milk, other dairy products, fish, and dark green vegetables are the major dietary sources of calcium in this country. One 8 oz glass of skim milk contains 300 mg of calcium, or 25 percent of the daily requirement for adult women who are not pregnant or nursing or postmenopausal. People who have difficulty digesting milk (as in lactase deficiency or lactose intolerance) might try low fat yogurt or skim milk that has been treated with the enzyme lactase so it can be digested. Some yogurts contain lactase naturally.

Other calcium-rich foods include fish and shellfish such as oysters, shrimp, and canned sardines and salmon (when edible bones are also consumed); and dark green vegetables such as collard, turnip and mustard greens, kale, and broccoli. Spinach is not a good source of calcium because, although it is high in calcium, it contains substances (oxalates) that diminish absorption of calcium.

What about Calcium Supplements?

For some people it may be difficult to reach optimum daily levels of calcium without taking supplements. If you are going to take supplements, make sure you read the labels because different formulations contain different amounts of elemental calcium. For example, some commonly available calcium compounds:

Calcium carbonate .... 40% calcium
Calcium lactate .... 13% calcium
Calcium gluconate .... 9% calcium

Further advice on taking supplements:

- Take supplements between meals and at bedtime. Absorption is better at those times.

- Absorption of calcium from calcium carbonate is impaired in people with little or no stomach acid, which is more common in people over age 60. For these people, taking supplements during meals is preferred.

- Bone meal and dolomite should not be taken as a calcium supplement. Although they are both high in calcium, they also tend to contain high amounts of lead and other toxic metals.

- Be alert to calcium supplements that have vitamin D added to them. Most people get enough of this vitamin in their diet or through sun exposure. Vitamin D becomes toxic at high doses.

- Avoid taking aluminum-containing antacids as a regular source of calcium. Instead, use ones which only contain calcium if you are taking them solely as calcium supplements.

- Drink a full glass of water when taking a calcium supplement.

Levels of calcium intake greater than those recommended can cause kidney stones in susceptible people. Thus, people with a history of kidney stones should take calcium supplements only with a doctor's guidance. These people should be especially careful to drink plenty of water.

Exercise Builds Bone as Well as Muscle

Research has shown that physically active women are less susceptible to broken bones.[33] This is partly because people who get exercise maintain better muscle tone, strength, and agility, all of which reduce both chances of falling and degree of injury.

But exercise—especially weight bearing exercise—does more than build muscle. It actually builds bone. Bone is an adaptive tissue which develops its structure and function in proportion to the mechanical and metabolic demands you put on it. The development of bone mass during the phase of bone growth, and its continued strength throughout your life, is partially a consequence of the amount of mechanical loading and muscular activity required of it.

There is a nearly constant ratio of bone to muscle in a woman's body. Women who have a subnormal amount of bone, (osteoporosis) have an equally subnormal amount of muscle. This association points to the importance of a lifelong program of vigorous physical activity.

This makes sense even in old age, even though few studies have been conducted on the benefits of exercise in preventing fractures in the elderly. In one study, nursing home volunteers aged 69 through 95 performed light physical activity that included arm exercises and running in place.[34] Three years later, forearm bone mineral content was higher in those who completed the regimen. Another study showed similar improvement in a slightly younger group of women.[35]

While there are only a few studies showing that exercise started very late in life will increase bone density in older women, it may just be that a lifetime of healthy exercise continued into old age maintains a basic level of physical conditioning that in itself reduces risk of fractures, and perhaps of falling. Delayed reflexes, weakened muscles, and reduced soft tissue padding may contribute to an inability to absorb the energy from a fall which in turn would result in a fracture. But even if you have not exercised enough when you were younger, starting when you are older will probably be of benefit.

═══ Safer Alternative to Estrogens for Osteoporosis ═══

A recently discovered alternative to estrogen in the treatment of postmenopausal osteoporosis is etidronate (trade name Didronel, marketed by Norwich-Eaton). In two well-designed studies, one Danish, one American, periodic therapy with etidronate for two to three years increased spinal bone mass, reduced spinal fractures, and decreased height loss in women with postmenopausal osteoporosis. In editorials the *New England Journal of Medicine* called etidronate "a welcome new option,"[36] while the British journal the *Lancet* said it "represents a new and effective therapeutic approach for osteoporosis."[37]

In a three-year Danish study, vertebral fractures were reduced to only 6 per 100 patient-years in women taking etidronate, compared with 54 per 100 patient-years in controls, a ninefold decrease. Etidronate, which is approved in the United States for the treatment of Paget's disease, was administered orally in doses of 400 mg/day for two weeks, followed by a free period of 13 weeks. Daily 500 mg calcium supplements were also part of the treatment. Side effects were minor (nausea, diarrhea), and the cost was comparable to estrogen therapy.[38]

Etidronate therapy appears to increase bone mass even after two years of therapy, although further study is needed to confirm its long-term effectiveness. Since gains from estrogen therapy level off after two years, this would be an advantage of the new agent.

HEART DISEASE AND HORMONE REPLACEMENT THERAPY

If hormone replacement therapy turned into the "wonder treatment" for preventing osteoporosis in the 1980s, it is quickly becoming the prescription against heart disease in the 1990s. Today estrogens are presented as a magic potion. Is this another frantic, profitable overpromotion of an arsenal of cholesterol-lowering drugs in this country, a pharmacologic quest to reduce the number of heart attacks in older women? In the 1990s, once again, we see another alleged "triumph of medical technology" in the form of another use for cheap-to-make and extremely profitable estrogens.

While many physicians are devoted to therapeutic hormones for preventing osteoporosis, others are convinced of their protective effects but don't agree that protecting against brittle bones is their mission. "The problem of osteoporosis is trivial compared to the problems of heart disease in older women," said physician Robert Marcus. Writing in a well-respected journal, Marcus may have voiced the thinking and indeed the practices of many gynecologists and other physicians across the country: "It could turn out that the most powerful thing a physician could do to protect a woman against heart disease after the age of menopause would be to place her on estrogen."[39]

The seriousness of heart disease as a killer of American women is clear. Heart disease costs an average of over 300,000 lives a year among women over 50 years old.[40] In older women, cardiovascular diseases also cause an incredible amount of disability and hospitalization. Unfortunately, while the devastating problems of heart disease in men have been studied for decades, the same attention has not been given to the problem in women. One possible explanation for the paucity of knowledge about females is that for the most part women don't get heart disease until later in life. While men are faced with the risk of heart attacks as young adults, women appear to be protected until after menopause. Within a few years after that, the rate of heart disease in women equals that in men 6 to 10 years younger. Women never catch up to men, but it is by far the leading cause of death of American women over 50.

Menopause and Heart Disease

Something that occurs in women during the complicated phys-iological changes of menopause leaves them more susceptible to heart disease than when they were younger. Currently some medical thinkers speculate that older women suffer more heart attacks and strokes than young women because they don't have the protection of estrogen after menopause. One of the many things estrogen does is help metabolize fat and this estrogenic contribution seems to keep unwanted cholesterol levels down in premenopausal women.

Cholesterol doesn't circulate in the bloodstream in pure form. With the help of proteins and fats it combines into mole-cules called lipoproteins. These not only circulate through the bloodstream, but they also pass through the delicate cell mem-branes into cells throughout the body. Two important choles-terol compounds are high density lipoproteins (HDLs) and low density lipoproteins (LDLs). HDLs have become known as "good cholesterol" because they seem to help rid cells of cholesterol. LDLs have been coined "bad cholesterol" and are seen as the main culprit in coronory heart disease.

Studies have shown that giving estrogens to women after menopause decreases the unwanted LDL level and increases the HDL level.[41] Remember, it's the HDLs which are believed to be the body's means of cleansing itself of cholesterol that might otherwise be deposited in arteries.

Much of the enthusiasm over using estrogen as a choles-terol- lowering drug in postmenopausal women comes from the assumption that women basically turn into men after menopause as far as their cardiovascular protection is concerned. So looking at the male model, studies have shown that high LDL levels in men increase their risk of coronary heart disease and high levels of HDLs in men reduce their risk.[42]

However, there is no direct data from properly conducted studies which shows that modifying lipid and lipoprotein concentrations in women will impact their risk of coronory heart disease, or cut down on the number of women who die each year from heart attacks. In fact, for reasons that are still unclear, women with comparable levels of cholesterol to men have much lower rates of coronary heart disease.[43] In one major study, women with cholesterol concentrations higher than 295 mg/dl (the most common units for measuring cholesterol: milligrams per tenth of a liter) had rates of heart attack the same or lower than for men with cholesterol concentrations of less than 204 mg/dl. The elevated risk in women occurs only at relatively high levels of total cholesterol (more than 260 mg/dl).[44]

Nonetheless, older women are dying of heart disease and once again medical science is looking for a drug to be the solution. The pharmacological approach to addressing cholesterol levels in women is in full swing, and today estrogen is the drug of choice.

Dr. Trudy Bush of Johns Hopkins University in Baltimore is a leading advocate of preventing heart disease through estrogen therapy after menopause. She has written that if women experience even a modest increase in HDL concentration it could theoretically have profound effects on risk of coronary disease. "At present HDL cholesterol appears to be the most important lipid for women."[45]

In her view, even if menopausal hormones double a woman's chances of getting breast cancer, it wouldn't come near canceling estrogen's lifesaving potential. She believes the risks associated with estrogen use in most cases don't compare to the benefits.

Mind you, these benefits are still very theoretical. Since there is little data to show that reducing lipid levels in women will reduce the incidence of death from heart disease, there is no evidence that long-term use of estrogens will ultimately provide this much acclaimed protection. Dr. Bruce Stadel, director of epidemiology for the drug division of the Food and Drug

Administration, is a cautious supporter of estrogen therapy but admits there are big unanswered questions. "There simply hasn't been any good, solid on-going surveillance of vascular disease in women to assess the real effects of hormone replacement therapy. It just hasn't been done."[46]

Estrogen and Male Heart Disease

As a matter of fact, estrogen therapy has been tried as a cholesterol-reducing drug on men. In the 1950s, after it was found that estrogen inhibited atherosclerosis in chicks fed cholesterol, long-term clinical studies of estrogen use in men were begun. Men were used as subjects for studying the effects of higher dose estrogen on heart disease because, researchers figured, it was the estrogen in young women that kept them from getting heart attacks. The hope that estrogen was the answer to male heart disease was dashed in the 1970s after these studies showed that high doses of estrogens increased cardiovascular disease in men. In two of the large multicenter trials, evidence showed that not only was there no protection against heart attacks from estrogen use, the incidence of nonfatal illness actually increased.[47]

Now, millions of women are entering long-term treatment using estrogen, albeit at lower doses, for much the same reason that failed in men. The results, in the form of data on whether or not estrogen actually reduces the incidence of heart attacks in older women, are simply not in yet. Although there are several studies suggesting a reduction in heart attacks in women, no properly done study designed to test the effectiveness of estrogens in preventing heart disease has been done. By contrast, such studies have been done in men to establish the effectiveness of cholesterol-lowering drugs in preventing heart attacks. Now that the rush of cholesterol-lowering drugs for men has peaked, attention has been focused on the role of proper diet and exercise as being the major ways men can lower their cholesterol and lessen their cardiovascular risk. The same approaches will clearly work for women.

What about Adding Progestins?

What we do know is that estrogen replacement therapy increases your risk of uterine cancer. Depending on the dose and duration of estrogen use, your risk of getting this slow growing cancer may increase from five- to fourteenfold.[48] To ameliorate that problem, progestin is added, which may have the effect of countering the constant stimulation of the uterine lining for 7 to 10 days. This may resolve the problem of uterine cancer, but it complicates the cardiovascular outcome. So far it looks as though progestins counteract the beneficial estrogenic effect on lipid levels. Some progestin formulations reduce HDL levels (good cholesterol) by as much as 31 percent.[49] If what researchers like Dr. Bush say about the importance of HDLs is true, then clearly taking progestins isn't a good idea.

How to Lower Your Cholesterol and Decrease Your Cardiovascular Risk Without Medication

Where does this leave you? Not, hopefully, looking to drugs such as estrogen and progestin to keep your cholesterol levels down. There are other things that determine lipid levels in women, namely, your genetic makeup, dietary cholesterol, dietary fat, total calorie intake, alcohol consumption, cigarette smoking, and physical exercise.

Lifestyle practices matter and probably the older you get the more they matter. Once again, smoking leads the list in damage potential to your heart, blood vessels, and vascular system. If you eat a diet high in fat and cholesterol, if you smoke cigarettes, have several alcoholic drinks a day, and don't get exercise, your chances of having a heart attack increase. While most women know that good health habits include watching the "consumption" factors listed above, it may be that benefits of exercise in older women have been overlooked. In both men and women, exercise will increase HDL cholesterol levels.[50] The good news is that you don't have to exercise strenuously to accomplish positive changes in your cholesterol level.

In a study published in 1989 researchers found significant benefits when previously sedentary women started walking. "Our study helps to resolve the uncertainty over the amount and type of exercise needed to diminish the risk of coronary heart disease. In these sedentary women a considerable progressive increase in high density lipoprotein cholesterol concentration resulted from a programme of brisk walking for one year."[51]

At an FDA meeting in June 1990 Wyeth-Ayerst tried to convince the government to approve the use of their estrogen product, Premarin alone, to prevent heart disease, but only for those women who have had hysterectomies. The idea was that these women would at least not be at risk for one of the well-documented dangers of Premarin, cancer of the uterus and would therefore not have to use progestins to neutralize this risk.

Reminding those at the meeting of the significantly increased rate of deaths from heart disease in women when they grow older and enter menopause, a doctor from Wyeth-Ayerst pointed out that the extraordinary drop in deaths from heart disease in the United States in women over the last 35 years was "consistent" with the increased use of Premarin in this country during the same period of time.[52]

What the company's doctor neglected to mention was that during the same several decades, there has been a similarly large decrease in deaths from heart disease in American men, even though they never started taking estrogens. He also forgot to point out that in the majority of other industrialized countries, with the exception of Eastern Europe, there were also similarly sharp decreases in deaths from heart disease even though only the smallest proportion of women in most of these countries use menopausal estrogens.

So, there is virtually no evidence that the 30 to 40 percent decreases in heart disease in women (or men) over the last 35 years can possibly be attributed to the use of menopausal estrogens.

It was also pointed out at that same FDA meeting that if we applied what *is* known today about the prevention of heart disease in women—increases in exercise, weight loss, eating less cholesterol and harmful fats, stopping smoking, and treating high blood pressure—we could reduce heart disease in women by 90 percent.

In a recent editorial explaining why focusing on the use of estrogens to prevent heart disease is not a panacea, Harvard Professor of Medicine Dr. Alexander Leaf stated that "The isolated management of one risk factor is poor medicine . . . all the major risk factors need attention if coronary disease is to be markedly reduced."[53]

But automatically prescribing estrogens is not only poor medicine if you could accomplish 90 percent of your goal by taking care of the other risk factors and not using Premarin or other estrogens. It is dangerous medicine, because for an unproven benefit, thousands of cases of breast cancer would be needlessly caused by widespread use of estrogens such as Premarin.

1. Testimony of Dianne Kennedy before the Fertility and Maternal Drug Advisory Committee. FDA, February 1–2, 1990.

2. Brett AS. Treating hypercholesterolemia. New England Journal of Medicine 1989; 321:676–80.

3. Cancer Statistics Review 1973–1987, National Cancer Institute 1990; I:8–9.

4. Willis J. Progress against breast cancer. FDA Consumer, May 1986; Cancer Statistics, op. cit.

5. Hoover R, Gray LA, Cole P, MacMahon B. Menopausal estrogens and breast cancer. New England Journal of Medicine 1976; 295:401–5; Ross RK, Paganini-Hill A, Gerkins VR, Mack TM, Pfeffer R, Arthur M, Henderson BE. A case-control study of menopausal estrogen therapy and breast cancer. Journal of the American Medical Association 1980; 243:1635–9; Brinton LA, Hoover RN, Szklo M, Fraumeni JF. Menopausal estrogen use and risk of breast cancer. Cancer 1981; 47:2517–22; Hoover R, Glass A, Finkle WD, Azevedo D, Milne K. Conjugated estrogens and breast cancer risk in women. Journal of the National Cancer Institute 1981; 67:815–20.

6. Hoover, Menopausal estrogens and breast cancer, op. cit.

7. Ross, op. cit.

8. Brinton, op. cit.

9. Brinton LA, Hoover R, Fraumeni JF. Menopausal oestrogens and breast

cancer risk: an expanded case control study. British Journal of Cancer 1986; 54:825–32.

10. Kaufman DW, Miller DR, Rosenberg L, Helmrich SP, Schottenfeld D, Shapiro S. Noncontraceptive estrogen use and the risk of breast cancer. Journal of the American Medical Association 1984; 252:63–7; Wingo PA, Layde PM, Lee NC, Rubin G, Ory HW. The risk of breast cancer in postmenopausal women who have used estrogen replacement therapy. Journal of the American Medical Association 1987; 257:209–15.

11. Testimony of Janet Daling, FDA hearings, op. cit.

12. FDA hearings, op. cit.

13. Smith DC, Prentice R, Thompson DJ, Herrmann WL. Association of exogenous estrogen and endometrial carcinoma. New England Journal of Medicine 1975; 293:1164–7; Ziel HK, Finkle WD. Increased risk of endometrial carcinoma among users of conjugated estrogens. New England Journal of Medicine 1975; 293:1167–70; Mack, TM, Pike MC, Henderson BE, Pfeffer RI, Gerkins VR, Arthur M, Brown SE. Estrogens and endometrial cancer in a retirement community. New England Journal of Medicine 1976; 294:1262–7.

14. Bergkvist L, Adami HO, Persson I, Hoover R, Schairer C. The risk of breast cancer after estrogen and estrogen-progestin replacement. New England Journal of Medicine 1989; 321:293–7.

15. Hoover R. Interview with author, November 1989.

16. Wilson RA. Feminine Forever. New York: M. Evans & Company, 1966.

17. Wentz AC. Management of the menopause. In Novak's Textbook of Gynecology. Eleventh Edition. Baltimore: Williams & Wilkins, 1988, 402–3.

18. Ibid.

19. Riggs BL. Pathogenesis of osteoporosis. American Journal of Obstetrics and Gynecology 1987; 156:1342–6.

20. Christiansen C, Christensen MS, Transbøl I. Bone mass in postmenopausal women after withdrawal of oestrogen/gestagen replacement therapy. Lancet 1981; 1:459–61; Ettinger B, Genant HK, Cann CE. Long-term estrogen therapy prevents bone loss and fractures. Annals of Internal Medicine 1985; 102:319–24; Horsman A, Jones M, Francis R, Nordin C. The effect of estrogen dose on postmenopausal bone loss. New England Journal of Medicine 1983; 309:1404–7.

21. Hutchinson TA, Polansky SM, Feinstein AR. Postmenopausal oestrogens protect against fractures of hip and distal radius: a case-control study. Lancet 1979; 2:705–9; Kiel DP, Felson DT, Anderson JJ, Wilson PWF, Moskowitz MA. Hip fracture and the use of estrogens in postmenopausal women, New England Journal of Medicine 1987; 317:1169–74.

22. Research Advances in Osteoporosis, summary statement. National Osteoporosis Conference; Arlington, VA, February 1990.

23. Lindsay R, Hart DM, MacLean A, Clark AC, Kraszewski A, Garwood J. Bone response to termination of oestrogen treatment. Lancet 1978; 1:1325–7.

24. Ernster VL, Bush TL, Huggins GR, Hulka BS, Kelsey JL, Schottenfeld D. Clinical perspectives: benefits and risks of menopausal estrogen and/or progestin hormone use. Preventive Medicine 1988; 17:201–23.

25. Riggs, op. cit.

26. Research Advances in Osteoporosis, op. cit.

27. Marcus R. Interview with author, February 1990.

28. Bohr H, Schaadt O. Bone mineral content of femoral bone and the lumbar spine measured in women with fracture of the femoral neck by dual photon absorptiometry. Clinical Orthopaedics and Related Research 1983; 179:240–5; Krølner B, Nielsen SP. Bone mineral content of the lumbar spine in normal and osteoporotic women: cross-sectional and longitudinal studies. Clinical Science 1982; 62:329–36; Elsasser U, Hesp R, Klenerman L, Wootton R. Deficit of trabecular and cortical bone in elderly women with fracture of the femoral neck. Clinical Science 1980; 59:393–5.

29. Riggs BL, Wahner HW, Seeman E, Offord KP, Dunn WL, Mazess RB, Johnson KA, Melton LJ. Changes in bone mineral density of the proximal femur and spine with aging: differences between the postmenopausal and senile osteoporosis syndromes. Journal of Clinical Investigation 1982; 70:716–23.

30. Riggs BL, Melton LJ. Involutional osteoporosis. New England Journal of Medicine 1986; 314:1676–86.

31. Melton LJ, Riggs BL. Epidemiology of age-related fractures. In Avioli LV, ed. The Osteoporotic Syndrome. New York: Grune & Stratton, 1983:45–72.

32. Heaney RP. Nutritional factors in causation of osteoporosis. Annales Chirurgiae et Gynaecologiae 1988; 77:176–9.

33. Kelsey JL. Risk factors for osteoporosis and associated fractures. In press.

34. Smith EL, Reddan W, Smith PE. Physical activity and calcium modalities for bone mineral increase in aged women. Medicine and Science in Sports and Exercise 1981; 13:60–4.

35. Block JE, Smith R, Black D, Genant HK. Does exercise prevent osteoporosis? Journal of the American Medical Association 1987; 257:3115–7.

36. Riggs BL. A new option for treating osteoporosis. New England Journal of Medicine 1990; 323:124–5.

37. New treatments for osteoporosis. Lancet 1990; 335:1065–6.

38. Storm T, Thamsborg G, Steiniche T, Genant HK, Sørensen OH. Effect of intermittent cyclical etidronate therapy on bone mass and fracture rate in women with postmenopausal osteoporosis. New England Journal of Medicine 1990; 322:1265–71.

39. Marcus R. Estrogen replacement therapy. Western Journal of Medicine 1989; 151:295.

40. Thom TJ. Cardiovascular disease mortality among U.S. women. In Eaker E, Packard B, Wenger N, Clarkson T, Tyroler HA, eds. Coronary Heart Disease in Women. New York: Haymarket Doyma, 1987:33–41.

41. Krauss RM, Lindgren FT, Wingerd J, Bradley DD. Effects of estrogens and progestins on high density lipoproteins. Lipids 1979; 14:113–8; Bain C, Willett W, Hennekens CH, Rosner B, Belanger C, Speizer FE. Use of postmenopausal hormones and risk of myocardial infarction. Circulation 1981; 64: 42–6.

42. Lipid Research Clinics Program. The lipid research clinics coronary primary prevention trial results I. Reduction in incidence of coronary heart disease. Journal of the American Medical Association 1984; 251:351–64; Lipid Research Clinics Program. The lipid research clinics coronary primary prevention trial results II. The relationship of reduction in incidence of coronary heart disease to cholesterol lowering. Journal of the American Medical Association 1984; 251:365–74.

43. Kannel WB, Wolf PA, Garrison RJ. The Framingham Study, Some risk factors related to the annual incidence of cardiovascular disease and death using pooled repeated biennial measurements: Framingham Heart Study 30-Year Followup. National Institutes of Health, April 1987, 31.

44. Ibid.

45. Bush TL, Fried LP, Barrett-Connor E. Cholesterol, lipoproteins and coronary heart disease in women. Clinical Chemistry 1988; 34:B60–B70.

46. Stadel B. Interview with author, February 1990.

47. Coronary Drug Project Research Group. The coronary drug project: initial findings leading to modifications of its research protocol. Journal of the American Medical Association 1970; 214:1303–13; The Coronary Drug Project Research Group. The coronary drug project: findings leading to discontinuation of the 2.5 mg/day estrogen group. Journal of the American Medical Association 1973; 226:652–7.

48. Smith, op. cit.; Ziel, op. cit.; Mack, op. cit.

49. Bush TL, Miller VT. Effects of pharmacologic agents used during menopause: impact on lipids and lipoproteins. In Mishell DR, ed. Menopause: Physiology and Pharmacology. Chicago: Year Book Medical Publishers, 1987:187–208.

50. Wood PD, Haskell WL. The effect of exercise on plasma high density lipoproteins. Lipids 1979: 14:417–27; Haskell WL, Taylor HL, Wood PD, Schrott H, Heiss G. Strenuous physical actitivity, treadmill exercise test performance and plasma high density lipoprotein cholesterol. The Lipid Research Clinics Program Prevalence Study. Circulation 1980; 62(Suppl IV):IV53–61.

51. Hardman AE, Hudson A, Jones PRM, Norgan NG. Brisk walking and plasma high density lipoprotein cholesterol concentration in previously sedentary women. British Medical Journal 1989; 299:1204–5.

52. Meeting of the Fertility and Maternal Health Drugs Advisory Committee, Center for Drug Evaluation and Research, FDA, June 14, 1990.

53. Leaf A. Management of hypercholesterolemia. Are preventive interventions advisable? New England Journal of Medicine 1989; 321:680–3.

ACCUTANE

Acne Treatment of Last Resort

> Accutane is a very effective treatment of last resort for severe acne. It can also have catastrophic effects on developing fetuses. When this highly potent drug is given to pregnant women, 40 percent of early exposures miscarry,[1] and 25 percent of pregnancies that continue result in major birth defects.[2]
>
> Incredibly, despite well-known dangers of this drug, tens of thousands of fertile women are taking it, many for nonjustifiable reasons.

*C*YSTIC acne is a disfiguring condition that can be difficult to treat. In the United States there are currently about 400,000–500,000 cases, but only about 70,000 are women, most young.[3] About 5,000 a year may be appropriately treated with Accutane (see box on page 225), those being the fraction of acne sufferers whose condition is unresponsive to less dangerous acne therapy.

From the time Accutane was first approved in 1982 for use in treating these extreme cases it has been grossly overprescribed, especially to young women who have mild acne problems. According to Hoffmann-LaRoche, the drug's manufacturer, about 50,000 to 100,000 women have been treated with it each year since 1982.[4] This is 10 to 20 times the number who should actually be using it.

As of 1990 Accutane had already caused hundreds of serious birth defects, including an unknown number of spontaneous and induced abortions. In the United States, 84 serious birth defects were actually reported to the FDA but, due to serious underreporting of adverse drug effects, it is likely that at least three times as many more actually occurred (about 237 serious

US birth defects). This is a stark contrast to the four birth defects that have been reported in all of Europe as of 1990, where regulatory authorities have placed much more stringent restrictions on the distribution of the drug.[5]

Typically, the FDA would ban a drug which caused anywhere near the number of birth defects that have been caused by Accutane. But Accutane is clearly a valuable drug when appropriately used.

Labels have identified the catastrophic effects on developing fetuses. The problem is not physician awareness. The problem is that too many physicans are prescribing the drug to women who don't need it, and a significant number of these women are getting pregnant. The future will bring more birth deformities, more miscarriages, and more induced abortions by women whose fetuses are at risk after exposure to Accutane.

Once again, the issue of safety is in your hands here. If you plan to be treated for acne or if you are on Accutane, take extra precautions not to get pregnant. The drug is as easy to get as penicillin and more destructive to fetuses than thalidomide.

1. Rosa F, Baum C, Graham SJ. Maternal exposure to Accutane. Memo prepared by the Division of Epidemiology and Biostatistics, FDA., February 11, 1988.

2. Lammer EJ, Chen DT, Hoar RM, Agnish ND, Benke PJ, Braun JT, Curry CJ, Fernoff PM, Grix AW, Lott IT, Richard JM, Sun SC. Retinoic acid embryopathy. New England Journal of Medicine 1985; 313:837–41.

3. Maternal exposure to Accutane, op. cit. and update May 8, 1990.

4. Presentation by Hoffman-LaRoche to Joint Fertility and Maternal Health and Dermatologic Drug Advisory Committee, FDA, May 21, 1990.

5. Data obtained from the Food and Drug Administration, Center for Drugs.

Accutane must not be used by women who are pregnant or who may become pregnant while in treatment. There is an extremely high risk that you will give birth to a deformed infant if you get pregnant while taking Accutane in any amount, even for short periods. If you are a woman of childbearing potential, Accutane is not recommended unless you meet *all* of the following conditions:

- you have severe disfiguring cystic acne that is recalcitrant to standard therapies.
- you understand and carry out the instructions relevant to Accutane.
- you have received both oral and written warnings of the hazards of taking Accutane during pregnancy and the risk of possible contraception failure and have acknowledged your understanding of these warnings in writing.
- you have had a negative *serum* pregnancy test within two weeks prior to beginning therapy. (It is also recommended that pregnancy testing and contraception counseling be repeated on a monthly basis.)
- you begin therapy only on the second or third day of the next normal menstrual period.

Major human fetal abnormalities related to Accutane administration have been documented. There is also an increased risk of spontaneous abortion.

Effective contraception must be used for at least one month before beginning Accutane therapy, during therapy and for one month following discontinuation of therapy. It is recommended that two reliable forms of contraception be used unless abstinence is the chosen method.

If pregnancy does occur during treatment, you should discuss with your physician the desirability of continuing the pregnancy.

Accutane should be prescribed only by physicians who have special competence in the diagnosis and treatment of severe recalcitrant cystic acne and are experienced in the use of these kinds of drugs and are aware of their dangerous effect during pregnancy.

PART III

Products

Weight Loss Products, Tampons, Tobacco

WEIGHT LOSS PRODUCTS

The Truth Is Hard to Swallow

Half of all women in this country are currently on a diet.

Ever intensifying cultural pressures on women to be thin in order to be "attractive" continue to spawn an industry of weight loss products and programs, which cost women hundreds of millions of dollars each year but free them from very few pounds. Women who want to lose weight try an average of five weight loss regimens per year.

- Increasing scientific evidence points to the possibility that our bodies are programmed to maintain a certain weight, which makes staying slim extremely difficult for many women.

- All currently available weight control products for suppressing appetite, numbing taste buds, or making you feel artificially full are only effective for a short period of time at best. They play no role in long-term weight loss. In addition, most are dangerous.

- Despite evidence that these products don't sustain weight loss, 20 million people used diet aid products in 1989.

- Nonprescription diet aids consistently appear prominently in official statistics of drug abuse problems reported from hospital emergency rooms.

- The vast majority of people who lose weight on their diets regain it within three years. This failure is not just the fault of diets themselves, but perhaps more the result of ineffective strategies for keeping weight off.

Recommendations

Despite all the sensational claims to the contrary, nothing but relentless, lifelong diligence to watching what you eat and getting regular exercise holds any promise for keeping your weight down permanently.

- If you are more than 20 percent heavier than you should be (see chart, page 232) and have a family history of diabetes, heart disease, or high blood pressure, weight loss is important, but see a physician first.

- You don't have to use artificial food substitutes or fad diets. Learn to cut back on foods containing large quantities of fats, oils, and sugar.

- Pay attention to the things that intensify stress in your life and seek alternatives to responding by overeating.

*I*N our society, women learn as girls to equate body shape with personal worth. The pressure to be thin begins to affect their self-image even before girls are old enough to shop for themselves. As adults, millions of women have swallowed the pervasive cultural message that pounds are to be loathed and shed, or at the very least covered up. Many slightly overweight women, who make up the vast majority of dieters in this country, have succumbed to the notion that being even a little heavy means there is something wrong with you, something you should change.

For women who are minimally overweight, it may be more useful to improve self-esteem and reconsider these damning cultural messages than to spend a lifetime trying to lose a few unwanted pounds.

This, however, is not the main focus of our chapter. We will not delve at length into the serious dilemma women face in a society that scorns obesity. In this chapter we will primarily discuss medical issues involved in carrying excessive weight, not the full array of psychological issues that are arguably as important. We deal with significant obesity as a medical problem, not with the equally serious fact of it as a particularly cruel cultural problem for women. We acknowledge the two cannot easily be separated, and that clearly the pressure on women to be thin may not only instill deep self-loathing, but may also fuel serious eating disorders.

Real obesity does carry clear health risks. In this chapter we will review when it is important to lose weight and how to do it safely. Whether you need to lose weight for medical reasons or not, there are safe and effective ways to do it, but there are also unhealthy, even dangerous methods to avoid.

LOSING WEIGHT SAFELY AND EFFECTIVELY

True obesity is a serious health problem. The fear of it is a national obsession. Together, the real and imagined conditions associated with unwanted weight have spawned a vast industry of products, programs, and promises that have remarkable failure rates. An estimated 90 percent of all patients who lose more than 25 pounds in a diet program regain that weight within three years.[1] Despite all the sensational claims to the contrary, nothing but relentless, lifelong diligence to watching what you eat and getting regular exercise holds any promise for keeping your weight down permanently. The truth is hard to accept.

It is estimated that 45 percent of women in this country between ages 35–64 are overweight.[2] Basically, you are probably overweight if you are 20 percent above your so-called "ideal weight," unless the reason you are heavy is because you're very muscular and/or large boned. "Severe obesity" is used to describe people who are 40 percent above their ideal weight.[3]

Medically speaking, ideal weight is based on weight tables. For purposes of this discussion, ideal weight is defined as the midpoint of the range for medium-frame people as shown in the 1983 Metropolitan Height and Weight Table (below). Tables like these are designed to give the weights which over time have resulted in the lowest mortality rates.

One problem with these tables is that they are mostly based on statistics derived from a relatively young, affluent population. Another problem is that they fail to adjust for the amount of muscle in the body: a highly muscular, well trained athlete appears overweight in the table although he or she is not, and a middle-aged person in poor muscular condition appears at the correct weight in the table although he or she may be overweight.

Ideal Weight Table (lbs)

Height (ft, in)	MEN Average	Acceptable		WOMEN Average	Acceptable	
4 10				102	92	119
4 11				104	94	122
5 0				107	96	125
5 1				110	99	128
5 2	123	112	141	113	102	131
5 3	127	115	144	116	105	134
5 4	130	118	148	120	108	138
5 5	133	121	152	123	111	142
5 6	136	124	156	128	114	146
5 7	140	128	161	132	118	150
5 8	145	132	166	136	122	154
5 9	149	136	170	140	126	158
5 10	153	140	174	144	130	163
5 11	158	144	179	148	134	168
6 0	162	148	184	152	138	173
6 1	166	152	189			
6 2	171	156	194			
6 3	176	160	199			
6 4	181	164	204			

[This table is adapted from a conference on obesity at the Fogarty International Center of the National Institutes of Health, and based on figures of the Metropolitan Life Insurance Company. It defines height without shoes, and weight without clothes.]

In a strict sense, obesity is determined by how much of total body weight is fat. This can be measured in a variety of ways, but probably the most accurate is an ordinary scale and an honest judgment about muscularity and body build.

To figure out whether you are 20 percent overweight, look at the table and find your height. Look across to the "acceptable weight" range column. Calculate the midpoint between those two numbers and add 20 percent. If you weigh more than that figure, you may want to consider losing weight.

However, you should also consider the "acceptable normal" range to be very wide, as much as 30 percent in some cases. For example, someone who has a stable weight for many years at the low part of the range and then suddenly gains 20 percent of her weight (after a pregnancy, say) might be uncomfortable at that new weight but would still be in the "normal" range .

While there is no specific number of extra pounds that universally results in increased health risks, people who are 20 percent or more above their ideal weight are more likely to develop any of the following health problems: coronary artery disease (progressive hardening of the blood vessels that carry blood to the heart muscle); heart failure; high blood pressure; diabetes; cancer of the uterus, cervix, breast, ovaries, colon, and gallbladder; irregular or nonexistent menstrual periods; inflammation of the gallbladder; gallstones; and varicose veins.[4] Of course, there is no magic about the 20 percent over ideal weight cutoff point. Even if you are slightly below it you still may need to lose weight because of adverse health consequences.

Besides the medical consequences, many obese individuals suffer socially and emotionally in a society that views fat as unattractive. Obese people earn less on average than their leaner associates and they are discriminated against in hiring, job promotions, applications for college admissions, and housing.[5]

Needless to say, there are real and present dangers in being obese. But you do have options for losing weight safely. If you are "moderately obese" (20 to 30 pounds overweight) and you want to lose the pounds by yourself, there is plenty of evidence that with patience and a willingness to change your habits you can do it. If you are seriously obese (50 or more pounds over-weight), you should be supervised, especially if you try some type of short-term modified fast.

There are a variety of weight loss products that appeal not only to obese individuals, but to the millions of dieters in this country who are not particularly overweight. A decade ago these products included body wraps to "melt off fat," vibrating rollers to pummel the fatty deposits, and even "slender baths" from which, it was claimed, you would walk out 10 pounds thinner. There was "slimming tea," the "diet that allows you to eat normally while losing weight," and "amazing exercise machines that remove weight effortlessly." Maybe those sound prehistoric and laughable, but in fact the torrent of fraudulent claims has not let up much in recent years.

In 1988 dieters spent over $314 million on over-the-counter appetite suppressants such as Acutrim, Prolamine, Dex-a-diet and Dexatrim.[6] These products temporarily reduce appetite, but since hunger alone is seldom the reason people gain and retain weight, these remedies are basically useless. There are candies and gum that dull taste sensation, but numbed mouths seldom quell the temptation to overeat. And there are fiber concoctions which make the stomach feel full, but feeling full is also not an adequate deterrent for most overeaters.

Despite the monotony and unpalatability of diet powders, their popularity has continued over the years, and while the content of these reconstitutable mixtures has improved, there are real dangers in using them without supervision. As always, there is the dizzying variety of diet books at the bookstore. Some of these diets are sensible, some nutritionally inadequate, others silly, and many are dangerous.

If you are seriously obese and you have failed traditional diet attempts, extreme diet approaches may be warranted, provided you are under close medical supervision and given other kinds of support as your body changes. But no product, pill, or program is the ultimate answer for anyone, obese or not. This is especially true for women (and, distressingly, girls too) who relentlessly pursue the lean body image they have learned to value, but are not physiologically predisposed to owning. For these women commercial hoaxes may be particularly insidious, not only because of the health risks of unsupervised dieting among the nonobese, but because of the millions of dollars they waste on products that ultimately don't work. No one has ever come up with a replacement for permanently restricting what you eat and getting regular exercise. It's that simple.

WHAT IS WRONG WITH BEING OVERWEIGHT?

If you weigh significantly more than the "ideal weight" for your height and frame, you are at an increased risk of developing a number of diseases. There is no precise threshold for obesity. However, even a small degree of excess fat above 20 percent over ideal weight can leave you in some danger of developing the health problems listed below.

- High blood pressure (hypertension) is especially prevalent among people who develop obesity late in life and accumulate the weight in the upper half of the body. Blood pressure is the amount of force exerted by the blood on the artery walls as it is pumped from the heart and through the circulatory system. If blood pressure is too high over an extended period of time, the arteries will become damaged, leading to increased risk of heart attack and stroke.

- Diabetes (non-insulin dependent or "Type II") is a disease which in most cases develops later in life and 90 percent of the time happens in obese individuals. In many cases, a weight loss program (even before the pounds come off) can improve the diabetic's blood sugar levels. Diet is a better and safer approach than medication in most non-insulin dependent diabetics.

- Coronary artery disease is the progressive narrowing of the blood vessels that carry blood to the heart muscle. Over time, these blockages can cause heart attacks.

- Other kinds of heart disease can be specifically aggravated by extra weight. Recent research has shown that just being over-weight makes the heart work harder and leads to a thickening of the heart muscle, which can increase the risk of dangerous heart rhythms or sudden death. This change is separate from the heart effects of high blood pressure and coronary heart disease, and can sometimes be reversed by weight loss. To-gether, obesity, high blood pressure, and coronary artery dis-ease are a very hazardous combination.

- Hypercholesterolemia (high levels of cholesterol in the blood) and hyperlipidemia (high levels of fat in the blood).

- Stroke (the blockage or rupture of blood vessels that supply the brain).

- Osteoarthritis (the most common arthritis, considered "wear and tear" arthritis). Strain on joints bearing body weight, such as the hips and knees, causes and worsens this joint destruc-tion. Excessive body weight increases this strain.

- Pulmonary disease (breathing difficulties). Obesity is associated with various respiratory problems, including sleep apnea (pe-riods of no breathing while asleep).

- Cancer risks for obese women are higher for cancer of the gallbladder, biliary passages (ducts connected to the liver and gallbladder), breast, uterus, and ovaries.

- Other diseases, including hormone imbalances, gallbladder disease, and kidney disease. Obesity also causes increased risks to pregnant women and male and female surgical patients, since it results in a higher probability of medical complica-tions. In addition, physical examination of very obese patients by doctors can be very difficult, making detection of other diseases more difficult.

Some of the conditions mentioned above may result not just from obesity itself, but from the kind of diet or sedentary lifestyle that leads to obesity. A sensible diet and activity plan which will help you lose weight will also help you reduce factors which may lead to other diseases.

WHAT INFLUENCES BODY WEIGHT?

Several factors influence your weight:

■ Food Intake

The more you eat, the more "fuel" you have for your body. Extra fuel which is not used in daily activities is stored in the form of fat or adipose tissue. Fat cells have tremendous storage capacity; each cell can expand to 100 times its normal volume in order to store fat. When adults gain weight, they usually do so by increasing the size of their fat cells. While the initial fat cell number is probably genetically determined, new fat cells are formed when existing cells reach maximum volume.

Food's energy content is measured in units of heat called calories. It is commonly believed that 3,500 calories equals a pound of body weight—a person who eats 3,500 calories too much will gain one pound. That is almost but not exactly true. Everyone handles calories differently. The same number of calories has been shown to create a weight gain in some people but not in others. Furthermore, not all calories are alike. Calories taken from fat in food can be stored by the body with practically no extra effort. But if extra calories come in the form of carbohydrates or proteins, the body must convert those substances into fat in order to store them. Like all body functions, that conversion requires energy. In other words, the body uses calories to store calories, more for nonfat carbohydrates and protein than for fat.

■ Activity

The more active you are, the more fuel (calories) you burn. That fuel may consist of recently eaten food or previously stored fat. Actually, increasing exercise alone will decrease body weight without alterations in your diet, except in severely obese people. While exercise does burn calories, it uses discouragingly few compared with the number of calories that you could eat in a single meal. While you could easily consume 1,000 calories in one sitting, you would have to ride a bike for two hours to burn up that many calories. However, the importance of exercise is not strictly an issue of burning calories. Daily regular exercise improves the efficiency of your body in metabolizing calories. Thus, someone who is in good physicial condition uses calories more quickly than someone who isn't. Furthermore, if you are attempting to lose weight, increasing physical activity combined with a weight reduction diet can help maintain muscle tissue during weight loss. Regular exercise is one of the few factors shown to predict successful long-term maintenance of weight loss.

■ Size and Body Type

The bigger and heavier you are, the more food you need just to maintain your weight. In addition, more fuel is required to maintain muscle mass and bone than to maintain fatty tissue. As a result, large boned, muscular people need to eat more just to maintain their weight than do small boned plump people.

■ Metabolism

This is the process by which food and stored fat are converted into energy. People with higher metabolic rates burn food and fat at a higher rate than do those with low metabolic rates. A quicker metabolism should mean faster weight loss. However, dieters know that over an extended period of caloric reduction, their weight loss tapers off. This is because resting metabolism rate (RMR) decreases as body cell mass diminishes (as pounds drop off).[7] Studies have shown that by incorporating physical exercise into a diet program, this decrease in metabolism can be reduced or prevented.[8]

■ Genetics

Studies have shown that the tendency to become fat sometimes runs in families.[9] It used to be believed that obesity in families was entirely due to eating habits and general environmental factors. Now it is clear that children of obese parents are much more likely to become obese adults, especially if the child has two obese parents. Studies of adopted children found their body size resembled that of their biological parents and bore no relationship to their adoptive parents.[10]

But even if your parents are overweight, you should not be overly discouraged by this information. Prevention of obesity may lie in acknowledging your risk and manipulating diet and exercise to help avoid a lifelong weight problem. Efforts to achieve a sound weight control program, including lifestyle changes as discussed later, need to start early and will require more work in obesity prone individuals.

Set Point Theory

One theory of weight control that has become widely accepted is the belief that our bodies "defend" a biologically predetermined weight, or "set point," through complex metabolic regulation. This theory says, in effect, that obesity may not be the result of a body's failure to expend calories properly, or of abnormal food intake; rather, each person has a biologically determined point at which the body regulates weight, fat, lean body mass, and other related variables. Any alteration of weight to above or below this point will result in a tendency to return to the regulated weight.[11]

Dr. Arthur Frank, a Washington D.C. physician who has been treating obesity for 20 years, believes strongly that part of the struggle to lose weight is based on the fact that you are bucking nature's design for your body.

Your body does defend a weight and there is every reason to believe it does that with tenacity. Weight has a very strongly held set point. If you lose weight, and then resume business as usual, you will gain the weight back, no matter what the reason for the original weight gain, no matter how you lost it. You have to sustain some kind of change in the way you conduct your eating habits or you'll gain it back, absolutely.[12]

The set point theory may be useful in understanding why weight is so hard to lose and keep off. However, it may also be discouraging for people who will see their weight problem as solely the result of a high "set point." This is counterproductive for people who need to lose weight to maintain good health.

Obviously, of all the factors influencing weight listed above, food intake and physical activity are the two over which you have the most direct control. A sensible weight reduction program should therefore begin with these.

WHEN TO SEEK MEDICAL ADVICE ABOUT LOSING WEIGHT

There is no magic number of pounds which once gained make it necessary to seek medical attention for treatment of obesity. In general, if you are 20 percent overweight (see weight table, page 232), physician supervision may be indicated. But this depends on several factors such as your age, whether you have obesity-associated disease, whether you have failed previous attempts to lose weight, how recently you accumulated the weight, if you're a smoker, and whether or not you are pregnant.

If you are over 60 or have heart disease, high blood pressure, diabetes, kidney disease, or other chronic conditions under medical care, or if your parents or other immediate family members have had heart attacks or diabetes, you should consider a checkup by a physician before starting a weight control program. The heavier and older you are, and the more stress factors you have, the more likely you are to need medical supervision, especially if you are over 45 and have not had a medical exam in over two years.

TRY TRADITIONAL DIETING FIRST

Most people losing weight need to shed only 5 to 20 pounds. Despite the unhappiness and impatience you may feel with this extra weight, the best approach to losing it safely and permanently is to take it off slowly and with painstaking attention to traditional diet principles, namely: *If more calories are eaten than burned, weight is gained; if fewer calories are eaten than burned, weight is lost.*

Unfortunately, as most who have tried to diet can attest,

losing weight is no easy task. Dieting must be a long-term process, involving permanent changes in eating habits and physical activity. In fact, experts agree that the best short-term solutions to moderate weight loss, namely the 1200 calorie diets, are the hardest to maintain. Why? Possibly because it is more difficult to choose what to eat within calorie limits than to be told what to eat. However, the critical issue in any diet attempt is that while you reduce your calories, you also work on permanently changing your eating habits.

Even if you are 20 pounds or so overweight, you may not need to go on an extreme diet to lose weight. You might be more successful just by being careful than by participating in any kind of prescribed diet or system. But once again we're talking about habits and choices: cutting down on what you eat, eliminating dessert, eliminating junk, selecting carefully, preparing food conscientiously, and restricting what you buy. By making conscious interventions in your life, it's possible you will be very successful over the long run.

Clearly, for many moderately overweight people, slow reduction and heightened self-awareness don't feel rewarding enough: such an approach might not get you into size 10 clothes in two weeks. There is always the temptation to take short cuts and try quick weight reduction schemes. However, any program which results in or promises short-term weight loss without any dietary or lifestyle changes will typically fail after the quick success. In fact, most people using so-called low calorie diets (discussed on page 247) regain weight back almost as quickly as they lose it.[13]

A REASONABLE PLAN: HOW TO LOSE A POUND A WEEK SAFELY

It is a considerable challenge to set a calorie adjustment which will result in permanent weight loss and allow you to integrate these changes into your life. The goal is to develop new, healthier diet and exercise habits, not just to lose weight fast only to gain it back. Minor or gradual alterations in diet are a more realistic approach to long-term weight loss than switching to a radically different diet.

A reasonable yet fairly ambitious program is to make a calorie adjustment of 3500 calories per week. This program will average about one pound lost each week, assuming that your weight is now fairly constant given your current diet and activity.

In a long-term program like this one, weight loss may be more pronounced in the early weeks. Actually, this is true in any weight reduction program. During this initial period there is significant water loss as well as other body adjustments. After the initial drop, your weight may level off (sometimes for a few weeks) before dropping again. This pattern of plateaus followed by drops in weight continues throughout a weight loss program.

A caloric adjustment of 3500 calories per week requires a net change of 500 calories each day. We recommend that you accomplish 400 calories of this through a decrease in dietary intake and 100 calories in increased activity each day.

Diet: How To Eat 400 Fewer Calories Per Day

Any effective weight control program involves changes in diet. We suggest that you design a reduction in calories that you can live with for good, not just for the short term.

To reduce your daily diet by 400 calories, review the foods you eat to see what you can eliminate. You may find a "calorie counter" book helpful; they are inexpensive and available in many supermarkets and bookstores. A few suggestions which may help are:

- **Make some sensible substitutions, using more low calorie foods in your regular daily diet.** For example, if you eat a lot of meat, substitute chicken, fish, or seafood for beef, lamb, and pork. They have less fat and generally fewer calories. Eat more vegetables and less meat. Tofu (bean curd), one of a variety of vegetable protein sources that have become widely available, has even fewer calories than chicken or seafood and is a good source of protein. Other simple substitutions can include: low fat cottage cheese rather than other cheese; nonfat skim milk rather than whole milk; fresh vegetables rather than sweet, salty, or fried snacks; and fresh fruit rather than sweet desserts.

■ **Eliminate "invisible calories"** (calories which do not add to the taste, quality, or appearance of food) by trying new methods of food preparation. Several excellent cookbooks now on the market will help you prepare flavorful meals with far less fat and sugar. You can eliminate calories that you will scarcely miss by trimming visible fat from meat, removing skin (a major source of fat) from poultry prior to cooking (or eating), cooking food in bouillon or broth instead of butter or oil, and using lemon juice or bouillon instead of butter or oil for basting or seasoning fish and vegetables.

■ **Learn to be calorie wise when dining out.** Ask the waiter or waitress to remove the tray of rolls or bread from the table, and, if possible, to bring some fresh celery or carrots. Enjoy a glass of club soda with a wedge of lime instead of a drink before dinner; alcohol is a major source of nonnutritional calories. Substitute a squeeze of lemon wedge for that heavy salad dressing, and avoid fried foods.

■ **Arrange for low calorie meals.** If your meals are prepared in a school dormitory, company cafeteria, or similar kind of institutional setting where you are not in control of food preparation, consult with the director of food services. Sometimes it is possible to work out a low calorie meal plan using the available food, or the school dietician can help you to obtain specially prepared meals, depending on the size and resources of the kitchen or food source. Most major airlines will serve low calorie meals if you request them a day before your trip.

■ **Keep a record of what you eat and when you eat—even checking out portion sizes with a small scale.** This will help you to learn what you should avoid in order to acquire and maintain your desirable weight. If you tend to be a fast eater, a constant snacker or someone who pays no attention to what you consume, a big part of your weight reduction program could be managed right here, through making yourself aware of all the little extras that add up in a day.

- **Learn to recognize and handle stress without responding by overeating.** Frequently people with weight problems use food as a way of coping with stress. Anxiety, anger, sadness, and even boredom are feelings that at times can be attributed to stressful situations. People sometimes handle these uncomfortable emotions by seeking comfort in food and consequently overeating. Then, after eating too much food, or the wrong kind of food, people frequently feel guilty or disappointed with themselves, which results in still more stress.

- **Seek help from others.** Losing weight can be a long and frustrating process. Find people in your life who can support your effort. Sometimes talking with a family member, friend, clergy, counselor, or psychotherapist will help. Choose people who understand the importance of what you are doing.

Proper Nutrition and Dieting

During a weight control program it is especially important to provide the body with proper nutrition. A program which involves only a slight change from past habits, as described in this chapter, should not result in nutritional deficiencies, as long as those past habits were nutritionally adequate.

The average American diet provides about 50 percent of its caloric intake from fats, 30 percent from carbohydrates and 20 percent from proteins—not an ideal mix.[14] We should, instead, obtain at least 50 percent of our calories from carbohydrates, 15 to 20 percent from proteins, and 20 to 30 percent from fats, preferably not animal fats like those in butter, cheese, and ice cream. Women require an average daily protein intake of 44 grams, which is roughly the equivalent of one serving of low fat yogurt, plus a half cup of cottage cheese, a piece of chicken (with skin removed) and two glasses of low fat milk. The nutritional goal of a well balanced diet is to increase the calories obtained from complex carbohydrates and decrease that amount of fat, sugar, cholesterol and salt. Many high fiber foods, whole grains, vegetables, and beans are also higher in complex carbohydrates, a better source of energy than simple sugars (such as cane sugar, honey, or molasses).

If you plan to lose weight on less than 1200 to 1500 calories a day, it is a good idea to take a multivitamin/mineral capsule daily.

There are a number of books of varying quality published on nutrition. *Jane Brody's Nutrition Book* is an up-to-date, sensible guide that we recommend as a source for further information.

Exercise: 100 Calories More Per Day

As anyone who has tried it knows, losing weight and keeping it off by dieting alone is very difficult.

As an example, a woman of 120 pounds in a sedentary job (burning about 1800 calories per day) would have to cut caloric intake by 28 percent to lose one pound per week through dieting alone. She would have to cut her meals back to spartan portions (which maintained minimally adequate nutrition), with little or no leeway for fattening "treats." If, however, she walked at a brisk pace for 20 minutes (such as to and from her job) each morning and evening, she would only have to cut back calories by 17 percent to lose the same amount.

Starting a serious exercise program after years of relative inactivity can be a strain on your body, especially your heart. If vigorous exercise has not been a part of your regular activities for some time, we recommend that you start slowly with walking rather than another more strenuous form of exercise.

You should seek medical advice before starting an exercise program if any of the following are true:

1. You are over 45 and have not had a checkup by a physician in the last two years, especially if you have been fairly inactive.

2. You have heart disease, high blood pressure, diabetes, or kidney disease, or are under the care of a physician for any other chronic disease.

3. You have a family history of heart attacks.

4. You experience any chest pain, dizziness, or shortness of breath with or without physical exertion.

We recommend that you use or burn at least an additional 100 calories every day. 100 calories is roughly equivalent to one of the following: 20 minutes of brisk walking (about 1 mile); 12 minutes of bicycle riding; 9 minutes of swimming; or 5 minutes of fast running. You should exercise hard enough to make yourself breathe faster. Any kind of new exercise should be preceded and followed by several minutes of stretching exercises, especially at the ankles and hips.

Depending on your physical condition, you may find that you are able to increase the amount of exercise, and hence improve upon your weight control program. Keep in mind that this increased activity should become a permanent daily activity.

Keep a log of your exercise. This can serve not only to keep you faithful to your new program, but also to encourage progress. With exercise, many people feel an increased sense of energy and a decreased desire for food.

BEYOND TRADITIONAL DIETS

For the Truly Obese, Outside Assistance May Be Necessary

Obesity experts have repeatedly acknowledged that permanent weight loss remains a dilemma for most really obese people (30 percent or more over your ideal weight). The best plan is not any one diet, traditional or fad, but a much more involved and comprehensive approach to the problem. In the last decade, researchers have modified and improved so-called behavior therapy techniques, with some promising results. They now advocate therapy that addresses not only eating behavior, but attitudes, social relationships, nutrition, exercise, and other factors. As one study reported: "Although obesity is classified most accurately as a chronic rather than an acute problem, most of our interventions have been oriented toward treating it in an acute manner."[15] The best approaches are programs that:

- combine dieting with behavior therapy (discussed below)
- provide regular medical supervision
- emphasize significant initial weight loss
- incorporate a structured exercise program
- provide instruction in relapse prevention
- exploit social networks for outside support
- offer continued support after weight loss is achieved
- include financial incentives[16]

The best programs require patience, commitment, and hard work. Not everyone is ready to get involved in counseling, but the benefits of it are directly related to how ready you are. One reason *not* to get involved in such an intensive weight loss program is that someone else is pressuring you to do it. The motivation has to come from you. Furthermore, if any of your family members are going to sabotage your hard work in any way, that problem should be dealt with first. The gains you make in therapy will be hard to sustain if someone at home is fighting your desire to lose weight.

Very Low Calorie Diets: Recommended Only for Truly Obese People

Evidence in recent years suggests increased success in long-term weight loss for obese people when the therapy begins with immediate, significant weight loss.[17] Experiencing initial dramatic physical changes can instill continued motivation, say researchers. To that end, the carefully supervised use of very low calorie diets has proven somewhat successful. These are only recommended for people who need to lose a minimum of 30 percent of their body weight and who are under the medical supervision of a physician who has had substantial extra training in nutrition and low calorie physiology. People on these plans should also be given psychological and nutritional counseling to improve their chances of keeping the lost weight off. Patients also need to be tested for heart problems, liver function abnormalities, cancer, diabetes, and significant psychiatric disorders.[18]

Currently the most popular low calorie diets are marketed through physicians and come in powdered form containing protein from egg or milk based sources. Others require that protein be obtained from lean meat, fish, or poultry. These diets are mixed with water and consumed three to five times a day and must be supplemented with vitamins and minerals.

Very low calorie diets have made a comeback in the American diet scene. Today they have a better reputation than they did in the 1970s and 1980s when liquid protein diets, inadequately supervised, caused an estimated 35 deaths.[19] The newer liquid diets usually provide 300 to 800 calories a day and are available through physicians or hospitals as part of packaged weight reduction programs. Weight losses of 2 to 5 pounds a week are common, as are losses of 40 to 60 pounds over a six month period.[20] Dieters typically stay on the plan for 12 to 16 weeks followed by a period of 3 to 6 weeks of "refeeding."

Scientists now claim these diets have improved for two reasons; they provide higher quality proteins and more essential nutrients, and their use is being supervised better by health professionals.[21]

Most studies on the safety of very low calorie diets have looked at their effects only on the severely obese, not people with milder weight problems. For these people, using very low calorie diets could mean the loss of lean body mass.[22] Large losses of this sort can have disastrous consequences, including damage to the heart and other organs. There is some evidence that very low calorie diets can be safe when used by people who have smaller amounts of weight to lose but this remains controversial. In general, these diets are more unpleasant than is necessary for people who only need to lose moderate amounts of weight.

Even as very low calorie diets offer dramatic and aggressive options for otherwise healthy but obese people, researchers warn they can be dangerous.

The recent and zealous marketing of various formula products to physicians, as well as the public's appetite for such diets, could lead to yet another round of complications and fatalities. We are particularly alarmed by the possible consumption of very-low-calorie diets by persons who are not severely overweight or who do not receive appropriate medical supervision. Moreover, the prescription of these diets by physicians untrained in their use is cause for anxiety.[23]

Extraordinary financial incentives abound for physicians to prescribe commercial very-low-calorie diets. In 1989, for example, a group called the Nutrition Institute of Maryland offered physicians quite a deal. If they enrolled 15 new patients on the Institute's MEDIFAST® diet plan, selling the diet powders at nearly twice what the doctor paid, and then followed the patients for an average of 3.8 months, the profits from these 15 patients alone could be $62,000 a year. In addition, the profits from the extra lab tests needed to assure that patients' health is maintained during this low calorie diet could add another $6,000 or more, for a total profit of more than $68,000 a year. This should illustrate the fact that the "business" of weight loss is not entirely driven by health considerations.

BEHAVIOR CHANGE: STILL THE ROOT OF SUCCESS

Psychologists and obesity experts criticize proponents of commercial weight loss products because seldom is the difficulty of using such products emphasized. Losing weight is hard, often depressing work. For years so-called behavioral programs have concentrated on day-to-day techniques to change eating habits. "Stimulus control," "self monitoring," and "reinforcement techniques" are the foundations of any behavior modification program. The stimulus control teaches people to reduce their exposure to food. The self monitoring promotes awareness of personal eating habits by requiring people to keep track of what they consume. And reinforcement techniques offer rewards (not food) along the way as goals are achieved.

While "managing behavior" is widely practiced and considered the basis of any good weight loss program, it requires a virtual obsession with eating and food, which many people eventually find impossible to sustain. One common response is to resort to commercial programs that take all choice away.

Furthermore, behavior training can fall short in other ways. Nutritional counseling can be limited to keeping a daily log of calories without including an awareness of sodium and fat, for example. Lowering salt and cholesterol not only helps weight loss but reduces the risks of some of the diseases associated with obesity. Also, while behavioral approaches emphasize energy intake (calories), they don't pay enough attention to energy output. Improving physical activity is too often glossed over in these programs. Daily exercise has both psychological and physical benefits.

The more sophisticated behavior modification programs screen participants carefully. Failing any program can leave the patient worse off than when she entered. Possible negative results of program failure include the following:[24]

- Losing and regaining weight can foster feelings of inadequacy.
- Initial weight loss followed by regain may lead to undesirable metabolic alterations.
- Failure may convince a patient that the problem is intractable, discouraging her from entering another program later.
- "Negative contagion" can occur in treatment groups, where a person who is not doing well can discourage others who are.

IS THE COMBINATION OF AGGRESSIVE DIETING AND BEHAVIORAL PROGRAMS THE ANSWER?

Here again, there's no panacea for long-term weight loss. One extensive study in 1986 separated 59 people who averaged 89 percent overweight into three groups: those receiving either a very low calorie diet alone, behavior modification therapy alone, or both. At the end of treatment, the first two groups on average lost around 31 pounds, and the people who had received combined therapy lost on average 42 pounds apiece. After one year the average losses were 10 pounds for diet alone, 21 pounds for behavior modification alone, and 28 pounds for the combination.[25]

After three years the participants were checked again. "At the 3-year follow-up, subjects in all three conditions had regained between 74 and 85 percent of their end-of-treatment weight loss."[26] One of the problems researchers cited was that participants waited too long to seek additional therapy when it became clear that they were regaining their weight.

It's important to note here that the quality of any behavior modification program is based largely on the quality of the therapist. Some are more skilled, compassionate, understanding, and sympathetic than others. The content of any behavior modification program can be standardized, but each therapist brings unique qualities and qualifications.

THE ROLE OF COUNSELING

Women who need to keep off 20 to 30 pounds probably need more support than is involved in learning tricks for eating more slowly or keeping records. Attitudes and beliefs about yourself have to be changed too. So-called cognitive methods of counseling attempt to replace irrational and destructive self concepts with more positive and reassuring ones.

> A person who sees herself as a "disgusting slob who fails at everything" when she looks in a mirror or overeats at a meal is less likely to continue her efforts than someone who can recognize that success or failure at weight control is only one aspect of her life and that failure at any one point does not make future failure inevitable.[27]

Dr. Ann Kearney-Cooke, a psychologist who specializes in body image problems, says women who want to overcome weight problems can learn how to respond to the prejudices that surround them. Through role playing, she helps patients learn how to react to bosses, boyfriends, family members, and coworkers who can inadvertantly reinforce low self-esteem with destructive comments like, "You're so pretty, you'd be so successful if you lost 30 pounds."[28]

Most weight specialists agree that counseling is critical and should continue in some form long after the weight loss has been achieved. "The work begins with the weight loss and then affects every other part of your life," says Washington D.C. physician and weight loss expert Dr. Arthur Frank. "People who lose a lot of weight have to deal with tremendous changes in their lives. Not only are their eating patterns different, their social patterns change, their career ambitions might change, their sexual patterns change. Support must be ongoing."[29]

Eating Disorders:
═══════ Anorexia Nervosa and Bulimia ═══════

Researchers predict that as thinness becomes more, not less desirable, the problem of eating disorders will worsen. The pressure on women to be slim, to be the model wife, mother, and working professional combine to make women especially vulnerable to irrational and sustained dieting. Over time, the rigidity of strict and often biologically unattainable weight standards creates a psychological and physical climate in which binge eating is a natural outcome.[30]

Bulimia

This may in part explain the high prevalence among young women of an eating disorder called bulimia. Bulimic behavior involves eating to excess followed by self-induced vomiting or use of laxatives to prevent weight gain. Bulimia can also be associated with another predominately female eating disorder, anorexia nervosa, characterized by a morbid fear of fat and the infliction of self starvation.

Anorexia Nervosa

Current medical literature describes anorexia nervosa this way:

- Self-inflicted weight loss accompanied thereafter by a sustained avoidance of mature body shape, which cannot be directly ascribed to other identifiable psychiatric causes, weight loss-inducing diseases, or externally imposed demands for reduced food intake
- A morbid and persistent dread of fat
- The manipulation of body weight through dietary restraint, self-induced vomiting, abuse of purgatives, or excessive exercise
- Disturbances in body image, manifest in the misrepresentations of actual body dimensions or extreme loathing of bodily functions
- Amenorrhea (cessation of menstruation) and the development of other behavioral-physiological consequences of starvation.[31]

Women who suffer from anorexia nervosa put themselves in a constant state of semistarvation and as a result are subject to a variety of dangerous physical and psychological complications. These include serious heart irregularities, liver failure, intestinal impairment, dental problems, anemia, dehydration, weakness, and hypothermia. Many women have died from extended periods of starving themselves. Anorexics commonly experience severe depression, low self-esteem, hopelessness, suicidal thoughts, insomnia, and reduced sex drive.

Both anorexia nervosa and bulimia are rare in men, but do occur. Bulimics are typically women in their 20s from upper socioeconomic groups. About 25 percent are married.[32]

Whereas women who are anorexic are typically extremely thin, many bulimic women maintain a weight within the normal range despite regular eating binges during which 5,000 to 10,000 calories may be consumed. Many bulimics practice self-induced vomiting immediately afterward to minimize the absorption of food. Laxatives, purgatives, and excessive exercise are also used by bulimics to counter the effects of binge eating. Bulimics complain they have lost control over their eating, and binging episodes usually follow periods of dieting. The episodes invariably occur in secret. This, along with the normal appearance of bulimics, makes the disorder hard to detect.

Both anorexia nervosa and bulimia result from a combination of psychological, physical, and environmental (family and social) disturbances. The common factor they share is usually an obsession with body shape and weight. No one explanation or treatment can be applied to these women, but one researcher expressed a view that seems appropriate for the young women today grappling with these problems:

> Today's young women are not the first generation to be exposed to this bias [preference for lean body type], but they are the first to be exposed to it in childhood and to be raised by mothers rejecting of their own bodies and concerned about the size of their daughter's body from the moment of birth. This is a heritage of anxiety and self-loathing.[33]

OVER-THE-COUNTER WEIGHT-LOSS DRUGS

American drug manufacturers have been quick to capitalize on and promote the public preoccupation with weight loss by filling neighborhood drugstores with prominent displays of diet aids of every description. Consumers, mostly women, have literally eaten it up, to the tune of $314 million in 1988.[34]

Over the past few decades, a parade of diet products has been placed on the market and disappeared unnoticed, while others have risen to take their place. For years a variety of capsules, tablets, powders, liquids, gums, candies, and canned low-cal meals, often with fantastic claims and prices, have been available for American consumers.

In 1982, a Food and Drug Administration advisory panel proposed rules for the marketing of over-the-counter weight control drug products. The only two ingredients approved for use in weight control were phenylpropanolamine hydrochloride (PPA) and benzocaine. All other drug products touted in any way for weight control lack evidence of safety, effectiveness, or both. Not until 8 years after this report, did the agency take further action in regulating this widely abused class of drugs.

Products Containing Phenylpropanolamine

Today, the most tempting items are those flat little boxes that dangle enticingly from drug store and supermarket shelves and promise "fast weight loss." These are the current stars of the profitable diet world, the products containing the drug phenyl-propanolamine hydrochloride, or PPA. This chemical is very similar to amphetamines, "speed," or "uppers." Originally marketed as a nasal decongestant, PPA is now the leading over-the-counter diet aid, accounting for most of the OTC diet pill sales. Products such as Control, Dexatrim (the sales leader), Dietac, Acutrim, Permathene, Prolamine, and Thinz-span contain PPA.

PPA was rated safe and effective by the FDA advisory panel for use as an anorectic (appetite suppressant) in weight control. Despite the panel's decision, it is our opinion that PPA poses a substantial hazard for its users, and has not succeeded in proving its long-term effectiveness. For this reason, WE RECOMMEND STRONGLY AGAINST THE USE OF ALL PRODUCTS CONTAINING PHENYLPROPANOLAMINE FOR USE IN WEIGHT LOSS.

No well controlled study has shown that PPA is effective as an aid in long-term weight control. It may help you lose weight for a few days, but you gain the pounds back when you stop taking it, and it won't help you make the changes in diet and exercise patterns which are needed to keep weight off.

Not only are there significant questions about PPA's effectiveness, but also serious doubts about its safety. PPA can cause hypertension (high blood pressure), even in young, healthy adults given amounts within the recommended dosage.[35]

The FDA acknowledges that PPA can be hazardous to a significant portion of the population (at least 20 percent).[36] You must avoid PPA if you have hypertension, heart disease, diabetes, or thyroid disease. This is serious because overweight individuals (the people who use PPA as an anorectic) are more likely to suffer from all these disorders, as discussed earlier. Additionally, it is estimated that 40 percent of all diabetics[37] and 30 percent of all hypertensives[38] are not aware of their disorders; for them products containing PPA pose an unknown and significant risk. There have been cases of potentially fatal heart problems,[39] kidney disease, and muscle damage[40] associated with the use of products containing phenylpropanolamine, although these effects have yet to be clearly shown in healthy subjects taking the recommended doses.

There have also been reports of amphetamine-like adverse reactions to products containing PPA. These include accelerated pulse rate, tremor, restlessness, agitation, anxiety, dizziness, and hallucinations.[41] These reactions may be aggravated by the presence of caffeine in many of these products.

As mentioned earlier, adverse reactions can occur with the use of PPA products in "recommended" doses. Reactions are often more severe or even life-threatening when these products are abused and overused. OTC diet aids consistently appear prominently in official statistics of drug abuse problems reported from hospital emergency rooms.[42] This fact, along with the hazards and ineffectiveness of PPA products in weight control, raises serious questions about the wisdom of making these products available at all.

In addition, phenylpropanolamine is a common ingredient in illicit amphetamine "look-alike" drugs.

Benzocaine And Other Weight Loss Drugs to Avoid

Benzocaine is an anesthetic like the novocaine you get at the dentist. Contained in lozenges, chewing gum, or candy (Ayds and Slim-line are examples), it is sold to be used immediately prior to a meal so as to reduce sensation in the taste buds and thus lessen the desire for food.

While benzocaine indeed produces a numbing of the tongue, there is little indication that this suppresses the appetite or promotes long-term weight loss in any other manner. There is also some question about the safety of the drug: it can sensitize some users, making them allergic to it and to other "caine" local anesthetics, such as novocaine and lidocaine.[43] This could pose problems in the event of future dental work or minor surgical procedures when these drugs are needed.

A number of other ingredients were evaluated by the FDA advisory panel and all others were found to lack evidence of safety, effectiveness, or both when used for weight control. Products containing the following ingredients should not be used as diet aids: alginic acid, carrageenan, carboxymethylcellulose sodium, chondrus, guar gum, karaya gum, methylcellulose, psyllium, sea kelp, sodium bicarbonate, and xanthan gum.

DOCTORS, WEIGHT CONTROL AND PRESCRIPTION DIET PILLS

As outlined above, certain people should consult a physician before beginning a weight control program. In all probability your doctor will approve of your decision to lose weight. The doctor may also have specific suggestions regarding your diet, and the type and amount of daily exercise you can safely handle.

In a few cases, you may still encounter a physician who prescribes "diet pills" to overweight patients although the number of prescriptions filled for antiobesity drugs has fallen precipitously in the last two decades. The decreased use of these prescription appetite suppressants represents a growing awareness on the part of doctors and patients of the capacity for addiction and abuse of these preparations, and their limitations as successful weight control agents. Unfortunately, the decrease in prescription diet pills has been more than compensated for by an increase in over-the-counter diet pills. All of these drugs can help in short-term weight loss. Any weight that is lost is regained quickly when the drug is stopped or tolerance is reached. In addition, these drugs can have serious side effects on the nervous system.

An ideal weight control drug would reduce the urge to overeat or alter the body's metabolism to allow weight loss, would maintain its effectiveness for the long-term, and would have few or no side effects. No such drug exists. All currently available weight control pills are appetite suppressants which are only effective for a short period of time and have many significant problems.

The only way to lose weight is for your body to use more calories than you consume. This involves either a reduction in calories consumed, an increase in energy expended, or—more likely to work—a combination of the two.

1. Friedman RB. Helping the patient fight fat. Postgraduate Medicine 1988; 83:106–11.

2. Manson JE, Colditz GA, Stampfer MJ, Willett WC, Rosner B, Monson RR, Speizer FE, Hennekens CH. A prospective study of obesity and risk of coronary heart disease in women. New England Journal of Medicine 1990; 322:882–9.

3. Van Itallie TB. Health implications of overweight and obesity in the United States. Annals of Internal Medicine 1985; 103(6 pt 2):983–8.

4. Garfinkel L. Overweight and cancer. Annals of Internal Medicine 1985; 103(6 pt 2):1034–6; Van Itallie TB. Obesity: adverse effects on health and longevity. American Journal of Clinical Nutrition 1979; 32(12 suppl):2723–33.

5. Brownell KD. Weight control and your health. World Book Encyclopedia 1989; 368–84.

6. What's ahead? The weight loss market. Obesity and Health 1989; 3: 51–4.

7. Donahoe CP, Lin DH, Kirschenbaum DS, Keesey RE. Metabolic consequences of dieting and exercise in the treatment of obesity. Journal of Consulting and Clinical Psychology 1984; 52:827–36.

8. Council on Scientific Affairs. Treatment of obesity in adults. Journal of the American Medical Association 1988; 260:2547–51.

9. Stunkard AJ, Sørensen TI, Hanis C, Teasdale TW, Chakraborty R, Schull WJ, Schulsinger F. An adoption study of human obesity. New England Journal of Medicine 1986; 314:193–8; Price RA. Genetics of human obesity. Annals of Behavioral Medicine 1987; 9:9–14.

10. Stunkard, op. cit.

11. Keesey RE. The body-weight set point. Postgraduate Medicine 1988; 83:114–23.

12. Frank A. Interview with author, March 1990.

13. Formula diets for obesity. The Medical Letter on Drugs and Therapeutics. New York: The Medical Letter Inc., 1989; 22–3.

14. Friedman RB. Fad diets; evaluation of five common types. Postgraduate Medicine 1986; 78:249–58.

15. Brownell KD, Kramer FM. Behavioral management of obesity. Medical Clinics of North America 1989; 73:185–201.

16. Brownell KD, Jeffery RW. Improving long-term weight loss: pushing the limits of treatment. Behavioral Therapy 1987; 18:353–74, as referenced in Brownell, op. cit.

17. Brownell, Behavioral management of obesity, op. cit.

18. Wadden TA, Stunkard AJ, Brownell KD. Very-low calorie diets: their efficacy, safety and future. Annals of Internal Medicine 1983; 99:675–84.

19. Sours HE, Frattali VP, Brand CD, Feldman RA, Forbes AL, Swanson RC, Paris AL. Sudden death associated with very low calorie weight reduction regimens. American Journal of Clinical Nutrition 1981; 34:453–61.

20. Friedman RB. Very low-calorie diets: how successful? Postgraduate Medicine 1988; 83:153–61.

21. Wadden TA, Van Itallie TB, Blackburn GL. Responsible and irresponsible use of very-low-calorie diets in the treatment of obesity. Journal of the American Medical Association 1990; 263:83–5.

22. Forbes GB. Lean body mass-body fat interrelationships in humans. Nutrition Reviews 1987; 45:225–31; Forbes GB, Drenick EJ. Loss of body nitrogen on fasting. American Journal of Clinical Nutrition 1979; 32:1570–74; Van Itallie TB, Yang M-U. Current concepts in nutrition: diet and weight loss. New England Journal of Medicine 1977; 297:1158–61.

23. Wadden, op. cit.

24. Brownell KD, Marlatt GA, Lichtenstein E, Wilson GT. Understanding and preventing relapse. American Psychologist 1986; 41:765–82.

25. Wadden TA, Stunkard AJ. Controlled trial of very low calorie diet,

behavior therapy and their combination in the treatment of obesity. Journal of Consulting and Clinical Psychology 1986; 54:482–8.

26. Wadden TA, Stunkard AJ, Liebschutz J. Three-year follow-up of the treatment of obesity by very low calorie diet, behavior therapy and their combination. Journal of Consulting and Clinical Psychology 1988; 56:925–8.

27. Brownell, Behavioral management of obesity, op. cit.

28. Kearney-Cooke A. Interview with author, March 1990.

29. Frank, op. cit.

30. Brownell KD, Foreyt JP. The eating disorders: Summary and Integration. In Brownell KD, Wadden TA, eds. Epilogue; Handbook of Eating Disorders: Physiology, Psychology and Treatment of Obesity, Anorexia and Bulimia. New York: Basic Books, 1986, 508.

31. Strober M. Anorexia Nervosa: History and psychological concepts. In Handbook op. cit., 237.

32. Fairburn CG, Cooper Z, Cooper PJ. The clinical features and maintenance of bulimia nervosa. In Handbook, op. cit., 390.

33. Wooley SC, Kearney-Cooke A. Intensive Treatment of Bulimia and Body-Image Disturbance. In Handbook, op. cit., 478.

34. What's ahead? op. cit.

35. Horowitz JD, Lang WJ, Howes LG, Fennessy MR, Christophidis N, Rand MJ. Hypertensive responses induced by phenylpropanolamine in anorectic and decongestant preparations. Lancet 1980; 1:60–1.

36. 47 Federal Register 8475; February 26, 1982.

37. Personal communication with author. Diabetes Clearinghouse, Department of Health and Human Services, September 14, 1982.

38. Hypertension in Adults, 25–74 years of age, USA, 1971–1975. DHHS, PHS, #81–1671, April 1982.

39. Pentel PR, Mikell FL, Zavoral JH. Myocardial injury after phenylpropanolamine ingestion. British Heart Journal 1982; 47:51–4.

40. Swenson RD, Golper TA, Bennett WM. Acute renal failure and rhabdomyolysis after ingestion of phenylpropanolamine-containing diet pills. Journal of the American Medical Association 1982; 248:1216

41. Dietz AJ. Amphetamine-like reactions to phenylpropanolamine. Journal of the American Medical Association 1981; 245:601–2.

42. Data from the Drug Abuse Warning Network, Annual Data 1988. U.S. National Institute on Drug Abuse, Series 1, Number 8, 1989.

43. Fisher A. Contact Dermatitis. 3rd edition. Philadelphia: Lea and Febiger, 1986; 42; North American Contact Dermatitis Group. Epidemiology of contact dermatitis in North America: 1972. Archives of Dermatology 1973; 108:537–40.

TAMPONS

High Absorbency Still
Means Needless Risk of
Toxic Shock Syndrome

Hundreds of people a year, mostly women, still get toxic shock syndrome (TSS), and some of them will die. About three-fourths are menstruating women, many of whom are using tampons which are needlessly dangerous.[1]

- TSS is a serious illness that can cause a sudden high fever, vomiting, diarrhea, a rash, a drop in blood pressure, and sometimes death.
- TSS most frequently afflicts women under age 30 who use tampons, particularly young women between ages 15 to 19.

Recommendations

If you choose to wear tampons:

- use the lowest absorbency product that works for you.
- during your period, alternate tampons with sanitary napkins.
- store tampons in a clean, dry place.
- wash hands with soap and water before and after inserting or removing a tampon.
- try a less absorbent variety if a tampon is irritating or difficult to remove.

WHEN was the last time you forgot to change your tampon and left it in all day? Luckily, you said to yourself, it

What You Can Do
═══════ To Prevent Toxic Shock Syndrome ═══════

1. Use the lowest absorbency tampon effective for you. It is safer to use a less absorbent style of tampon and change tampons frequently than to use highly absorbent types.
2. Alternate use of tampons with sanitary pads.
3. Wash hands with soap and water before and after inserting or removing a tampon.
4. If symptoms of TSS appear, remove your tampon if you are using one and seek medical attention promptly. Tell your doctor what your symptoms are, when your period began, what absorbency of tampon you use, and whether you have ever had TSS.
5. People who have had TSS in the past are at higher risk of TSS and should consult their physician before using tampons.

was a "super plus" tampon, so you got away with it. After seven hours it was still absorbing.

The benefit of high absorbency tampons is something any woman who uses them appreciates from time to time, but it is a benefit that comes with risks. The longer a tampon lasts, the greater your chances of developing TSS. The flu-like condition was first identified over 10 years ago as possibly being caused by a toxin-producing strain of bacteria.

The exact link between TSS and tampon use is not completely known. It is believed that the illness requires the presence of a bacterium that is commonly found on the body in such areas as the nose, skin, or vagina. The bacterium usually causes no problem, but in rare instances it can lead to serious infection after tampon use, a deep wound, or surgery. Up to 25 percent of TSS cases occur in men, or in women who are not menstruating.[2]

TOXIC SHOCK AND THE TAMPON CONNECTION

TSS first gained widespread attention in 1980 when Procter & Gamble's super absorbent Rely brand tampons were linked to TSS and removed from the market after two studies found that Rely increased the risk of TSS.[3] Since a link with other brands was not detected, it led some to conclude that the danger was in the composition of Rely and not its high absorbency.

However, hopes of this easy solution were dashed when the subsequent removal of Rely tampons from the market did not eliminate the occurrence of TSS. Further definitive scientific studies revealed that Rely was not the only culprit and that any high absorbency tampon increased a woman's risk of getting TSS.[4]

In 1982 the Food and Drug Administration (FDA) required tampon manufacturers to place a warning on tampon labeling about the threat of TSS and advise women to use the minimum absorbency necessary to control their menstrual flow. However, the regulations issued in 1982[5] were largely useless because the tampon packages did not give women enough information to heed this advice.

While labels read "regular" or "super," the terms did not have uniform meanings: one brand of "regular" may have been more absorbent than another brand's "super." In fact, at one time o.b. Regular tampons were more absorbent than Tampax Super.

The FDA admitted that the labels were grossly inadequate and in 1989 (under a court order from a lawsuit brought by Public Citizen Health Research Group)[6] issued the new regulations to help standardize the absorbency of tampon products.[7] Unfortunately, while it was a step in the right direction, it did not go far enough.

THE NEW LABELS

The government has finally required tampon manufacturers to add absorbency information and arrive at some consistency among their products. Tampon labels today tell you several things. The outer package must display one of the following terms representing the corresponding absorbency range:

Absorbency Range (grams)	Corresponding Term
6 and under	Junior absorbency
6 to 9	Regular absorbency
9 to 12	Super absorbency
12 to 15	Super plus absorbency

The word *absorbency* was added to alert consumers of the changes.

The 1989 regulation lists two other absorbency ranges, "15 to 18" and "above 18," but doesn't designate absorbency terms for these ranges.[8] There are no currently existing products for these ranges. Unfortunately, allowing for ultrahigh absorbency in the regulation may well encourage manufacturers to once again market tampons that are known to carry a significant risk of TSS.

The improvement in the labels is that now *all* brands that say "junior absorbency" mean the same thing. They conform to specific ranges of absorbencies that are uniform from brand to brand. So if you switch brands, say from one super to another, the range now remains consistent.

Unfortunately, the ranges and the nomenclature still do not tell you exactly what you need to know, namely, the specific absorbency of each tampon product. For example, you know that a sunscreen with a 15 rating will protect you. Would you feel as sure about one labeled "10 to 15"? Single numbers let a woman know exactly what she is buying, because she can select tampons with a particular, known absorbency. If you consider your risk of getting toxic shock syndrome when you buy tampons, it would be better if this critical safety information were available in a more precise form.

Right now tampon products are tested for absorbency using a "syngyna test," which simulates normal conditions of tampon use. In this test, every gram of fluid that is absorbed is measured. This is a very important test because studies have shown that for every gram of absorbency, the risk of TSS goes up 37 percent.[9]

Unfortunately, instead of offering this very useful single digit information, the labels describe ranges and there is a significant difference in absorbencies among products within the same range. With present labeling, women do not know if they are purchasing products at the low or high end of a given range. Thus, women could unwittingly use tampons with higher absorbencies than they care to expose themselves to, and increase their risk for illness.

WHERE DOES THIS LEAVE YOU?

First, remember that what is now labeled "regular absorbency" is not necessarily the same as your old "regular." Under the new labeling system, these terms have changed. While "regular absorbency" products are now comparable in terms of their absorbency ranges, remember that these are ranges, and tampons can still vary as much as three grams in their absorbency values. In other words, you could buy a "regular absorbency" at the low end and a "super absorbency" at the high end, and while they may sound like they are fairly similar, they may be very different products differing by as much as six grams (one having *twice* the risk of TSS as the other). For this reason, it is as important as ever to use the lowest range possible and change your tampon frequently.

1. Reduced incidence of menstrual toxic shock syndrome—United States 1980–1990. Morbidity and Mortality Weekly Report 1990; 39:421–3.

2. Ibid.

3. Kehrberg MW, Latham RH, Haslam BT, Hightower A, Tanner M, Jacobson JA, Barbour AG, Noble V, Smith CB. Risk factors for staphylococcal toxic-shock syndrome. American Journal of Epidemiology 1981; 114:873–9; Centers for Disease Control. Follow-up on toxic shock syndrome. Morbidity and Mortality Weekly Report 1980; 29:441–5.

4. Petitti DB, Reingold A, Chin J. The incidence of toxic shock syndrome in Northern California 1972 through 1983. Journal of the American Medical Association 1986; 255:368–72. Institute of Medicine; Toxic Shock Syndrome: Assessment of current information and future research needs. Washington, DC: National Academy Press, 1982.

5. 47 Federal Register 26982-90, June 22, 1982.

6. Public Citizen Health Research Group et al. v. Commissioner, Food and Drug Administration et al., U.S. District Court for the District of Columbia, C.A. # 88-1492, August 28, 1989.

7. 54 Federal Register 43766–72, October 26, 1989.

8. Ibid.

9. Berkley SF, Hightower AW, Broome CV, Reingold AL. The relationship of tampon characteristics to menstrual toxic shock syndrome. Journal of the American Medical Association 1987; 258:917–20.

TOBACCO

A Women's Issue

Tobacco-related diseases kill an estimated 125,000 women a year.

- In one generation, there has been a fivefold jump in the rate of lung cancer in women.

- If you smoke as few as one to four cigarettes a day, you've doubled your risk of heart attack. If you also take birth control pills, your risk of having a heart attack is ten times that of women who don't smoke.

- If you're pregnant and smoke, you increase your risk of delivering a low birthweight infant by 54 to 130 percent. In fact, smoking now surpasses poor nutrition as the primary cause for underweight newborns in industrialized nations. Low birthweight dramatically increases health risks to newborns.

- Smoking also increases your risk of premature delivery, spontaneous abortion, and stillbirth. About 4,000 infants die each year from problems caused by their mothers' smoking.

- Smoking doubles your risk of cervical cancer.

- Nicotine is passed through breast milk as long as five hours after the last puff.

- Far from insuring attractiveness and sophistication, cigarettes cause bad breath, gum disease, dental problems, hoarse voice, cough, decreased senses of smell and taste, stained teeth and hands, yellow fingernails, stale smelling clothing, and wrinkled skin.

Recommendations

- If you smoke, stop.

- If you've tried before and relapsed, try again until you succeed.

- If you're pregnant, don't smoke and don't let others smoke around you. If you have children, don't let anyone smoke around them.

- There are many ways to stop smoking. Use the method that makes the most sense for you. Many people stop smoking without any formal help. Others use stop-smoking clinics or classes. The nonprofit clinics such as the American Lung Association, American Cancer Society, American Heart Association or the Seventh Day Adventist Five Day Plan are effective and less expensive than for-profit clinics.

- If you are a parent, be aware that new generations of youngsters are now the targets of tobacco advertisers. Remember that 60 percent of smokers start before they turn 15. Advertisements appeal to youthful impression-ability. Talk with your children about the dangers of smoking to counteract the impact of these messages. Without your intervention, these ads and peer pressure may silently ensnare your child in a lifelong addiction.

- Nicotine is an addictive chemical compound. You may need help getting over your tobacco addiction, just as you would need treatment for any other addiction. Some people benefit from the use of nicotine gum which is available by prescription only. Education, counseling, physician's assistance, and nicotine gum may be the most successful combination for treating your nicotine addiction. The pros and cons of each of these methods are discussed below.

NICOTINE is a dangerous, addictive, incredibly fast acting chemical compound, only 1 of 4,000 contained in the smoke of burning tobacco.[1]

Every year, new evidence demonstrates still more dangers of inhaling many of these substances. For women the health consequences are greater than for men. Women suffer the same tobacco-related diseases as men: cancer, heart disease, chronic obstructive lung disease, and stroke. But women also suffer from a variety of other smoking-induced problems which are uniquely female: increased risk of osteoporosis, fertility problems, cervical cancer, and early onset of menopause.

Furthermore, smoking while pregnant has unfortunate consequences for future generations as well. It dramatically increases a woman's chances of having:

- placental abnormalities
- stillbirth
- premature delivery
- a low birthweight infant
- a baby with congenital malformations[2]

If you are a smoking mother, your infant is certainly not out of the woods after birth. Your baby runs a higher risk of sudden infant death syndrome (SIDS), respiratory infections, and conditions resulting from retarded prenatal growth. Sadly, if you keep smoking your child eventually will be more likely to pick up your habit, risking other smoking-related health problems later in life.

For these reasons, smoking has been aptly labeled "a women's issue." It is also a women's issue because the tobacco industry is playing a sophisticated and sinister game with young girls through cigarette advertising. The industry is managing to induce thousands of girls each year to start smoking.

The latest data from the U.S. Office of Smoking and Health show that 26.8 percent of all women over 20 smoke, 30 percent of whom are between 25 and 34 years old, the prime childbearing years. As the tobacco marketers well know, 90 percent of smokers start before their 20th birthday. Today, more of those smokers are female than male. For example, among high school seniors, female smoking rates exceed males' by two to six percent since 1977. In 1985, 26 percent of college women and 19 percent of college men reported having smoked during the past 30 days. Women under age 23 represent the fastest growing segment of new smokers.[3]

Images of slimness, glamour, fitness, and strong-minded independence portrayed in most cigarette advertising aimed at women are tailor-made to appeal to the insecurities of teenage girls. Says researcher Ellen Gritz:

> Young adolescent females have been characterized by cognitive and emotional immaturity, hypersensitivity to peer rejection, vulnerability to impulsive behavior, and difficulty in acquiring a positive body image. It is along these very few dimensions that the teenage female is exquisitely vulnerable to the seductive allure of taking up smoking.[4]

Everything, of course, is ludicrous about the glamorous message women receive. Far from insuring attractiveness and sophistication, cigarettes cause bad breath, gum disease, dental problems, hoarse voice, cough, decreased sense of smell and taste, stained teeth and hands, yellow fingernails, stale smelling clothing, and even wrinkled skin.[5]

WOMEN WHO SMOKE LIKE MEN, DIE LIKE MEN[6]

In other words, a large number of tobacco-related diseases don't discriminate between the sexes. Men and women smokers alike increase their risk of:

- heart attacks
- cancer of the oral cavity, larynx, and esophagus
- lung cancer
- bronchitis and emphysema
- peptic ulcers
- bladder, kidney, and pancreatic cancer

LUNG CANCER IN WOMEN

Lung cancer is the most preventable cancer killer of women. By the mid-1980s, 30 years after an explosion in the number of women smokers in this country, lung cancer was killing more American women than breast cancer. In 1987 the disease killed 44,000 American women.[7] Almost two-thirds of all female lung cancer deaths occur among women who currently smoke one pack or more daily, or who have quit within the last five years. Nine out of 10 lung cancer deaths occur in women with some history of regular cigarette use.[8]

CERVICAL CANCER

It has been clear for some time that women who smoke are at greater risk for cervical cancer. The most widely assumed cause of cervical cancer is that it comes from an infectious agent that is transmitted sexually. Therefore, women who have many sexual partners are likely to run a higher risk of getting cervical cancer.

However, tobacco smoke itself is known to contain mutagens and carcinogens (cancer-causing agents) that may either cause or promote the growth of already existing cancer of the cervix. Relatively high levels of nicotine have been found in the cervical mucus of smokers. Research suggests that carcinogenic factors in cigarette smoke might concentrate in the cervix and play a direct role in the development of cervical cancer.[9] This possibility means that a dangerous reproductive cancer must be added to the list of tobacco-related diseases.

HEART DISEASE

Tobacco kills more women through heart disease than through all the cigarette-related cancers combined. While this has been known to be true for men, recent studies have confirmed the tragedy in women. A study published in 1987, which had followed 119,404 nurses (ages 30 to 55 at the beginning of the study) for several years, found that smoking even a few cigarettes a day significantly increased women's risk of heart attack or other serious heart disease. Specifically, smokers of 25 or more cigarettes a day were more than 5 times as likely to have heart disease as nonsmokers. Even women who only smoked between one and four cigarettes a day doubled their risk of heart disease. The evidence was much worse for women who smoked heavily (more than 45 cigarettes a day). Cigarette smoking accounted for 91 percent of the heart attacks in this group of nurses.[10]

The lethal effect of cigarette smoke multiplies for women who also take oral contraceptives. If you smoke more than 15 cigarettes a day and you currently take the pill, you may be 21 times more likely to have a heart attack than a nonsmoker.[11]

One group of researchers describes the overall risk of heart attack among smokers using oral contraceptives this way: "Overall, smoking was the most important independent risk factor and had a strong influence on risks associated with other factors."[12]

The good news in these statistics is that if you stop smoking, you will reduce your risk of heart attack. In a report published in 1990, it was found that although ex-smokers still had an elevated risk of heart attack two years after they quit, the risk of a first heart attack is largely dissipated after two or three years.[13]

PREGNANCY

There is good reason to believe that tobacco use affects every aspect of fertility: it's harder to get pregnant, and it threatens the success of a pregnancy and the health of the baby once born. At the other end of fertility, it causes premature menopause.

To get pregnant in the first place, all hormones have to be present at the right time and in the proper amounts to trigger the release of an egg with normal chromosomes. Studies have shown that nicotine disrupts the fine tuning of hormones designed to maximize the chances for successful ovulation and implantation. This may explain why smokers are 3.4 times more likely than nonsmokers to take more than one year to conceive.[14]

One of the ways this may occur is that with nicotine present, the egg itself may have a tougher time making the critical journey through the fallopian tube. The trip is a complicated one, but normally the egg is assisted by wavelike motions from the tube which push it along to its destination, a receptive uterus. Cigarette smoking can alter tubal motility by increasing the resting period between wavelike contractions within the fallopian tube. It may be this abnormal contractability of the tubes which accounts for a greater than twofold increase in ectopic pregnancy (pregnancy located outside the normal body of the uterus) among women who have smoked during pregnancy compared to women who have never smoked.[15]

Conception is also threatened if your partner smokes, because nicotine also affects the quality of sperm. Studies have shown that male smokers have fewer sperm, and that the sperm they have are more likely to be abnormally shaped and slower moving than those of nonsmokers.[16] Since miscarriage is often nature's way of eliminating genetically aberrant embryos, perhaps this is one explanation for the higher incidence of spontaneous abortion among smokers. One study showed the odds of miscarriage increased by 46 percent for the first 10 cigarettes smoked per day and by 61 percent for the first 20 cigarettes smoked.[17]

ENDANGERED BABIES

Between 20 and 40 percent of United States women are smokers at the time they become pregnant. About 35 percent quit while they are pregnant, but most resume after the birth of their baby.[18]

It is estimated that if all pregnant women stopped smoking, the number of fetal and infant deaths in this country would drop by about 10 percent. In the United States, this would result in about 4,000 fewer infant deaths each year.[19]

What kills the babies of smoking moms? Undoubtedly it's the impact of toxic ingredients in smoke that pass through the mother's bloodstream, altering the heart rate, blood pressure, oxygen supply, and acid balance of the developing fetus.

A pregnant woman who smokes two packs a day cuts out the equivalent of 25 percent of the fetal oxygen supply. Oxygen deprivation and increased levels of carbon monoxide from smoking are blamed for another factor that endangers the health of newborn infants, namely their size. On average, a smoker's baby is shorter and weighs less than babies of nonsmoking moms (smokers' babies average 1/2 inch shorter). Low birth-weight raises the baby's chances of developing future health problems.[20]

SMOKING AND THIN BONES

Osteoporosis (bone thinning, discussed on pages 193–222) leading to fractures, especially of the hip, wrist, and spine, can cause disability and death, predominantly among older postmenopausal women. Several studies have shown that female smokers seem to lose bone faster than nonsmokers.[21] In the past few years there has been considerable debate about the connection between bone loss and smoking.

Some researchers argue that the problem begins in adolescence, when most of a woman's bone density is established. It is thought that young smokers may consume less calcium during adolescence and young adult life, possibly because cigarettes replace good nutrition during this period when maximum bone mineral mass is reached.[22]

A further finding is that women who smoke tend to have an earlier menopause than nonsmokers.[23] Early menopause means a premature drop in estrogen levels. Estrogen plays an important role in the metabolism of calcium and thus in maintaining strong bones. During and after menopause, estrogen production slows down naturally over a period of years, causing a bone loss in postmenopausal women. It's possible that a premature and accelerated menopause is a major cause of the higher incidence of abnormal bone loss, or osteoporosis, among women who smoke.

WHY WOMEN DON'T QUIT

Most women who smoke want to give it up.[24] Many women are quitting, but not nearly as quickly as men; there was a 19 percent drop in the rate of male smokers in this country between 1965 and 1987, but for women, the drop was only five percent.[25] Why are women slow to quit?

There is the pain of withdrawal, for one thing. The intensity of nicotine's addictive nature results in withdrawal problems that make many attempts to quit short-lived.[26] However, researchers who have studied this found that the symptoms of withdrawal are no worse for women than they are for men.[27]

Women may have additional problems in quitting due to social and behavioral factors associated with smoking. The fear of gaining weight is one of the often quoted reasons women give for not wanting to stop smoking, and is frequently an obstacle to permanent success.[28]

Unfortunately, for decades tobacco advertisers have nurtured these fears, beginning with the Lucky Strike ads of the 1930s that advised women to "reach for a Lucky instead of a sweet."[29] While it's true that some women will gain weight when they stop smoking, most often it is a smaller amount than feared and can be controlled by increasing the amount of exercise in your life as you cut out the cigarettes. Even a little weight gain is insufficient to counteract the enormous health benefits of quitting smoking.[30]

For many women, smoking offers a way to relax, concentrate, or handle stress. Studies have shown that people who smoke to handle stress have a more difficult time quitting than smokers who light up, say, to look glamorous or sophisticated.[31]

Researchers have observed that women smoke to suppress anger more than men.[32] Since it has always been less acceptable for women to express anger in our society, this outlet for dealing with stress may be particularly hard for women to learn to live without.

RANKING CESSATION PROGRAMS

Stopping smoking is hard work. However, you need not do it alone. There are a variety of options, programs which offer support and information. Shop around and see which one might suit your needs. Remember, if you've relapsed after trying a program or after trying all by yourself, that doesn't mean you'll never stop smoking.

Below are brief descriptions of the types of programs available, together with general information about how successful they are.

Self-help Programs: 16 to 20 Percent Success Rate after One Year[33]

These programs provide educational materials without personal counseling. Many nonprofit organizations often provide self-help booklets with information on the dangers of smoking, tips for setting a quit date, changing behavior, and providing encouragement. Examples include the American Lung Association's *Freedom From Smoking* brochure, the American Cancer Society's *FreshStart* pamphlet, and the National Cancer Institute's *Cleaning the Air* book. These are available for a nominal fee from local chapters of these organizations. Addresses and phone numbers are readily available in local phone books. The National Cancer Institute has a toll free number (1-800-4-CANCER) to get more information. Materials can be ordered without charge by writing the Office of Cancer Communications Bldg. 31, Room 10A18, Bethesda, MD, 20892.

If motivated smokers follow the programs outlined in the booklets, 16 to 20 percent can expect to be "smoke free" after one year. These programs are especially helpful for smokers who want to quit on their own but do not feel comfortable attending group sessions or "quit clinics".

Interventional Programs: Average 27 Percent Success Rate in One Year.[34]

Nonprofit service organizations such as the American Cancer Society, the American Lung Association, and the Seventh Day Adventists sponsor group quitting clinics for smokers who need extra support. Led by a trained facilitator, usually a former smoker, the groups meet on variable schedules and cost between $25 and $75. The basic therapy involves a review of the reasons for quitting smoking, setting a quit date, positive reinforcement, and skills training. Smokers learn to recognize situations which lead to smoking. Sometimes a "buddy system" is established to offer support against relapse.

For-profit Cessation Clinics: Claims of High Success Rates Are Unsubstantiated

Many for-profit smoking cessation companies claim incredibly high "quit" rates, but their claims are rarely substantiated by objective outside evaluators. The programs themselves keep records, but quit rates are generally confined to graduates. Obviously, proprietary programs have a strong incentive to claim high success rates. Unfortunately, objective assessments are not done very often and the public cannot accurately know how successful they really are.[35]

It is generally believed by smoking cessation experts that these for-profit interventional clinics have about the same success rate as nonprofit ones. The only real difference is the cost.

ONE OPTION FOR BREAKING THE ADDICTION

Some smokers suffer withdrawal from nicotine addiction, which significantly hampers their attempts to stop permanently. For these smokers it makes sense to deal with the physical and psychological aspects of addiction simultaneously. To that end, nicotine gum can help.

In the early 1980s, reports of nicotine polacrilex gum (Nicorette) as an aid to smoking cessation were published in Britain.

In 1984 the prescription gum was approved for sale in the United States. Now it looks as though nicotine gum used in conjunction with some form of supportive therapy may be a very successful cessation program. This approach appears to treat both the physical addiction to nicotine and the behavioral attachment to cigarettes. However, using gum alone doesn't seem to be any more successful than self-help programs.

Nicotine gum works best in heavy smokers who are more dependent on nicotine.[36] These people smoke more cigarettes, smoke early in the day, cannot go long periods without smoking, and suffer noticeable withdrawal symptoms when forced to forgo cigarettes.

Nicotine gum has problems, however. Many doctors hand out the gum with little or no instruction or follow-up counseling. In some cases, patients expect a miracle cure for their smoking and are gravely disappointed when they find out more effort on their part is needed. The gum is also expensive: it can cost more than $500 for a three month supply.

The gum has adverse effects as well. In large doses, palpitations, dizziness, mouth sores, and ulcers can occur. Another serious possible outcome is that some people who use it can't stop taking the gum.

Still, the combination of proper use of the gum and effective, caring counseling may be the most promising development in smoking cessation to date for those people who are highly addicted.

TIPS FOR HELPING YOURSELF QUIT

Studies have shown that 90 percent of people who successfully quit smoking do it on their own.

The following advice is provided by the National Cancer Institute in Washington D.C. as part of a manual for helping physicians help their patients to quit.[37] The book is called *How To Help Your Patients Stop Smoking*. More information on quitting is available by calling the Cancer Information Service at 1-800-4-CANCER.

Tips for Preparing to Stop

- Decide positively that you want to stop. Try to avoid negative thoughts about how difficult it might be.
- Develop strong personal reasons in addition to your health and obligations to others. For example, think of all the time you waste taking cigarette breaks, rushing out to buy a pack, hunting for a light, etc.
- Begin to condition yourself physically: start a modest exercise program; drink more fluids; get plenty of rest; and avoid fatigue.

Know what to expect:

- Have realistic expectations—stopping isn't easy, but it's not impossible either. More than 3 million Americans stop smoking every year.
- Understand that withdrawal symptoms are temporary and are healthy signs that the body is repairing itself from its long exposure to nicotine. Withdrawal symptoms may appear within 24 hours of abrupt smoking cessation, as the body begins its healing process.
- Know that most relapses occur in the first week or two after stopping, when withdrawal symptoms are strongest and your body is still dependent on nicotine. Be aware that this will be your hardest time, and use all your personal resources—willpower, family, friends, and any tips that work for you—to get you through this critical period successfully.

Involve someone else:

- Bet a friend you can stop on your target date. Put your cigarette money aside every day, and forfeit it if you smoke. (But if you do, don't give up; simply strengthen your resolve and try again.)
- Ask your spouse or a friend to stop with you.
- Tell your family and friends that you're stopping and when.

They can be an important source of support both before and after you stop.

Tips for Just Before Stopping

- Practice going without cigarettes.
- Don't think of never smoking again. Think of stopping in terms of one day at a time.
- Stop carrying cigarettes with you at home and at work. Make them difficult to get to.
- Don't empty your ashtrays. This will remind you of how many cigarettes you've smoked each day and the sight and smell of stale butts will be very unpleasant.
- Collect all your cigarette butts in one large glass container as a visual reminder of the mess smoking represents.

Tips for the Day You Stop

- Throw away your cigarettes and matches. Hide your lighters and ashtrays.
- Clean your clothes to rid them of the cigarette smell, which can linger a long time.
- Develop a clean, fresh, nonsmoking environment around your-self—at work and at home. Buy yourself flowers—you may be surprised how much you can enjoy their scent now.
- Visit the dentist and have your teeth cleaned to get rid of tobacco stains. Notice how nice they look and resolve to keep them that way.
- Make a list of things you'd like to buy for yourself or someone else. Estimate the cost in terms of packs of cigarettes and put the money aside to buy these presents.
- Keep very busy on the big day. Go to the movies, exercise, take long walks, or go bike riding.
- Buy yourself a treat or do something special to celebrate.
- Stay away from other smokers if they could weaken your resolve (this need only be a temporary measure).
- Remember that one cigarette could ruin a successful attempt.

- Remember that alcohol will weaken willpower.
- Refuse to allow anything to change your mind.

Tips to Help You Cope with the Urge to Smoke

- First, remind yourself that you've stopped and you're a non-smoker. Then, look closely at your urge to smoke and ask yourself:
  - Where was I when I got that urge?
  - What was I doing at the time?
  - Who was I with?
  - What was I thinking?
- Think about why you've stopped:
  Repeat to yourself (aloud if you are alone) your three reasons for stopping. Write down your three main reasons for stopping, then three reasons for smoking.
- Anticipate triggers and prepare to avoid them:
  Keep your hands busy—doodle, knit, type a letter; avoid people who smoke; spend more time with nonsmoking friends; find activities that make smoking difficult (gardening, exercise, washing the car, taking a shower).

  Put something other than a cigarette in your mouth. Keep oral substitutes handy—try carrots, sunflower seeds, apples, celery, or raisins instead of a cigarette. Cut a drinking straw into cigarette-sized pieces and inhale air. Use a mouthwash.

  Change your surroundings when an urge hits; get up and move about, or do something else.

  Avoid places where smoking is permitted. Sit in the nonsmoking section of restaurants, trains, and planes.

  Look at your watch whenever the urge to smoke hits you. You'll find the urge will only last a few minutes.

  Wear a rubber band around your wrist. When you really feel like you want a cigarette, snap the rubber band a few times and in your mind say STOP. While you do this, picture in your mind a red stop sign. You might try this at home aloud a few times and then do it silently when in public.

Be prepared for "first times" as a nonsmoker: your first vacation, first time home alone, first long car ride, first period of boredom. If you know you will be in a high risk situation, plan how you will get through it without smoking.

- Change your daily routine in order to break your habits and patterns:

After meals, get up from the table, brush your teeth or take a walk.

Change the order in which you do things, particularly your morning routine.

Don't sit in your favorite chair.

Eat your lunch in a different location.

- Use positive thoughts:

If self-defeating thoughts start to creep in, remind yourself again that you're a nonsmoker, that you don't want to smoke and that you have good reasons to stop.

Keep a daydream ready to go. For example, start planning a perfect vacation; work on that plan when thoughts about cigarettes start to give you trouble.

Look around at all the people who don't smoke, including children. Remind yourself that they feel normal and healthy without cigarettes.

- Use relaxation techniques:

Breathe in deeply and slowly, while you count to five; breathe out slowly, counting to five again.

Take 10 deep breaths and hold the last one while lighting a match. Exhale slowly and blow out the match. Pretend it's a cigarette and crush it out in an ashtray.

If you can't concentrate, don't worry. You'll be able to when you need to, when the adrenalin flows.

Tips for Coping with Relapse

- Stop smoking immediately.
- Get rid of any cigarettes you may have.
- Write down three reasons why you ought not become a regular smoker again.
- Recognize that you've had a slip. A slip means you've had a

small setback and smoked a cigarette or two. But your first cigarette or two didn't make you a smoker to start with and a small setback doesn't make you a smoker again.

- Don't be too hard on yourself. One slip doesn't mean you're a failure or that you can't be a nonsmoker, but it's important to get yourself back on the nonsmoking track immediately.
- Realize that most successful former smokers stop for good only after more than one attempt.
- Identify the trigger. Exactly what was it that prompted you to smoke? Be aware of the trigger and decide now how you cope with it when it comes up again.
- Sign a contract with yourself to remain a nonsmoker.

1. Silva OC. Metabolic effects of tobacco and cannabis. In Principles and Practices of Endocrinology and Metabolism. Philadelphia: JB Lippincott Co, 1990.

2. The health consequences of smoking for women, a report of the Surgeon General. Washington DC: U.S. Department of Health and Human Services, 1980.

3. Reducing the health consequences of smoking, a report of the Surgeon General 1989. Washington DC: Department of Health and Human Services Publication # CDC 89–8411; 1989, 269. Also testimony at Hearings of Senate Labor and Resources Committee on the Tobacco Education and Control Act of 1990, February 20, 1990.

4. Not Far Enough Network: Women vs. Smoking. Final Report for Contract no. No1 CN 65012, The Advocacy Institute, April 1, 1988, 42.

5. Dorfman SF. Tobacco, women and health. As presented at the Advocacy Institute workshop entitled "Not Far Enough: Women vs. Smoking." February 4, 1987.

6. Quote from Joseph Califano, former Secretary of Health and Human Services, as quoted in Not Far Enough, op. cit., 41.

7. Cancer Statistics Review 1973–1987. National Cancer Institute 1990.

8. Surgeon General, Reducing the health consequences of smoking, 1989, op. cit., 125.

9. Slattery ML, Robison LM, Schuman KL, French TK, Abbott TM, Overall JC, Gardner JW. Cigarette smoking and exposure to passive smoke are risk factors for cervical cancer. Journal of the American Medical Association 1989; 261:1593–8.

10. Willett WC, Green A, Stampfer MJ, Speizer FE, Colditz GA, Rosner B, Monson RR, Stason W, Hennekens CH. Relative and absolute excess risks of

coronary heart disease among women who smoke cigarettes. New England Journal of Medicine 1987; 317:1303–9.

11. Croft P, Hannaford PC. Risk factors for acute myocardial infarction in women: evidence from the Royal College of General Practitioners' oral contraception study. British Medical Journal 1989: 298:165–8.

12. Ibid.

13. Rosenberg L, Palmer JR, Shapiro S. Decline in the risk of myocardial infarction among women who stop smoking. New England Journal of Medicine 1990; 322:213–7.

14. Reducing the health consequences of smoking 1989, op. cit., 75.

15. Handler A, Davis F, Ferre C, Yeko T. The relationship of smoking and ectopic pregnancy. American Journal of Public Health 1989; 79:1239–42.

16. Ablin, RJ. Cigarette smoking and quality of sperm. New York State Journal of Medicine 1986; 2:108.

17. Reducing the health consequences of smoking 1989, op. cit., 73.

18. Windsor RA, Orleans CT. Guidelines and methodological standards for smoking cessation intervention research among pregnant women: improving the science and art. Health Education Quarterly, Summer 1986; 13:131–61.

19. Reducing the health consequences of smoking, op. cit., 73.

20. Ibid.

21. Daniell HW. Osteoporosis of the slender smoker. Archives of Internal Medicine 1976; 136:298–304; Paganini-Hill A, Ross RK, Gerkins VR, Henderson BE, Arthur M, Mack TM. Menopausal estrogen therapy and hip fractures. Annals of Internal Medicine 1981; 95:28–31; Williams AR, Weiss NS, Ure CL, Ballard J, Daling JR. Effect of weight, smoking and estrogen use on the risk of hip and forearm fractures in postmenopausal women. Obstetrics and Gynecology 1982; 60:695–9.

22. Sandler RB, Slemenda CW, LaPorte RE, Cauley JA, Schramm MM, Barresi ML, Kriska AM. Postmenopausal bone density and milk consumption in childhood and adolescence. American Journal of Clinical Nutrition 1985; 42:270–4.

23. Willett W, Stampfer MJ, Bain C, Lipnick R, Speizer FE, Rosner B, Cramer D, Hennekens CH. Cigarette smoking, relative weight and menopause. American Journal of Epidemiology 1983; 117:651–8.

24. Senate hearings, op. cit.

25. Reducing the health consequences of smoking, op. cit., 269.

26. Benowitz NL. Pharmacologic aspects of cigarette smoking and nicotine addiction. New England Journal of Medicine 1988; 319: 1318–30.

27. Svikis DS, Hatsukami DK, Hughes JR, Carroll KM, Pickens RW. Sex differences in tobacco withdrawal syndrome. Addictive Behaviors 1986; 11:459–62.

28. The health consequences of smoking; nicotine addiction: a report of the Surgeon General 1988. Department of Health and Human Services CDC Publications # 88–8406:439.

29. Rigotti NA. Cigarette smoking and body weight, New England Journal of Medicine 1989; 320: 931–3.

30. Ibid.

31. Pomerleau O, Adkins D; Pertschuk M. Predictors of outcome and recidivism in smoking cessation treatment. Addictive Behaviors 1978; 3:65–70.

32. Bozzetti LP. Group psychotherapy with addicted smokers. Psychotherapy Psychosom. 1972; 20:172–5.

33. Review and Evaluation of Smoking Cessation Methods: The United States and Canada, 1978–1985, Department of Health and Human Services, NIH Publication # 87–2940, April 1987.

34. Ibid.

35. Ibid.

36. Ibid.

37. Glynn TJ, Manley MW. How to help your patients stop smoking. National Cancer Institute, National Institutes of Health, NIH Publication 89–3064, March 1989.

Epilogue

Regulation of the pills, procedures, and products detailed in this book occurs simultaneously at three important levels: government, common law, and at the patient level.

Government Regulation: There will always be a need to protect the most vulnerable in our society. Government regulation occurs via the Congress and regulatory agencies such as the Food and Drug Administration. If they determine a drug or a medical device to be generally unsafe, it is taken off the market. It is too dangerous to assume that everyone who is at risk of serious injury will be able to become aware enough of the problem to avoid it. The increased vulnerability due to barriers of language, intelligence and age—especially for children and teenagers—make a theoretical market/information-driven approach too risky.

Besides removing a product from the market, government regulatory agencies can require stronger warnings on the labelling of drugs for doctors and patients. Such an approach maximizes consumer information and the possibility of real "informed consent." In 1981, a patient package information program, which would have required pharmacists to automatically give patients an information sheet when many major classes of drugs were dispensed—amounting to one-seventh of all prescribed drugs—was arbitrarily cancelled by the Reagan administration under pressure from doctors, pharmacists, and drug companies. However, government action, albeit always delayed in deference to industry, has resulted in warnings on menopausal estrogens, Accutane, tampons, cigarettes, and other products and a succession of stronger but currently still inadequate warnings on the birth control pill.

As alluded to above, there is inordinate pressure from the pharmaceutical and medical device industries to confound, weaken, or delay governmental action on their products, either in the form of bans or stronger warnings. The well-documented information and evidence upon which the government eventually acts is usually available months or, more typically, years before action is taken. In addition, even when the label on a prescription drug, for example, is strengthened so that the doctor is more aware of the risks, except for the Pill, estrogens, and other hormones (progestins), there is no mandatory written patient information on any prescription drug or device. Although many intelligent and conscientious doctors do adequately inform patients about the benefits as well as the risks, many do not, implying "doctor knows best," "trust me," and "do you think I would prescribe anything for you that was not safe?"

Thus, there is no way to effectively keep one step ahead of the marketeers. While warning labels on some drugs and products have improved over the past few years, the system designed to protect the public is grossly inadequate. A wide array of medical devices, including breast implants, have never been proven safe inside the human body. Further, in May 1990, a government report showed that 102 of the 198 drugs approved for marketing between 1976 and 1985 by the Food and Drug Administration actually had serious enough side effects that they should be removed from the market or their labels changed substantially to warn of these dangers.

Common Law Regulation. Whereas drugs and devices and other products are at least theoretically regulated by various federal agencies, doctors, once licensed, are grossly under-regulated. Few states do an adequate job disciplining even the one or two percent of doctors who are practicing dangerous or otherwise unacceptable medicine and few hospitals have effective quality assurance or risk prevention programs to prevent unnecessary deaths or injuries.

A recent study done by Harvard University of hospitalizations in New York State at a representative sample of hospitals concluded that over 51 percent of patients who died in the hospital as a result of their interaction with the medical care they received in the hospital were killed as a result of negligence by doctors or other health care providers. Projected nationally, this means that approximately 90,000 patients a year are killed in American hospitals as a result of negligence.

Amongst the more common kinds of negligence are unnecessary surgery and the lack of informed consent as to risks and benefits of various treatments. There is little question that civil litigation has been an important factor in bringing about an improvement in written informed consent for surgical and diagnostic procedures and has at least started many hospitals down the path of better control over the quality of care they deliver.

In the area of product liability, litigation concerning the Dalkon Shield, certain heart valves, and many other drugs and devices has started sending a message to industries that if they are grossly negligent and their products injure or kill people, they are going to have to pay.

Across the country, doctors and insurance companies are attempting to make it very difficult for injured patients to recover for damages suffered as a result of negligent medical care by trying to get state legislators to overhaul the current malpractice system. Similarly, drug and device companies are lobbying heavily to be relieved of having to pay the full costs for deaths and injuries they cause, even when they are grossly negligent. Legislation introduced in many states and in the federal Congress would immunize companies from having to pay punitive damages in product liability lawsuits as long as the drug or device had been approved by the FDA. For example, Pfizer was grossly negligent in causing the deaths of over 750 people due to a defectively designed and manufactured heart valve (Bjork-Shiley convexo-concave heart valve). Such legislation would prevent recovery for punitive damages because the FDA had approved the valve, even though it was eventually taken off the market because it was killing so many people.

Regulation by Patients. In the end, regulation by consumers is necessary because, even in the best of all possible worlds, government regulation will never be responsive enough or thorough enough to meet your needs, and not everybody has the resources to sue a company. The control that the government and the courts exercise over the behavior of doctors or drug companies will always need to be supplemented by an ever-increasing amount of control by consumers. Empowered with more information (such as that found in *Women's Health Alert*), women will be able to weigh important questions more accurately:

- Should I have a hysterectomy or try a nonsurgical approach to my problem?
- Even if I've had two cesarean section deliveries, why can't I try a vaginal birth for my third?
- Why am I still taking estrogen replacement pills at age 60?
- Am I taking the lowest dose birth control pill I can?
- I prefer high absorbency tampons, but do they still increase my risk of toxic shock syndrome?
- What else can I do besides take tranquilizers to reduce my nagging anxiety?
- Should I buy this new weight-loss plan?

It comes down to a matter of deciding for and protecting ourselves.

Appendix A

Hospital Cesarean Section Rates

Arizona 1-1-89 to 6-30-89

Name of Facility	Total Deliveries	Cesarean Rate	Name of Facility	Total Deliveries	Cesarean Rate
Arrowhead Community	60	21.7%	Navapache	249	22.1%
Bullhead Community Med. Ctr.	54	46.3%	Phoenix Baptist	504	16.1%
Casa Grande Regional Med. Ctr.	153	20.3%	Phoenix General Hosp. Deer Valley	172	24.4%
Chandler Regional	933	21.1%	Phoenix Mem.	1021	14.7%
Community Hosp. Phoenix	176	12.5%	Pinal General	230	17.4%
Desert Samaritan	2295	27.2%	Scottsdale Mem.	615	24.2%
Flagstaff Med. Ctr.	455	15.2%	Scottsdale Mem. Hosp. North	446	19.7%
Gila Co. General	77	18.2%			
Good Samaritan	2945	20.7%	Sierra Vista Community	285	22.1%
Havasu Samaritan	252	23.4%	Southeast Arizona	212	12.7%
Humana Desert Valley	347	29.4%	*St. Joseph's Hosp. Phoenix	2000	21.5%
Humana Phoenix	138	20.3%	St Joseph's Hosp. Tucson	1039	23.0%
John C. Lincoln	427	23.7%	Thunderbird Samaritan	1245	19.9%
Kingman Regional	286	24.8%	Tucson General	248	14.9%
Kino Community	579	13.1%	Tucson Med. Ctr.	2258	27.4%
Marcus J. Lawrence	194	18.0%	*University Med. Ctr.	1323	18.6%
*Maricopa Med. Ctr.	2573	12.9%	Yavapai Regional Med. Ctr.	336	23.8%
Maryvale Samaritan	812	19.7%	Yuma Regional Med. Ctr.	1007	18.0%
Mesa General	397	22.7%			
Mesa Lutheran	762	18.4%	**STATE TOTALS**	**27105**	**20.6%**

Source: Arizona Department of Health Services, from hospital discharge data. Data on neonatal intensive care units from the American Hospital Association "1988 Guide to the Health Care Field."

California 1987

Name of Facility	Total Deliveries	Cesarean Rate	Name of Facility	Total Deliveries	Cesarean Rate
Alameda	435	30.8%	*Cedars-Sinai Med. Ctr.	7105	29.7%
Alexian Brothers	1571	22.7%	*Centinela Hosp. Med. Ctr.	1917	24.2%
*Alta Bates	3679	29.8%	Chapman General	1023	31.3%
Alta Hosp. District	253	23.7%	Charter Suburban	1349	32.2%
Amador	232	19.4%	*Children's Hosp. of San Francisco	2919	24.2%
American River	1180	21.8%			
Ami-Valley Med. Ctr.	450	18.7%	Chinese	276	37.7%
Anaheim General	470	37.0%	Chowchilla District Mem.	36	25.0%
Antelope Valley Hosp. Med. Ctr.	2775	23.8%	Circle City	693	38.4%
			Clovis Community	288	28.8%
Auburn Faith Community	630	28.9%	Coastal Communities	1144	35.3%
*Bakersfield Mem.	2303	32.1%	Colusa Community	115	34.8%
Barstow Community	532	30.1%	Community	3171	22.3%
Barton Mem.	697	18.2%	Community Hosp. of Santa Cruz	1005	22.4%
Bay Harbor	675	33.8%			
Bear Valley Community	136	11.0%	Community Hosp. of The Monterey Peninsula	1901	27.0%
Bellflower Doctors	637	26.7%			
Bellwood General	524	36.8%	*Community Hosp. & Rehab Ctr. - Los Gatos	704	25.7%
Beverly	1757	31.0%			
Brookside	923	22.0%	Community Mem. Hosp. of San Buena Ventura	1698	26.4%
Brotman Med. Ctr.	816	32.6%			
Burbank Community	481	14.3%	Corcoran District	126	32.5%
*California Med. Ctr. - Los Angeles	2822	28.4%	Corona Community	824	36.2%
			Coronado	722	24.7%

Name of Facility	Total Deliveries	Cesarean Rate	Name of Facility	Total Deliveries	Cesarean Rate
Dameron	2770	21.9%	Humana Hosp. Westminister	592	24.7%
Del Puerto	117	21.4%			
Delano Regional Med. Ctr.	777	18.4%	*Huntington Mem.	3920	38.2%
Delta Mem.	606	25.4%	Inter-Community Med. Ctr.	568	36.3%
Desert	1811	23.4%	John C. Fremont	59	0.0%
Doctors Hosp. of Lakewood	750	23.3%	John F. Kennedy Mem.	1783	23.2%
			John Muir Med. Ctr.	1654	31.6%
Doctors Hosp. of Lodi	254	24.0%	Kaiser Foundation DBA Santa Teresa Community	2724	16.8%
Doctors Hosp. of Manteca	273	28.2%			
Doctors Hosp. of Montclair	1916	27.9%	*Kaiser Foundation Anaheim	2913	16.2%
Doctors Med. Ctr.	1374	27.1%			
Dominguez Med. Ctr.	2268	22.0%	*Kaiser Foundation Bellflower	4734	22.4%
*Dominican Santa Cruz	1239	20.6%			
*Donald N. Sharp Mem. Community	6964	30.8%	*Kaiser Foundation Fontana	4004	21.0%
			*Kaiser Foundation Harbor City	2033	19.6%
Downey Community	623	21.7%			
East Los Angeles Doctor's	489	29.9%	*Kaiser Foundation Hayward	2791	21.5%
Eastern Plumas	48	8.3%			
Eden Hosp. Med. Ctr.	1077	28.6%	*Kaiser Foundation LA	4248	17.3%
El Camino	3329	23.9%	*Kaiser Foundation Oakland	2849	20.3%
*El Centro Regional Med. Ctr.	1092	37.4%			
			*Kaiser Foundation Panorama City	2097	21.4%
Emanuel Med. Ctr.	1055	25.5%			
Fallbrook Hosp. District	985	28.2%	Kaiser Foundation Redwood City	1641	17.1%
Feather River	684	20.9%			
FHP Hosp. - Fountain Valley	1961	23.0%	*Kaiser Foundation Sacramento	4295	18.2%
Foothill Presbyterian	478	36.4%	*Kaiser Foundation San Diego	4143	20.6%
*Fountain Valley Regional	4477	26.2%			
Fremont Med. Ctr.	1901	24.5%	*Kaiser Foundation San Francisco	2784	21.6%
French Hosp. of Los Angeles	1942	22.8%			
			*Kaiser Foundation Santa Clara	3273	18.4%
Fresno Community Hosp. & Med. Ctr.	5233	28.0%			
			Kaiser Foundation Vallejo	2582	17.2%
*Garfield Med. Ctr.	3079	33.3%	Kaiser Foundation Walnut Creek	3055	25.2%
*General	724	28.0%			
George L. Mee Mem.	219	18.7%	Kaiser Foundation Woodland Hills	1351	21.8%
*Glendale Adventist Med. Ctr.	2343	29.2%			
			*Kaiser Foundation West LA	2129	19.4%
Glendale Mem. Hosp. and Health Ctr.	460	28.7%	*Kaweah Delta District	1989	25.7%
			*Kern Med. Ctr.	3425	14.0%
Glendora Community	905	34.7%	*LA Co. Harbor-UCLA Med. Ctr.	6438	18.6%
Goleta Valley Community	524	22.7%			
Granada Hills Community	1269	28.0%	*LA Co. Martin Luther King, Jr./Drew Med. Ctr.	6921	15.6%
Greater El Monte Community	909	31.1%			
			LA Co. Olive View Med. Ctr.	304	13.5%
*Grossmont District	3873	24.5%			
Hanford Community Med. Ctr.	1071	22.2%	*LA Co. USC Med. Ctr.	16181	18.3%
			La Palma Intercommunity	632	32.6%
Hazel Hawkins Mem.	355	29.9%	Lassen Community	258	22.1%
Healdsburg General	179	19.0%	Lincoln Hosp. Med. Ctr.	495	23.4%
Hemet Valley Hosp. District	1038	29.9%	Lindsay Hosp. Med. Ctr.	719	24.3%
Henry Mayo Newhall Mem.	1174	28.5%	Little Company of Mary	2297	29.2%
Highland General	2074	17.4%	Lodi Mem.	877	23.1%
*Hoag Mem. Hosp. Presbyterian	2487	26.9%	*Loma Linda University Med. Ctr.	1904	24.9%
			Lompoc District	411	16.3%
Hollywood Presbyterian Med. Ctr.	2837	32.2%	Long Beach Community	2891	21.2%
			Los Alamitos Med. Ctr.	796	24.7%
Holy Cross Med. Ctr.	2376	31.7%	LA Community	781	30.6%
Humana Hosp. Huntington Beach	573	32.1%	Los Banos Community	310	34.5%
			*Los Medanos Community	477	23.5%
Humana Hosp. San Leandro	571	40.1%	Los Robles Regional Med. Ctr.	1243	34.4%
Humana Hosp. West Anaheim	896	28.9%	Mad River Community	410	18.8%
			Madera Community	715	31.0%
*Humana Hosp. West Hills	1200	35.5%			

*indicates this facility has a neonatal intensive care unit

Name of Facility	Total Deliveries	Cesarean Rate	Name of Facility	Total Deliveries	Cesarean Rate
Marian Med. Ctr.	1130	33.9%	Pioneer	1620	28.4%
*Marin General	1642	25.9%	Pioneers Mem. Hosp. District	1102	29.9%
Marina Hills	845	23.1%			
Mark Twain	65	20.0%	Placentia-Linda Community	235	23.0%
Marshall	669	19.4%	Pleasant Valley	613	22.5%
*Martin Luther Hosp. Med. Ctr.	2404	31.1%	Plumas District	111	23.4%
			Pomerado	1329	23.1%
Mayers Mem.	99	22.2%	*Pomona Valley Hosp. Med. Ctr.	3521	25.5%
*Med. Ctr. of Garden Grove	594	22.9%			
Med. Ctr. of La Mirada	2477	14.7%	*Presbyterian Intercommunity	2007	30.6%
*Med. Ctr. of Tarzana	2295	38.3%			
Mem. Hosp. At Exeter	39	28.2%	Providence Hosp. of Oakland	446	18.2%
Mem. Hosp. Modesto	1580	27.4%			
Mem. Hosp. of Gardena	946	30.4%	Queen of Angels Med. Ctr.	2148	30.2%
*Mem. Med. Ctr. of Long Beach	5127	30.7%	*Queen of The Valley Hosp. West Covena	4152	23.2%
Mendocino Coast District	258	15.5%	*Queen of The Valley Hosp. Napa	825	27.7%
Merced Community Med. Ctr.	1705	26.0%			
			Redbud Community	161	2.5%
Mercy General	1841	18.5%	Redlands Community	1811	21.1%
*Mercy	844	22.2%	Redwood Mem.	542	18.6%
Mercy Hosp. and Med. Ctr.	2880	28.9%	Ridgecrest Community	496	24.6%
*Mercy Med. Ctr., Redding	998	38.6%	Rio Hondo	589	19.5%
Mercy Med. Ctr. Mount Shasta	188	25.0%	Riverside Community	2486	27.6%
			*Riverside General	2611	17.2%
Mercy San Juan	1329	23.7%	Roseville	1468	22.8%
Merrithew Mem.	986	19.3%	Sacred Heart	611	18.0%
Methodist Hosp. of Sacramento	753	22.3%	Salinas Valley Mem.	2310	29.2%
			Samuel Merritt	499	21.3%
Methodist Hosp. of Southern California	990	32.5%	San Antonio Community	1950	30.5%
			San Bernardino Community	1787	34.6%
*Mills Mem.	1165	29.6%			
Mission Hosp. Regional Med. Ctr.	2424	36.3%	*San Bernardino County Med. Ctr.	5742	12.0%
Mission Hosp. Huntington Park	1636	35.0%	San Clemente General	2283	33.0%
			San Dimas Community	1788	30.7%
Modoc Med. Ctr.	63	11.1%	San Francisco General Hosp. Med. Ctr.	2881	16.2%
Monterey Park	1384	28.8%			
*Mount Zion Hosp. and Med. Ctr.	1028	21.8%	San Gorgonio Pass Mem.	2839	23.5%
			San Joaquin Community	1704	28.4%
Mountains Community	126	20.6%	*San Joaquin General	1932	22.3%
Mt Diablo Hosp. Med. Ctr.	964	34.3%	San Jose Med. Ctr.	654	27.6%
Natividad Med. Ctr.	1574	26.7%	San Luis Obispo General	735	27.6%
Needles Desert Communities	108	22.2%	San Pedro Peninsula	2113	28.8%
			Sanger	361	28.2%
*North Bay Med. Ctr.	1144	23.3%	Santa Ana Hosp. Med. Ctr.	1590	22.6%
*Northern Inyo	370	18.9%	*Santa Barbara Cottage	2215	24.8%
*Northridge Hosp. Med. Ctr.	2436	40.0%	*Santa Clara Valley Med. Ctr.	1581	21.6%
Novato Community	111	27.9%	Santa Marta	802	20.0%
Nu Med Regional Med. Ctr.	213	39.4%	*Santa Monica Hosp. Med. Ctr.	788	36.3%
N.T. Enloe Mem.	1443	15.9%			
Oak Valley Hosp. District	90	16.7%	Santa Paula Mem.	447	28.2%
Ojai Valley Community	245	18.0%	*Santa Rosa Mem.	1370	21.6%
Oroville	546	20.3%	Santa Teresita	2000	26.6%
O'Connor	2696	21.0%	Scripps Mem. Hosp. Chula Vista	2764	18.9%
Pacific Hosp. of Long Beach	731	19.7%	Scripps Mem. Hosp. La Jolla	1461	37.3%
Pacific Presbyterian Med. Ctr.	923	22.4%	Selma District	2023	26.1%
			Seneca	386	48.6%
Pacifica Hosp. of The Valley	927	26.0%	Sequoia Hosp. District	1169	27.4%
Palo Verde	371	25.3%	Seton Med. Ctr.	685	25.9%
Palomar Med. Ctr.	2247	25.1%	Sierra Kings District	3774	26.7%
Paradise Valley	1480	22.2%	Sierra Nevada Mem.	2060	15.8%
Parkview Community Hosp. Med. Ctr.	1790	26.1%	Sierra View District	487	20.4%
			Sierra Vista	72	28.5%
*Peninsula Hosp. & Med. Ctr.	912	20.4%	Simi Valley Adventist	1057	32.5%
Petaluma Valley	351	29.6%	Siskiyou General	880	19.2%
Physicians' Community	421	32.3%	Sonoma Valley Hosp. District	529	27.1%

*indicates this facility has a neonatal intensive care unit

Name of Facility	Total Deliveries	Cesarean Rate	Name of Facility	Total Deliveries	Cesarean Rate
Sonora Community	652	24.4%	*Torrance Mem. Hosp. Med. Ctr.	3049	33.2%
South Bay	775	28.1%	Tracy Community Mem.	423	26.0%
South Coast Med. Ctr.	1040	26.1%	Trinity	76	14.5%
Southern Humboldt Community Hosp. District	701	18.8%	Tri-City Hosp. District	3611	23.8%
			Tulare District	803	39.9%
*Stanford University	193	20.4%	Twin Cities Community	459	38.1%
St. Agnews Med. Ctr.	181	31.2%	*UCLA Med. Ctr.	2504	18.7%
St. Bernardine Med. Ctr.	599	26.9%	UCSD Med. Ctr.	4125	21.3%
St. Elizabeth Community	2000	24.8%	Ukiah General	884	17.5%
St. Francis	495	26.5%	*University of California Davis Med. Ctr.	1590	15.8%
*St. Francis Med. Ctr.	85	30.1%			
St. Helena Hosp. & Health Ctr.	83	26.7%	*University of California Hosp.s & Clinics	1485	25.5%
St. John's Hosp. and Health Ctr.	1565	32.2%	*University of California Irvine Med. Ctr.	4127	17.8%
St. John's Regional Med. Ctr.	3419	24.7%	Valley Community	926	32.7%
			Valley Hosp. Med. Ctr.	761	17.5%
St. Joseph Hosp. of Orange	2488	29.7%	*Valley Med. Ctr. of Fresno	3359	16.1%
*St. Joseph Med. Ctr.	333	29.3%	Valley Mem.	988	26.2%
St. Joseph's Med. Ctr. of Stockton	1685	23.8%	Valley Presbyterian	3047	37.4%
			*Ventura County Med. Ctr.	2664	22.1%
St. Jude Hosp. Yorba Linda	1477	19.3%	Verdugo Hills	1012	35.4%
St. Jude Hosp. Fullerton	793	22.7%	Victor Valley Community	713	29.9%
St. Luke's	1404	23.5%	Visalia Community	753	29.3%
St. Mary Desert Valley	1569	22.1%	Washington	1855	25.0%
*St. Mary Med. Ctr.	2105	28.2%	Watsonville Community	1222	26.9%
*St. Mary's Hosp. & Med. Ctr.	747	20.2%	West Covina	665	35.2%
			West Side District	81	22.2%
St. Rose	1043	26.3%	*Western Med. Ctr.	2011	34.0%
Sutter Coast	233	28.3%	Westlake Community	747	30.1%
*Sutter Mem.	5717	26.1%	Wheeler	574	34.5%
Sutter Solano Med. Ctr.	369	27.9%	*White Mem. Med. Ctr.	4784	18.5%
Tahoe Forest	325	23.1%	Whittier Hosp. Med. Ctr.	2512	18.9%
The Good Samaritan Hosp. of Santa Clara Valley	3923	28.4%	Woodland Mem.	1569	15.7%
			STATE TOTALS	**479902**	**25.0%**

Source: California Office of Statewide Health Plan Development. Data on neonatal intensive care units from the American Hospital Association "1988 Guide to the Health Care Field."

Colorado 7-1-87 to 12-31-87

Name of Facility	Total Deliveries	Cesarean Rate	Name of Facility	Total Deliveries	Cesarean Rate
Arkansas Valley Med. Ctr.	198	18.7%	Porter Mem.	72	20.8%
Boulder Community	1008	21.0%	Poudre Valley	998	18.9%
Delta County	51	13.7%	Presbyterian Aurora	440	26.8%
*Denver General	1524	11.7%	Prowers Med. Ctr.	44	20.5%
Eisenhower Med. Ctr.	87	19.5%	Rocky Mountain	49	26.5%
Grand Junction Community	124	20.2%	*Rose Med. Ctr.	1747	22.3%
Humana Hosp. Aurora	842	27.2%	Salida	97	11.3%
Humana Hosp. Mountain View	419	23.6%	San Luis Valley	257	12.5%
			Southwest Mem.	135	19.3%
Longmont United	390	21.8%	St. Anthony Central	627	21.5%
*Lutheran Med. Ctr.	851	21.5%	St. Anthony Hosp. North	401	23.7%
McKee Med. Ctr.	295	24.7%	St. Francis	256	24.6%
*Mem. Hosp. Colorado Springs	1065	21.6%	*St. Joseph Hosp. Denver	2490	16.6%
			St. Luke's	711	17.7%
Mercy Hosp. Durango	376	19.7%	*St. Mary Corwin	568	16.7%
Montrose Mem.	131	17.6%	*St. Mary's	560	23.8%
Mount San Rafael	83	18.1%	St. Thomas More	104	14.4%
North Colorado Med. Ctr.	789	19.8%	*Swedish Med. Ctr.	1400	26.4%
Parkview Episcopal	324	27.8%	*University	1366	7.5%
Penrose Community	1597	18.0%	Valley View Glenwood Springs	355	20.3%
Platte Valley Med. Ctr.	227	14.5%			
			STATE TOTALS	**23058**	**19.4%**

Source: Colorado Health Data Commission, from hospital discharge data. Data on neonatal intensive care units from the American Hospital Association "1988 Guide to the Health Care Field."

Connecticut 1989

Name of Facility	Total Deliveries	Cesarean Rate	Name of Facility	Total Deliveries	Cesarean Rate
*Bridgeport	2801	24.9%	New Milford	448	23.0%
Bristol	879	24.1%	*Norwalk	1710	24.9%
Charlotte Hungerford	684	23.5%	Park City	685	14.9%
*Danbury	2606	21.4%	Rockville General	691	26.2%
Day Kimball	760	18.9%	Sharon	444	20.3%
Greenwich	1164	28.9%	Stamford	1926	22.1%
Griffin	825	26.2%	*St. Francis Hosp. & Med.	2788	21.1%
*Hartford	4864	24.4%	Ctr.		
*Hosp. of St. Raphael	1494	16.7%	St. Joseph's	563	24.3%
Lawrence & Mem.	2053	23.4%	St. Mary's	1590	25.3%
Manchester Mem.	1337	25.2%	St. Vincent's Med. Ctr.	1544	20.1%
Meriden-Wallingford	1200	24.8%	Waterbury	1474	17.1%
Middlesex Mem.	1138	24.3%	William W. Backus	1264	20.6%
Milford	649	29.7%	Windham Community	481	27.9%
Mt. Sinai	1786	24.0%	Mem.		
*New Britain General	2421	21.4%	*Yale-New Haven	5289	19.4%
			STATE TOTALS	**47558**	**22.6%**

Source: State of Connecticut Commission on Hospitals and Health Care 1989 hospital discharge data. Data on neonatal intensive care units from American Hospital Association "1988 Guide to the Health Care Field."

Florida 7-1-89 to 12-31-89

Name of Facility	Total Deliveries	Cesarean Rate	Name of Facility	Total Deliveries	Cesarean Rate
Alachua General	1059	26.1%	*Humana Hosp. Brandon	933	30.7%
AMI Med. Ctr. Orlando	368	43.2%	Humana Hosp. Ft. Walton	569	29.5%
AMI Palm Beach Gardens	465	37.0%	Humana Hosp. Kissimmee	862	22.4%
Med. Ctr.			Humana Hosp. Lucerne	458	34.3%
Baptist Hosp. Miami	1845	35.3%	Humana Hosp. Orange	649	32.0%
Baptist Hosp. Pensacola	613	28.1%	Park		
*Baptist Med. Ctr.	1420	30.3%	Humana Hosp. Pasco	146	28.8%
Jacksonville			Humana Hosp. Sebastian	98	21.4%
Bartow Mem.	156	28.8%	Humana Hosp. South	305	26.6%
Bay Med. Ctr.	549	27.9%	Broward		
Bayfront Med. Ctr.	2389	28.0%	*Humana Women's Hosp.	2671	35.1%
*Bethesda Mem.	1652	25.9%	Tampa		
*Broward General Med.	2869	26.4%	Indian River Mem.	512	25.0%
Ctr.			Jackson Hosp. Marianna	284	27.1%
Cape Canaveral	509	19.6%	*Jackson Mem.	8337	18.4%
Cape Coral	472	24.2%	James Archer Smith	182	16.5%
Citrus Mem.	389	26.5%	James E. Holmes Regional	1138	27.4%
Coral Springs Med. Ctr.	1058	28.4%	Med. Ctr.		
Desoto Mem.	270	22.6%	Lake Shore	191	25.1%
East Pasco Med. Ctr.	266	32.3%	Lake Wales	197	19.8%
Everglades Mem.	696	26.4%	Lakeland Regional Med.	1070	26.6%
Flagler	289	24.2%	Ctr.		
*Florida	2871	25.2%	Lawnwood Regional Med.	898	30.2%
Florida Keys Mem. Hosp.**	408	27.0%	Ctr.		
Gadsden Mem.	244	31.1%	*Lee Mem.	1879	19.7%
*Good Samaritan Hosp. W.	1006	28.7%	Leesburg Regional Med.	375	16.0%
Palm Beach			Ctr.		
Halifax Hosp. Med. Ctr.	1386	23.8%	Lykes Mem.	279	29.7%
Hamilton Co. Mem.	201	13.4%	L.W. Blake Mem.	429	33.6%
HCA Central Florida	605	19.0%	Manatee Mem	765	24.8%
Regional			Martin Mem.	816	20.7%
HCA Gulf Coast	457	33.0%	Mease Hosp. & Clinic	763	33.2%
HCA Northwest Regional	373	38.9%	Mem. Hosp. Hollywood	2223	30.5%
HCA Putnam Community	252	14.3%	*Mem. Med. Ctr.	1425	32.8%
HCA Tallahassee	371	31.8%	Jacksonville		
Community			Mercy Hosp.**	957	39.8%
HCA West Florida Regional	448	31.7%	Morton F. Plant	1270	21.4%
Med. Ctr.			Mt. Sinai Med. Ctr.	916	45.2%
Hialeah	1549	47.8%	Munroe Regional Med. Ctr.	1215	20.2%
*Holy Cross	738	35.6%	Naples Community	1101	26.0%

Name of Facility	Total Deliveries	Cesarean Rate	Name of Facility	Total Deliveries	Cesarean Rate
Nassau General	125	34.4%	Southeast Volusia Hosp. District	145	30.3%
North Miami Med. Ctr.	332	41.6%			
*North Shore Med. Ctr.	1495	34.2%	St. Anthony's	304	41.4%
Orlando General	249	29.3%	St. Francis	116	28.4%
*Orlando Regional Med. Ctr.	2584	27.0%	St. Joseph Hosp. Port Charlotte	514	27.6%
Palms West	132	22.7%	*St. Mary's	2438	22.2%
Parish Med. Ctr.	410	34.4%	St. Vincent's Med. Ctr.	872	21.2%
Pembroke Pines General	308	35.1%	Sun Coast	384	26.0%
Plantation General	1382	42.6%	*Tallahassee Mem. Regional Med. Ctr.	1730	25.3%
Polk General Hosp.**	1178	29.1%			
Riverside Hosp. Jacksonville	570	24.7%	*Tampa General	3601	15.6%
			*University Hosp. Jacksonville	2779	9.0%
Riverside Hosp. Pasco Co.	682	38.3%	Walker Mem.	429	25.6%
*Sacred Heart Hosp. Pensacola	1353	35.9%	Waterman Med. Ctr.	434	27.4%
Santa Rosa Med. Ctr.	472	26.3%	West Orange Mem.	217	18.0%
*Sarasota Mem.	1528	21.5%	West Volusia Mem.	637	20.4%
*Shands Teaching Hosp. & Clinics	1957	21.9%	Winter Haven	718	22.4%
			Winter Park Mem.	955	24.1%
South Florida Baptist	150	26.0%	Women's Med. Ctr.	127	26.8%
*South Miami	1620	42.6%	Wuesthoff Mem.	523	24.7%
			STATE TOTALS	**95606**	**26.7%**

Source: Florida Health Care Cost Containment Board, from hospital discharge data. Data on neonatal intensive care units from the American Hospital Association "1988 Guide to the Health Care Field."

** indicates this facility has not yet certified its discharge data as complete and accurate for the third quarter of 1989.

Georgia 1989

Name of Facility	Total Deliveries	Cesarean Rate	Name of Facility	Total Deliveries	Cesarean Rate
Appling General	88	17.0%	*Georgia Baptist	3188	29.7%
*Athens General	1399	22.5%	Gilman	302	21.9%
Bacon Co.	51	25.5%	Glynn-Brunswick Mem.	1261	30.2%
Baldwin Co.	529	26.7%	Gordon Co.	335	37.0%
Banks-Jackson Commerce	267	18.4%	*Grady Mem.	8185	16.6%
Barrow Med. Ctr.	161	22.4%	Griffin-Spalding Co.	986	3.7%
Bulloch Mem.	823	24.1%	Gwinnett Med. Ctr.	1945	27.1%
Burke Co.	269	32.7%	Habersham Med. Ctr.	265	27.9%
Candler Co.	90	4.4%	*Hamilton Mem.	1730	19.9%
Candler General	2043	34.6%	Hart Co.	65	20.0%
Clayton General	1701	21.8%	Henry Co.	429	37.1%
Clinch Mem.	70	2.9%	*Houston Co. Med. Ctr.	890	28.0%
Cobb General	1275	21.8%	Humana Hosp. Augusta	651	26.1%
Cobb Mem.	281	24.9%	Humana Hosp. Bartow	451	22.8%
Coffee General	691	27.8%	Humana Hosp. Gwinnett	1276	27.2%
Coliseum Park	1421	36.7%	Humana Hosp. Newnan	628	17.4%
Colquitt Reg. Med. Ctr.	383	21.7%	Hutcheson Med. Ctr.	722	20.1%
*Crawford Long Mem.	1798	30.1%	Hutchinson Mem.	311	25.7%
Crisp Co.	380	28.9%	Jeff Davis Co.	128	14.8%
Dekalb General	2731	40.2%	Jenkins Co.	38	36.8%
Doctors Hosp. Tucker	187	22.5%	John D. Archbold Mem.	1151	18.4%
Dodge Co.	169	16.0%	John M. Meadows Mem.	487	22.4%
Donalsonville	86	9.3%	*Kennestone	3895	30.7%
Dorminy Med. Ctr.	275	31.6%	Liberty Mem.	275	26.2%
Douglas General	728	20.5%	Louis Smith Mem.	80	28.7%
Early Mem.	139	7.9%	*Med. College of Georgia	2283	12.3%
Elbert Co.	144	20.8%	Med. Ctr. Columbus City	3566	31.9%
Emanuel Co.	124	28.2%	*Med. Ctr. of Central GA	2718	19.7%
Evans Mem.	93	21.5%	Mem. Hosp. Adel	470	17.7%
Fairview Park	967	29.4%	Mem. Hosp. Decatur Co.	456	36.0%
Fannin Regional	58	29.3%	Mem. Hosp. Ware Co.	862	21.2%
Floyd Med. Ctr.	2349	22.9%	Mem. Med. Ctr. Chatham	2564	22.5%
Fort Benning	1295	25.0%	Meriwether Mem.	100	8.0%
Fort Gordon Station	695	7.5%	Miller Co.	98	7.1%

*indicates this facility has a neonatal intensive care unit

Name of Facility	Total Deliveries	Cesarean Rate	Name of Facility	Total Deliveries	Cesarean Rate
Minnie G. Boswell Mem.	147	0.7%	Southwest Community	438	30.1%
Mitchell Co.	92	0.0%	Stephens Co.	309	27.5%
Moody AFB	221	27.6%	*St. Joseph's Hosp. Augusta	1075	26.1%
Morgan Mem.	66	31.8%	St. Joseph's Hosp. Dahlonega	360	28.1%
Newnan	270	27.4%			
Newton Co.	763	15.3%	St. Joseph's Hosp. Savannah	343	24.8%
*North Fulton Med. Ctr.	759	22.0%	*St. Mary's Hosp. Athens	937	30.4%
Northeast GA Med. Ctr.	2073	26.3%	Sumter Regional	805	22.1%
Northside	6295	31.9%	Tanner Med. Ctr.	252	24.2%
Parkway Regional	863	26.1%	Tanner Mem.	1081	28.8%
Patterson	157	12.1%	Tattnall Mem.	94	13.8%
Peach Co.	174	25.9%	Three Rivers	44	13.6%
Perry Houston Co.	307	37.1%	Tift General	908	28.1%
*Phoebe Putney Mem.	2845	22.8%	Towns Co.	53	1.9%
Pickens General	98	1.0%	Union General	142	23.9%
Piedmont	2720	27.0%	*University	3650	27.6%
Robins AF Base	365	24.7%	Upson Co.	923	19.1%
Rockdale Co.	804	22.5%	US Army	1111	17.6%
R.T. Jones Mem.	395	21.0%	Watkins Mem.	36	22.2%
R. J. Taylor Mem.	131	26.7%	Wayne Mem.	391	18.4%
*Shallowford Community	1925	23.4%	*West GA Med. Ctr.	612	15.5%
Smith	119	15.1%	*West Paces Ferry	1735	19.5%
South Fulton	1305	29.8%	Wills Mem.	38	28.9%
South GA Med. Ctr.	1223	20.8%	Worth Co.	166	19.3%
			STATE TOTALS	**106171**	**24.9%**

Source: Georgia Department of Human Resources "Births by Method of Delivery 1987-88." Data on neonatal intensive care units from the American Hospital Association "1988 Guide to the Health Care Field."

Hawaii 1989

Name of Facility	Total Deliveries	Cesarean Rate	Name of Facility	Total Deliveries	Cesarean Rate
Castle Med. Ctr.	694	27.8%	Kona	570	28.1%
Hilo	1210	26.2%	Maui Mem.	1482	20.4%
*Honokaa	38	0.0%	Molokai General	82	0.0%
Kahuku	161	19.3%	*Queens Med. Ctr.	1885	17.7%
Kaiser	2174	15.8%	Tripler Army	3451	18.3%
Kapiolani Med. Ctr.	6046	24.2%	Wahiawa General	544	20.0%
Kauai Veterans	107	23.4%	Wilcox	679	20.8%
			STATE TOTALS	**19123**	**21.2%**

Source: State of Hawaii Department of Health "C-Section Births by Hospital." Data on neonatal intensive care units from the American Hospital Association "1988 Guide to the Health Care Field."

Illinois 1988

Name of Facility	Total Deliveries	Cesarean Rate	Name of Facility	Total Deliveries	Cesarean Rate
Abraham Lincoln Mem.	283	21.9%	Community Hosp. of Ottawa	297	25.3%
Alexian Bros Med. Ctr.	971	17.8%			
Alton Mem.	749	27.5%	Community Mem. Hosp. Monmouth	157	31.8%
Bethany	1123	18.7%			
Blessing	897	23.0%	Community Mem. of Staunton	34	5.9%
Brokaw	1249	16.9%			
*Carle Foundation	1012	24.5%	Condell Mem.	1219	24.9%
Central Dupage	3182	23.1%	*Cook Co.	5841	15.6%
Centreville Township	1270	28.7%	Copley Mem.	1679	22.1%
*Chicago Osteopathic	1057	19.5%	Covenant Med. Ctr. Champaign	687	25.5%
*Christ	4062	18.3%			
Clay Co.	136	18.4%	Covenant Med. Ctr. Urbana	1252	21.7%
*Columbus Hosp. Chicago	1391	26.2%	Crawford Mem.	71	29.6%
Community General Hosp. Sterling	681	21.7%	Decatur Mem.	75	20.0%
			Delnor Hosp. St. Charles	1166	23.6%

*indicates this facility has a neonatal intensive care unit

Name of Facility	Total Deliveries	Cesarean Rate	Name of Facility	Total Deliveries	Cesarean Rate
Douglas City Jarman	69	18.8%	Morris	267	27.7%
Dr. John Warner	51	23.5%	Morrison Community	43	4.7%
Edgewater	130	16.2%	*Mt. Sinai Hosp. Med. Ctr. Chicago	2461	12.0%
Edward A. Utlaut	155	23.2%			
Edward Hosp. Assoc.	754	28.8%	N Illinois Med. Ctr.	655	27.9%
Elmhurst Mem.	1689	22.1%	Northwest Community	2722	26.5%
Eureka	186	19.4%	*Northwestern Mem.	4575	23.1%
*Evanston	3277	19.6%	*Norwegian-American	3030	27.0%
*F. G. McGaw/Loyola U.	1347	27.5%	Oak Park	199	18.1%
Fairbury	48	25.0%	Oliver C. Anderson	647	28.9%
Fairfield Mem.	99	23.2%	Olympia Fields Osteo Ctr.	686	21.7%
Fayette Co.	39	17.9%	Our Lady of Resurrection	202	29.2%
Franciscan Med. Ctr.	922	18.9%	Palos Community	1984	17.3%
Freeport Mem.	763	26.3%	Passavant Area	533	18.0%
Galesburg Cottage	291	25.4%	Pekin Mem.	516	19.8%
Gibson Community	32	25.0%	Perry Mem.	223	26.9%
Glenoaks Med. Ctr.	207	30.0%	Proctor Community	647	24.3%
Good Samaritan Hosp. Mt. Vernon	690	15.9%	Ravenswood	2165	27.1%
			Resurrection	1269	30.8%
Good Samaritan Hosp. Downers Grove	2316	24.5%	Richland Mem.	526	15.0%
			Riverside Med. Ctr. Kankakee	1248	20.4%
Good Shepard	1411	18.9%			
Gottlieb Mem.	497	28.2%	Rochelle Community	181	18.8%
Graham Hosp. Assoc.	202	17.8%	*Rockford Mem.	1807	31.6%
Grant Hosp. of Chicago	968	24.3%	Roseland Community	952	25.2%
Hammond Henry District	204	27.5%	Rush North Shore Med. Ctr.	306	37.6%
Harvard Community Mem.	100	16.0%	*Rush Presbyterian St. Luke's	2616	23.1%
Herrin	316	23.1%			
Highland Park	1026	17.9%	Sandwich Community	88	23.9%
Hillsboro	176	25.6%	Sara Culbertson Mem.	111	10.8%
Hinsdale	2453	23.1%	Sarah Bush Lincoln	950	24.0%
Holy Cross	287	16.4%	Savanna City	37	13.5%
Holy Family	672	18.6%	Sherman Hosp. Assoc.	1768	19.3%
Humana Hosp./Suburban Med. Ctr.	2284	24.7%	Silver Cross	1099	30.5%
			Sparta Community	182	24.7%
IL Community Hosp. Pittsfield	88	9.1%	St. Anne's Hosp. Chicago	371	22.9%
			St. Anthony Hosp. Chicago	726	20.7%
IL Masonic Med. Ctr.	1830	22.5%	St. Anthony Med. Ctr.	782	18.5%
IL Valley Community	194	16.5%	St. Anthony's Hosp. Alton	184	23.9%
Illini	516	26.2%	St. Anthony's Mem.	812	20.8%
Ingalls Mem.	2485	24.2%	St. Bernard Hosp. Chicago	826	16.2%
Iroquois Mem.	210	24.3%	St. Cabrini Hosp. Chicago	1401	14.7%
Jackson Park	102	19.6%	St. Clement	183	26.2%
Jersey Community	348	16.4%	St. Elizabeth Med. Ctr. Granite City	790	27.3%
Katherine S. Bethea	402	18.2%			
Kewanee Public	220	25.5%	St. Elizabeth's Hosp. Belleville	1003	27.5%
Kishwaukee Community	789	22.7%			
LaGrange Mem.	1183	22.2%	St. Francis Hosp. Blue Island	1170	25.6%
Lake Forest	1949	28.1%			
Lawrence Co. Mem.	133	21.8%	St. Francis Hosp. Evanston	989	13.3%
LGH-Lincoln Park	204	31.9%	St. Francis Hosp. Litchfield	306	27.8%
*Little Co. of Mary	2062	30.4%	*St. Francis Med. Ctr. Peoria	2493	27.4%
Louis A. Weiss	555	25.6%			
*Lutheran General	3571	24.1%	St. James Hosp. Pontiac	424	23.6%
MacNeal	1489	19.5%	*St. James. Hosp. Chicago Hts.	1351	17.5%
Marion Mem.	204	17.2%			
Marshall Browning	135	21.5%	*St. John's Hosp. Springfield	2633	18.2%
McDonough District	465	30.1%			
Mem. Hosp. Woodstock	751	26.2%	St. Joseph Hosp. Bloomington	724	17.5%
Mem. Hosp. Belleville	1628	38.5%			
*Mem. Hosp. Carbondale	1367	23.3%	St. Joseph Hosp. Breese	484	21.3%
Mem. Hosp. Carthage	136	28.7%	St. Joseph Hosp. Chicago	1246	24.6%
Mem. Hosp. Chester	120	22.5%	St. Joseph Hosp. Elgin	475	18.5%
Mem. Med. Ctr. Springfield	1390	18.4%	St. Joseph Hosp. Highland	484	27.1%
Mendota Community	135	16.3%	St. Joseph Med. Ctr. Joliet	1762	29.2%
Mercer Co.	101	29.7%	St. Joseph Mem. Hosp. Murphysboro	163	13.5%
Mercy Ctr. Health Care Aurora	723	20.7%			
			St. Margaret	202	21.3%
Mercy Hosp. & Med. Ctr. Chicago	1933	18.8%	St. Mary Hosp. Quincy	429	18.9%
			St. Mary of Nazareth	1131	21.1%
Methodist Med. Ctr. Peoria	1774	28.7%	St. Mary's Hosp. Centralia	674	19.9%
*Michael Reese	4223	16.8%	St. Mary's Hosp. Decatur	1224	21.7%

Name of Facility	Total Deliveries	Cesarean Rate	Name of Facility	Total Deliveries	Cesarean Rate
St. Mary's Hosp. Galesburg	518	22.0%	*University of IL 1740 Taylor	3517	20.2%
St. Mary's Hosp. Kankakee	377	19.6%			
St. Mary's Hosp. Streator	357	23.5%	United Med. Ctr. W.	809	23.5%
St. Therese Med. Ctr.	1164	22.3%	United Samaritans Danville	609	20.9%
St. Vincent Mem. Hosp. Taylorville	247	25.9%	United Samaritans Sager	261	25.3%
			Victory Mem.	1321	29.3%
*Swedish American	1877	19.2%	Wabash General	105	24.8%
Swedish Covenant	785	28.3%	Washington Co.	78	34.6%
S. Chicago Community	1695	21.0%	Westlake Community	626	23.2%
S. Suburban	851	19.7%	Wood River Township	250	32.0%
*U of Chicago Hosp. & Clinics	3038	15.5%	W. Suburban Hosp. Oak Park	1161	18.6%
			STATE TOTALS	**167400**	**22.4%**

Source: Illinois Health Care Cost Containment Council "Cesarean Deliveries in Illinois Hospitals: 1988." Data on neonatal intensive care units from the American Hospital Association "1988 Guide to the Health Care Field."

Indiana 1988

Name of Facility	Total Deliveries	Cesarean Rate	Name of Facility	Total Deliveries	Cesarean Rate
Adams Co. Mem.	302	16.6%	Jasper Co.	218	13.3%
*Ball Mem.	1761	23.0%	Jay Co.	195	21.0%
Bartholomew Co.	1242	23.5%	Johnson Co. Mem.	610	19.3%
Bedford Med. Ctr.	464	17.7%	Kings Daughters	426	18.8%
Blackford Co.	90	23.3%	Kingwood	528	20.1%
Bloomington	1696	26.1%	Kosciusko Community	678	24.8%
Cameron Mem. Community	319	24.5%	*Lafayette Home	1922	15.1%
Caylor-Nickel	380	20.3%	Lagrange	331	22.7%
Clark Co. Mem.	576	24.0%	Laporte	672	21.6%
Clay Co.	193	28.5%	*Lutheran Hosp. Indiana	1564	18.1%
Clinton Co.	273	16.1%	Major	304	16.4%
Community Hosp. Anderson & Madison Co.	837	23.4%	Margaret Mary Community	345	24.1%
			Marion General	963	17.2%
Community Hosp. Bremen	130	0.8%	Mary Sherman	223	19.7%
			McCray Mem.	358	13.4%
Community Hosp. Indpls - North	771	20.5%	Mem. Hosp. Jasper	524	21.8%
			Mem. Hosp. Logansport	553	13.7%
Community Hosp. Indpls - Ritter	1794	16.4%	Mem. Hosp. Michigan City	323	27.2%
			*Mem. Hosp. South Bend	3262	20.8%
Community Hosp. Munster	2468	37.6%	Mercy	143	14.0%
			Methodist Hosp. Gary - Northlake	1574	21.9%
Culver Union	378	24.9%			
Daviess Co.	395	21.8%	Methodist Hosp. Gary - Southlake	1305	27.4%
Deaconess	1061	23.9%			
Dearborn Co.	381	26.2%	*Methodist Hosp. Indianapolis	4039	17.2%
Decatur Co.	212	26.9%			
Dekalb Mem.	428	22.2%	Michiana Community	446	17.3%
Dukes Mem.	300	16.3%	Morgan Co. Mem.	378	18.8%
Dunn Mem.	294	22.1%	Orange Co.	153	23.5%
Elkhart General	1833	19.1%	*Parkview Mem.	3112	15.6%
Fayette Mem.	242	21.1%	Perry Co. Mem.	78	12.8%
Floyd Mem.	828	21.1%	Porter Mem.	1457	23.6%
George Ade Mem.	41	14.6%	Pulaski Mem.	177	25.4%
Gibson General	189	16.9%	Putnam Co.	246	19.9%
Good Samaritan	544	36.9%	Randolph Co.	126	16.7%
Goshen General	1328	17.8%	Reid Mem.	1046	22.8%
Greene Co. General	145	26.2%	Riverview	508	22.0%
Hancock Mem.	338	17.2%	Rush Mem.	60	23.3%
Harrison Co.	196	17.9%	Scott Co. Mem.	129	16.3%
Hendricks Community	430	23.7%	Starke Mem.	159	22.0%
Henry Co. Mem.	465	18.9%	St. Anthony	711	24.2%
Holy Cross Parkview	308	17.2%	St. Catherine East Chicago	493	27.6%
Howard Community	441	28.3%			
*Humana Womens	2006	27.2%	St. Elizabeth Hosp. Med. Ctr.	609	13.1%
Huntington Mem.	399	22.6%			
*Indiana University	993	28.4%	*St. Francis	2161	16.7%
Jackson Co. Schneck Mem.	604	18.7%	St. Johns Health Care Corp	617	20.7%

Name of Facility	Total Deliveries	Cesarean Rate	Name of Facility	Total Deliveries	Cesarean Rate
St. Joseph's Hosp. Kokomo	1043	16.0%	Union City Mem.	39	2.6%
St. Joseph's Hosp. Mishawaka	808	12.5%	*Union	1669	24.3%
			Vermillion Co.	201	23.4%
St. Joseph's Hosp. Huntingburg	300	14.7%	Wabash Co.	376	27.1%
			Washington Co. Mem.	182	15.4%
St. Joseph's Med. Ctr. Fort Wayne	1137	13.4%	*Welborn Mem. Baptist	981	36.9%
			Wells Community	256	19.5%
*St. Margaret Hosp. and Health Ctr.	1547	34.4%	White Co. Mem.	193	9.3%
			Whitley Co. Mem.	383	29.0%
St. Mary's Med. Ctr. - Evansville	2312	26.2%	Wirth Osteopathic	47	6.4%
			Wishard Mem.	3251	10.7%
St. Vincent	3505	21.7%	Witham Mem.	144	21.5%
Terre Haute Regional	443	28.9%	Woodlawn	187	33.7%
Tipton Co. Mem.	90	14.4%	**STATE TOTALS**	**80895**	**21.3%**

Source: Indiana State Board of Health "1988 Births by Type of Delivery by Indiana Hospital of Occurrence." Data on neonatal intensive care units from the American Hospital Association "1988 Guide to the Health Care Field."

Kentucky 1988

Name of Facility	Total Deliveries	Cesarean Rate	Name of Facility	Total Deliveries	Cesarean Rate
Allen Co. War Mem.	38	5.3%	*Med. Ctr. at Bowling Green	1639	25.3%
Audubon	1848	26.4%	Mem. Hosp. Clay Co.	319	18.2%
*Baptist Hosp. East	1875	29.4%	*Methodist Evangelical	1439	24.7%
Caverna Mem.	68	0.0%	Methodist Hosp. Pike Co.	1099	19.8%
*Central Baptist	3053	24.7%	Middlesboro App. Regional	376	17.0%
Clark Co.	216	24.5%	Muhlenberg Community	479	16.5%
Community Hosp. Mayfield	280	27.1%	Murray-Calloway Co.	655	18.9%
*Community United Methodist	839	31.8%	*Norton	3218	21.2%
Crittendon Co.	112	19.6%	Ohio Co.	111	13.5%
Cumberland Co.	92	0.0%	Our Lady of the Way	253	36.0%
Ephriam McDowell Mem.	547	36.4%	Owensboro-Daviess Co.	1742	22.3%
Flaget Mem.	187	29.9%	Pattie A. Clay	666	23.6%
Franklin-Simpson Mem.	46	30.4%	Paul B. Hall Regional Med. Ctr.	305	34.4%
Ft. Logan	205	12.7%	Pineville Community	271	28.0%
Good Samaritan	390	17.2%	*Regional Med. Ctr. Madisonville	880	29.9%
Grayson Co. War Mem.	257	24.5%			
Hardin Mem.	885	25.1%	Scott General	123	21.1%
Harlan App. Regional	464	25.2%	Southeastern Baptist	795	24.7%
Harrison Mem.	125	13.6%	Southwest Jefferson Community Hosp	228	24.6%
Hazard App. Regional	451	39.9%			
Highland Regional Med. Ctr.	472	53.4%	Spring View Hosp./Mary Imac.	285	20.0%
*Humana	861	25.6%	St. Anthony's	1358	18.6%
James B. Haggin Mem.	173	20.8%	St. Claire Med. Ctr.	723	23.0%
*Jennie Stuart Mem.	559	32.9%	*St. Elizabeth Hosp. North	459	23.5%
*King's Daughters Hosp. Ashland	1028	25.7%	St. Elizabeth Hosp. South	2318	23.9%
			St. Luke Hosp. Ft. Thomas	1328	25.5%
King's Daughters Hosp. Shelby	244	20.9%	Suburban	287	25.8%
King's Daughters' Mem.	448	35.5%	Taylor Co.	455	20.9%
Knox Co. General	168	20.8%	Tri-Co. Community	124	31.5%
Lake Cumberland Med. Ctr.	1535	20.3%	T. J. Sampson Community	861	23.1%
Logan Co.	204	37.7%	*University Hosp. Lexington	2051	17.6%
Louisa Community	208	24.0%			
Marshall Co.	179	33.5%	University Hosp./LGH	2451	13.5%
Mary Breckinridge	344	21.8%	U.S. Army	1027	11.5%
Mary Chiles	498	16.9%	Western Baptist Hosp. Paducah	1553	21.9%
Marymount	208	29.3%			
Meadowview Hosp. Maysville	461	15.0%	Whitesburg App. Regional	395	26.8%
			Williamson App. Regional	128	23.4%
			STATE TOTALS	**49969**	**23.4%**

Source: Kentucky Cabinet for Human Resources, Department for Health Services, Health Data Branch/Data Development, from births statistics file. Data on neonatal intensive care units from the American Hospital Association "1988 Guide to the Health Care Field."

*indicates this facility has a neonatal intensive care unit

Maine 1989

Name of Facility	Total Deliveries	Cesarean Rate	Name of Facility	Total Deliveries	Cesarean Rate
Aroostook Med. Ctr.	315	11.7%	Miles	126	21.4%
Bath	366	20.2%	Millinocket	88	34.1%
Blue Hill	253	13.4%	Mt. Desert	122	17.2%
Calais	99	35.4%	North Cumberland	94	36.2%
Cary	265	22.3%	North Maine	86	18.6%
Central Maine Med. Ctr.	1151	22.6%	Osteopathic Hosp. of	443	23.0%
C.A. Dean Mem.	42	9.5%	Maine		
Down East	201	11.9%	Parkview	836	18.2%
Eastern Maine Med. Ctr.	1934	20.1%	Penobscot Bay Med. Ctr.	477	25.8%
Franklin	515	20.0%	Penobscot Valley	116	24.1%
Goodall	348	21.8%	Red-Fairview	266	27.1%
Houlton	228	33.3%	Rumford	161	19.9%
Kennebec Valley Med. Ctr.	747	20.2%	Southern Maine Med. Ctr.	540	20.6%
*Maine Med. Ctr.	3033	25.4%	Stephens	354	27.1%
Maine Coast	219	19.6%	St. Mary's	432	26.4%
Mayo Regional	214	17.3%	Waldo	198	18.2%
Mercy	620	19.5%	Waterville Osteopathic	181	21.5%
Mid-Maine Med. Ctr.	1054	14.6%	York	168	13.7%
			STATE TOTALS	**16292**	**21.5%**

Source: Maine Health Care Finance Commission "Obstetric Deliveries by Type, & Rate of Cesarean Deliveries by Hospitals, 1988 & 1989." Data on neonatal intensive care units from the American Hospital Association "1988 Guide to the Health Care Field."

Maryland 1989

Name of Facility	Total Deliveries	Cesarean Rate	Name of Facility	Total Deliveries	Cesarean Rate
Anne Arundel General	2833	30.4%	*Mercy	2638	24.8%
Calvert Mem.	685	28.2%	Montgomery General	1054	28.3%
Carroll Co. General	451	25.7%	Peninsula General	2192	26.2%
Dorchester General	313	32.3%	Physician's Mem.	507	30.8%
*Francis Scott Key Med. Ctr.	1136	19.5%	Prince George's	2996	25.1%
Franklin Square	3778	23.5%	Sacred Heart	676	19.5%
Frederick Mem.	1815	21.1%	Shady Grove Adventist	3814	27.9%
Garrett Co. Mem.	376	15.4%	*Sinai	3746	21.6%
*Greater Baltimore Med. Ctr.	4355	24.0%	South Baltimore General	2255	23.8%
			Southern Maryland	1432	38.8%
Greater Laurel Beltsville	205	32.2%	*St. Agnes	2520	19.7%
Harford Mem.	741	19.4%	St. Joseph	2322	25.2%
Holy Cross	6385	25.2%	St. Mary's	810	33.5%
Howard Co. General	2379	23.2%	Union Hosp. of Cecil Co.	432	18.3%
*Johns Hopkins	3255	22.3%	Union Mem.	1699	21.1%
Kent & Queen Anne's	206	43.2%	*U. of Maryland	1992	20.3%
Maryland General	920	14.0%	Washington Adventist	1932	31.6%
Mem. Hosp. at Easton	990	18.3%	Washington Co. Hosp	1484	21.2%
Mem. Hosp. Cumberland	636	18.9%	**STATE TOTALS**	**65960**	**24.5%**

Source: 1989 Maryland Hospital Discharge Data. Data on neonatal intensive care units from the American Hospital Association "1988 Guide to the Health Care Field."

Massachusetts 1988

Name of Facility	Total Deliveries	Cesarean Rate	Name of Facility	Total Deliveries	Cesarean Rate
Addison Gilbert	270	32.2%	Burbank	1071	12.8%
Anna Jacques	844	19.2%	Cambridge	674	14.8%
Atlanticare	976	25.6%	Cape Cod	1267	27.8%
*Bay State Med. Ctr.	6021	25.3%	Charlton Mem.	2048	22.4%
Berkshire Med. Ctr.	1390	25.1%	Cooley Dickenson	1072	24.9%
Beth Israel	5449	22.1%	Emerson	2022	18.8%
Beverly	1361	24.2%	Fairview	121	21.5%
*Boston City	1485	17.5%	Falmouth	627	31.6%
*Brigham & Women's	9982	27.2%	Framingham Union	2133	26.4%
Brockton	1203	16.6%	Franklin Med. Ctr.	914	19.5%

Name of Facility	Total Deliveries	Cesarean Rate	Name of Facility	Total Deliveries	Cesarean Rate
Goddard Mem.	2155	23.2%	New England Mem.	760	33.7%
Hale	701	20.4%	Newton-Wellesley	3027	21.6%
Harrington Mem.	615	24.1%	North Adams Regional	393	20.9%
Henry Heywood Mem.	350	18.3%	Norwood	1162	21.5%
Holy Family	1223	30.4%	Providence	1524	16.7%
Hunt Mem.	767	21.6%	Quincy City	1074	30.7%
Jordan	749	23.2%	Salem	1595	24.0%
Lawrence General	1893	22.3%	South Shore	2072	29.2%
Leominster	1289	22.1%	Sturdy Mem.	1014	28.4%
Leonard Morse	748	23.4%	St. Elizabeth's	1259	24.6%
Lowell General	2403	21.8%	St. Joseph's	601	36.6%
Malden	1947	25.4%	St. Luke's	2127	25.4%
Martha's Vineyard	160	37.5%	*St. Margaret's	3302	30.5%
Mary Lane	158	24.7%	St. Vincent's	2121	14.4%
Melrose-Wakefield	1207	33.0%	Tobey	475	19.6%
Milford-Whitinsville	564	32.1%	Waltham	672	22.8%
Morton	700	31.0%	Winchester	1664	27.5%
Mount Auburn	1308	24.0%	Worcester Hahnemann	1076	25.1%
Nantucket Cottage	89	20.2%	*Worcester Mem.	3559	27.0%
			STATE TOTALS	**89433**	**24.4%**

Source: Massachusetts Department of Public Health "Occurrence and Cesarean Births by Licensed Maternity Facility." Data on neonatal intensive care units from the American Hospital Association "1988 Guide to the Health Care Field."

Minnesota 1988

Name of Facility	Live Births	Cesarean Rate	Name of Facility	Live Births	Cesarean Rate
Abbott Northwestern	3216	25.7%	Holy Trinity	33	24.2%
Aitkin Community	68	14.7%	Hutchinson Community	377	19.1%
Albany Community	82	12.2%	Immanuel-St. Joseph's	1103	19.9%
Arlington Municipal	59	18.6%	Itasca Mem.	382	25.1%
Bethesda Lutheran	377	10.6%	Johnson Mem.	30	13.3%
Buffalo Mem.	418	19.9%	Kanabec	184	18.5%
Canby Community	52	9.6%	Karlstad Mem.	32	15.6%
Cannon Falls Community	67	6.0%	Lake City	103	23.3%
Central Mesabi Med. Ctr.	321	26.8%	Lake Region Hosp. Otter Tail	417	18.2%
Chippewa Co. Montevideo	156	18.6%			
Chisago Lakes	271	13.3%	Lakeview Mem.	59	6.8%
Clearwater Co. Community	47	4.3%	Lakeview Mem. Hosp. Washington	498	19.1%
Community Hosp. Rock Co.	156	14.7%			
Community Hosp. & HCC	117	21.4%	Long Prairie Mem.	135	15.6%
Community Mem. Hosp. Carlton Co.	153	17.6%	Madelia Community	63	11.1%
			Madison	38	31.6%
Community Mem. Hosp. Winona Co.	501	9.8%	Mahnomen Co. & Village	34	11.8%
			Meeker Co. Mem.	111	22.5%
Community Mem. Hosp. & Homestead	74	24.3%	Melrose Hosp. & Pine Villa	98	21.4%
			Mem. Hosp. Isanti Co.	415	35.7%
Community Mercy	78	24.4%	Mercy Hosp. & C & NC	87	9.2%
Cuyuna Range District	106	25.5%	Mercy Med. Ctr.	2054	17.8%
District Mem. Hosp. Washington	162	23.5%	Methodist Hosp. Hennepin	3523	19.5%
			Metropolitan Med. Ctr.	866	18.8%
Divine Redeemer Mem.	360	8.1%	Midway	961	23.0%
Douglas Co.	556	17.8%	Milaca Area	59	11.9%
Ely Bloomenson Community	60	15.0%	Minnesota Valley Mem.	51	13.7%
			Monticello Big Lake Comm.	195	24.1%
Fairmount Community	317	16.4%	Municipal Hosp & Granite Manor	86	39.5%
Fairview Princeton	212	15.1%			
Fairview Ridges	2293	18.1%	Murray Co. Mem.	45	26.7%
Fairview Southdale	2396	22.0%	Naeve	558	20.3%
Fairview & Deaconness	2770	22.7%	North Country	860	20.7%
Falls Mem.	131	26.0%	*North Mem. Med. Ctr.	3460	18.3%
Fosston Municipal	61	14.8%	Northfield City	271	17.7%
Glacial Ridge	63	14.3%	Northwestern Med. Ctr.	246	25.2%
Glencoe Area Health Ctr.	97	16.5%	Olmstead Community	934	19.1%
Hendricks Community	44	20.5%	Ortonville Municipal	91	25.3%
*Hennepin Co. Med. Ctr.	1974	11.0%	Owatonna Health Care Ctr.	399	17.5%

*indicates this facility has a neonatal intensive care unit

Name of Facility	Live Births	Cesarean Rate	Name of Facility	Live Births	Cesarean Rate
Paynesville Community	129	17.8%	St. Luke's Hosp. St. Louis	833	17.5%
Perham Mem.	132	8.3%	St. Mary's Hosp. Hennepin	1534	13.6%
Pipestone Co. Med. Ctr.	127	17.3%	Co.		
Queen of Peace	216	17.6%	St. Mary's Hosp. Detroit	395	18.7%
Redwood Falls Municipal	146	14.4%	Lakes		
Regina Mem.	329	22.8%	*St. Mary's Med. Ctr. St.	1472	23.5%
*Renville Co.	96	15.6%	Louis		
Rice Co. District 1	318	27.7%	St. Michael's	59	27.1%
Rice Mem.	874	19.9%	St. Olaf	474	22.4%
Riverview	194	20.6%	St. Paul Ramsey Med. Ctr.	1065	11.8%
Rochester Methodist	1831	20.5%	Swift County Benson	53	15.1%
Roseau Area	235	15.7%	Trinity Hosp. Lake of	57	17.5%
Rush City	49	20.4%	Woods		
Sanford Mem.	105	15.2%	Tri-County Hosp. Wadena	197	29.4%
Sioux Valley	401	23.7%	*U of Minnesota	465	27.7%
Sleepy Eye Municipal	58	37.9%	United District Hosp.	135	24.4%
Springfield Community	65	16.9%	Wadena		
Stevens Co. Mem.	128	12.5%	United Hosp. Blue Earth	97	24.7%
St. Cloud	2177	18.8%	United Hosp. Ramsey	3571	14.3%
St. Elizabeth's	81	27.2%	Unity Med. Ctr.	1974	20.3%
St. Francis Med. Ctr. Wilkin	352	33.2%	Virginia Regional Med. Ctr.	334	40.4%
St. Francis Regional Med.	765	19.3%	Waconia Ridgeview	838	16.9%
Ctr.			Waseca Area Mem.	178	23.6%
St. Gabriel's	367	21.8%	Watonwan Mem.	75	22.7%
St. John's Hosp. Red Wing	420	21.2%	Weiner Mem. Med. Ctr.	394	26.1%
St. John's Northeast Comm.	2096	12.4%	Wheaton Community	68	17.6%
St. Joseph's Hosp. Hubbard	169	21.9%	Windom Area	91	22.0%
Co.			Worthington Regional	410	17.8%
St. Joseph's Hosp. Ramsey	1633	8.7%	Zumbrota Community	32	0.0%
St. Joseph's Med. Ctr.	633	17.4%	**STATE TOTALS**	**65600**	**18.9%**

Source: Minnesota Department of Health, Center for Health Statistics. Data on neonatal intensive care units from the American Hospital Association "1988 Guide to the Health Care Field."

Missouri 1989

Name of Facility	Live Births	Cesarean Rate	Name of Facility	Live Births	Cesarean Rate
Audrain	228	22.8%	Jefferson Mem.	522	35.1%
A. M. Keller	69	2.9%	Jewish	1942	25.8%
Baptist Mem.	599	24.9%	J. Fitzgibbon	189	15.3%
Barnes	2404	20.0%	Kirksville	282	21.6%
Barton Co.	114	37.7%	Lafayette Regional	210	18.1%
Bates Co.	40	55.0%	Lake Ozark	491	26.5%
Boone Co.	1550	21.9%	Lakeside	278	19.4%
Bothwell	569	24.8%	Liberty	64	20.3%
Callaway Community	172	23.3%	Lincoln Co. Mem.	104	18.3%
Cass Co.	109	16.5%	Lucy Lee	812	19.1%
Cedar Co.	106	19.8%	Lutheran	288	25.3%
Christian	1605	28.2%	*L. E. Cox. Med. Ctr. South	3472	28.4%
Citizens Mem.	212	20.3%	Madison Co.	109	35.8%
C. E. Still	305	21.6%	Med. Ctr. Independence	829	22.8%
De Paul	1489	28.6%	Menorah Med.	1266	18.4%
Deaconess	2861	19.9%	Mercy	186	16.7%
Doctors	655	22.9%	Metro Med.	884	22.5%
Excelsior	89	12.4%	Mineral Area	561	28.9%
Fairfax Community	140	10.7%	MO Baptist Hosp. Sullivan	168	42.3%
Farmington Community	243	27.6%	MO Baptist Hosp. Twin Co.	984	24.9%
Freeman	1692	22.0%	MO Baptist Hosp.	149	24.8%
Gentry Co.	71	12.7%	Wentzville		
Golden Valley	347	31.1%	MO Delta	717	32.2%
Grim-Smith	317	35.3%	Moberly Regional Med. Ctr.	361	25.5%
G. L. Wood	492	17.5%	Nevada City	253	19.4%
G. Pershing	125	13.6%	*N. Kansas City Mem.	1569	31.2%
Hannibal Regional	505	17.4%	Oak Hill	624	14.4%
Heartland	1643	14.9%	Ozarks Med. Ctr.	579	23.0%
Hedrick Med.	388	14.7%	Pemiscot Co. Mem.	218	11.5%
Hermann	80	22.5%	Perry Co.	111	26.1%
Independence Regional	631	26.1%	Phelps Co. Mem.	1041	20.1%
Med. Ctr.			Pike Co.	79	11.4%

Name of Facility	Live Births	Cesarean Rate	Name of Facility	Live Births	Cesarean Rate
Putnam Co.	43	32.6%	St. Joseph Hosp. West	287	18.8%
*Research	1883	21.5%	St. Louis Regional Med. Ctr.	3346	10.7%
Reynolds Co.	40	37.5%	*St. Luke Hosp. Kansas City	3174	19.3%
Sac-Osage	88	25.0%	St. Luke Hosp. W. Chesterfield	2033	30.3%
Sale Mem.	59	11.9%			
Samaritan	44	13.6%	St. Mary Hosp. Jefferson City	1076	21.3%
Skaggs Community	121	31.4%			
*Southeast MO CP	1606	31.0%	St. Mary Hosp. Blue Springs	490	22.7%
Spelman Hosp. Smithville	359	24.0%			
Spelman St. Lukes	216	26.4%	St. Mary Hosp. Richmond Hts.	2800	27.9%
Springfield General	425	18.4%			
Ste. Genevieve Co.	94	25.5%	St. Peters Community	635	31.3%
St. Anthony	1282	26.8%	Texas Co.	173	27.7%
St. Francis Hosp. Mtn. View	67	11.9%	Truman M	2822	15.7%
St. Francis Hosp. Myville	273	15.0%	Truman Med. Ctr. East	1178	16.1%
*St. John Hosp. Springfield	1599	24.1%	Twin Rivers Regional	321	26.5%
*St. John's Hosp. C. Coeur	6227	28.8%	*U MO Hosp. & Clinics	1762	28.4%
*St. John's Hosp. M. Wash	595	21.8%	USAF Knob Noster	284	20.4%
*St. Joseph Hosp. Kansas City	1512	25.5%	Western MO Med. Ctr.	264	28.8%
			Wright Mem.	214	27.1%
St. Joseph Hosp. Kirkwood	998	25.3%	**STATE TOTALS**	**35663**	**23.4%**
St. Joseph Hosp. St. Charles	1516	28.1%			

Source: Missouri Department of Health "1988 & 1989 Missouri Recorded Live Births by C-Section." Data on neonatal intensive care units from the American Hospital Association "1988 Guide to the Health Care Field."

Nevada 1988

Name of Facility	Total Deliveries	Cesarean Rate	Name of Facility	Total Deliveries	Cesarean Rate
Boulder City	56	33.9%	St. Rose Dominican	446	24.7%
Carson-Tahoe	470	28.5%	Univ. Med. Ctr.	2750	18.1%
Churchill	221	27.1%	Valley	431	28.8%
Elko	420	31.2%	*Washoe Med. Ctr.	1994	26.7%
Humana Sunrise	2366	32.3%	Women's	2191	28.7%
Humboldt	53	39.6%	W. B. Ririe	97	20.6%
*St. Mary's	2456	25.3%	**STATE TOTALS**	**13951**	**26.3%**

Source: Nevada Department of Human Resources, Division of Health Resources and Cost Review "Personal Health Choices." Data on neonatal intensive care units from the American Hospital Association "1988 Guide to the Health Care Field."

New Hampshire 1-1-89 To 6-30-89

Name of Facility	Live Births	Cesarean Rate	Name of Facility	Live Births	Cesarean Rate
Alice Peck Day	152	24.3%	*Mary Hitchcock Med. Ctr.	619	22.1%
Androscoggin	113	31.0%	Memorial	175	19.4%
Catholic Med.	409	29.3%	Monadnock	245	25.7%
Cheshire	360	16.1%	Nashua Mem.	1073	17.8%
Concord	918	17.8%	Parkland Med.	310	27.4%
Elliot	1048	18.8%	Portsmouth	485	21.2%
Exeter	485	26.6%	Speare Mem.	52	34.6%
Franklin Regional	75	22.7%	St. Joseph	478	25.5%
Frisbie Mem.	341	21.1%	Upper Connecticut Valley	30	26.7%
Huggins	41	22.0%	Valley Regional	184	16.8%
Lakes Region	369	18.7%	Weeks Mem.	66	18.2%
Littleton	152	13.2%	Wentworth-Douglass	507	16.0%
			STATE TOTALS	**8687**	**20.8%**

Source: New Hampshire Hospital Association. Data on neonatal intensive care units from the American Hospital Association "1988 Guide to the Health Care Field."

*indicates this facility has a neonatal intensive care unit

New Jersey 1988

Name of Facility	Total Deliveries	Cesarean Rate	Name of Facility	Total Deliveries	Cesarean Rate
Anthony Yelencsics Community	1878	34.3%	Mountainside	1041	29.9%
			Muhlenberg	1939	18.1%
*Atlantic City Med. Ctr.	2678	28.2%	*Newark Beth Israel Med. Ctr.	2909	24.4%
Barnert Mem.	1052	38.2%			
Bayonne	415	44.6%	Newcomb	1406	21.8%
Burdette Tomlin Mem.	830	24.0%	Newton Mem.	1094	21.0%
Chilton Mem.	1530	22.6%	*Our Lady of Lourdes	2015	20.5%
Christ	1201	40.2%	*Overlook	2505	28.0%
Clara Maass Med. Ctr.	1441	31.4%	Palisades General	673	27.9%
Columbus	1143	36.5%	Pascack Valley	1493	28.9%
Community Med. Ctr.	1581	33.7%	Rahway	906	24.8%
*Cooper Med. Ctr.	2208	23.8%	Raritan Bay-Perth Amboy Div.	1319	29.3%
Dover General	1002	27.6%			
Elizabeth General	1766	34.2%	Riverview	2448	24.6%
Englewood	2260	22.6%	Robert Wood Johnson Univ.	1281	31.5%
Freehold Area	1178	32.3%			
General Hosp. Ctr. Passaic	1151	26.3%	Shore Mem.	1242	30.6%
*Hackensack Med. Ctr.	2356	35.4%	Somerset Med. Ctr.	1161	25.7%
Hackettstown Community	628	29.1%	*St. Barnabas Med. Ctr.	4404	31.4%
Helene Fuld Med. Ctr.	840	33.1%	*St. Clare Riv. Med. Ctr.	1562	27.8%
Holy Name	1422	23.1%	*St. Elizabeth	1100	27.5%
Hosp. Ctr. Orange	915	32.3%	St. Francis Med. Ctr.	660	24.1%
Hunterdon Med. Ctr.	1029	23.7%	St. James	532	48.5%
*Jersey City Med Ctr.	3067	30.4%	*St. Joseph's	2642	24.5%
*Jersey Shore Med. Ctr. Fitkin	1075	25.5%	St. Mary's Hosp. Hoboken	904	32.4%
			St. Mary's Hosp. Passaic	684	26.6%
Kennedy Mem. Hosp. Cherry Hill	2334	27.2%	St. Peter's Med. Ctr.	5106	30.7%
			S. Jersey Hosp. Syst. Bridgeton	916	16.5%
*Kimball Med. Ctr.	1049	23.1%			
Meadowland Hosp. Med. Ctr.	2018	40.3%	Underwood Mem.	1514	24.0%
			University	3862	18.3%
Med. Ctr. Princeton	1998	27.6%	Valley	3011	33.7%
Med. Ctr. Ocean Co. Brick	1408	25.1%	Warren	643	30.2%
Mem. Hosp. Burlington Co.	2078	36.1%	Wayne General	877	35.7%
Mem. Hosp. Salem Co.	512	23.8%	*West Jersey Hosp. East. Div.	4223	24.0%
Mercer Med. Ctr.	2881	21.8%			
*Monmouth Med. Ctr.	3514	26.4%	Zurbrugg Mem. Hosp. Rancocas Div.	1901	27.5%
*Morristown Mem.	2971	26.7%			
			STATE TOTALS	**113382**	**27.9%**

Source: New Jersey Department of Health from hospital discharge data. Data on neonatal intensive care units from the American Hospital Association "1988 Guide to the Health Care Field."

New York 1988

Name of Facility	Live Births	Cesarean Rate	Name of Facility	Live Births	Cesarean Rate
Hospital Service Area 1: Allegany, Cattaraugus, Chautauqua, Erie, Genesee, Niagara, Orleans, and Wyoming Counties.			*Medina Mem.	261	23.8%
			Mercy	2314	26.8%
Arnold Gregory Mem.	112	21.4%	Millard Fillmore Sub.	2392	27.7%
Bertrand Chaffee	561	26.2%	Mt. St. Mary's Niagara Falls	411	30.7%
Brooks Mem.	541	23.1%	Niagara Falls Mem. Med. Ctr.	836	31.1%
Buffalo General	1776	27.0%			
*Children's	4856	29.0%	Olean General	399	23.3%
Degraff Mem.	328	21.6%	Sisters of Charity	2448	26.5%
Genesee Mem.	593	26.6%	St. Francis	501	22.8%
Inter-Community Mem.	298	28.2%	Tri-Co. Mem.	85	14.1%
Jones Mem.	368	20.7%	Westfield Mem.	182	12.1%
Kenmore Mercy	632	20.1%	Women's Christian Assoc.	1068	17.5%
Lockport Mem.	366	34.4%	Wyoming Co. Community	443	27.5%

*indicates this facility has a neonatal intensive care unit

Name of Facility	Live Births	Cesarean Rate
Hospital Service Area 2: Chemung, Livingston, Monroe, Ontario, Schuyler, Seneca, Steuben, Wayne, and Yates Counties.		
*Arnot-Ogden Mem.	1588	24.2%
Corning	392	20.4%
F. F. Thompson	489	18.8%
Genesee	2792	18.2%
Geneva General	1047	17.7%
Highland	2926	14.5%
Ira Davenport Mem.	265	20.8%
Lakeside Mem.	472	18.2%
Myers Community Hosp. Fdtn.	277	31.4%
Newark-Wayne Community	379	32.2%
N.H. Noyes Mem.	369	24.9%
*Rochester General	2294	23.5%
Schuyler	127	28.3%
*Strong Mem.	3721	21.6%
St. James Mercy	467	35.5%
St. Joseph's	60	8.3%
St. Mary's	1212	17.7%
Hospital Service Area 3: Cayuga, Cortland, Herkimer, Jefferson, Lewis, Madison, Oneida, Onondaga, Oswego, St. Lawrence, and Tompkins Counties.		
Auburn Mem.	802	27.1%
A. Barton Hepburn	564	22.7%
Canton-Potsdam	402	16.7%
Carthage Area	189	42.9%
Community General	1484	34.2%
Community Mem.	315	20.6%
Cortland Mem.	692	27.0%
Crouse-Irving Mem.	4516	30.4%
E.J. Noble Hosp. Gouverneur	140	27.9%
House of Good Samaritan	1439	29.3%
Lewis Co. General	280	28.2%
Little Falls	346	25.4%
Massena Mem.	190	26.8%
Mercy Hosp. of Watertown	599	22.4%
Mohawk Valley General	355	40.8%
Oneida City	368	38.3%
Oswego	924	21.6%
Rome Hosp. & Murphy Mem.	661	24.5%
St. Elizabeth's	1009	34.7%
*St. Joseph's Hosp. Health Ctr.	3028	19.1%
St. Luke's Mem. Hosp. Ctr.	1454	28.7%
Tompkins Co.	1149	24.8%
Hospital Service Area 4: Broome, Chenango, and Tioga Counties.		
Charles S. Wilson Mem.	2101	30.2%
Chenango Mem.	449	16.7%
Our Lady of Lourdes Mem.	1722	22.2%
Hospital Service Area 5: Albany, Clinton, Columbia, Delaware, Essex, Franklin, Fulton, Greene, Hamilton, Montgomery, Otsego, Rensselaer, Saratoga, Schenectady, Schoharie, Warren, and Washington Counties.		
*Albany Med. Ctr	2538	34.3%
Alice Hyde Mem.	348	20.1%
Amsterdam Mem.	177	35.6%
Aurelia O. Fox Mem.	528	28.6%
Bellevue Maternity	1840	32.7%
Champlain Valley Phys.	1537	23.1%
Columbia Mem.	642	18.4%

Name of Facility	Live Births	Cesarean Rate
Community Hosp. Schoharie Co.	197	22.3%
Delaware Valley	131	30.5%
Ellis	716	26.8%
General Hosp. Saranac Lake	291	27.1%
Glens Falls	1555	28.7%
Mary Imogene Bassett	418	28.0%
Mary McClellan	215	17.7%
Mem. Hosp. Greene Co.	171	24.0%
Moses-Ludington	103	18.4%
Nathan Littauer	567	24.9%
Samaritan	1272	29.8%
Saratoga	804	27.6%
St. Clare's	894	29.9%
St. Mary's Hosp. Amsterdam	492	16.9%
St. Peter's	2796	24.2%
The Hosp.	277	18.8%
Hospital Service Area 6: Dutchess, Orange, Putnam, Rockland, Sullivan, Ulster, and Westchester Counties.		
Arden Hill	965	34.0%
Benedictine	1095	20.9%
Community General Hosp. Sull Co.	784	19.0%
E. A. Horton Mem.	1313	25.5%
Good Samaritan	1671	25.8%
Julia Butterfield Mem.	217	27.6%
Kingston	355	36.9%
Lawrence	1333	32.6%
Mercy Community	362	27.1%
Mt. Vernon	1052	25.3%
New Rochelle Hosp. Med. Ctr.	917	29.7%
Northern Dutchess	822	11.8%
Northern Westchester	1909	28.2%
Nyack	1880	31.4%
Peekskill Community	540	27.2%
Phelps Mem. Hosp. Assoc.	815	26.3%
Putnam Hosp. Ctr.	524	18.7%
St. Agnes	1022	30.8%
St. Anthony Community	429	31.9%
St. Francis Hosp. Beacon Div.	154	22.1%
St. John's Riverside	1649	31.2%
St. Lukes Hosp. Newburgh	1214	21.5%
United	745	26.3%
Vassar Brothers	2761	23.7%
*Westchester Co. Med. Ctr.	850	43.1%
White Plains Hosp. Med. Ctr.	1246	36.0%
Hospital Service Area 7: (New York City) Bronx, Kings, New York, Queens, and Richmond Counties.		
*Bellevue Hosp. Ctr.	1975	18.1%
*Beth Israel Med. Ctr.	4795	12.7%
Booth Mem. Med. Ctr.	3029	25.4%
*Bronx Municipal Med. Ctr.	3233	11.7%
*Bronx-Lebanon Hosp. Ctr.	2793	15.4%
Brookdale Hosp. & Med. Ctr.	4680	13.8%
*Brooklyn Hosp.-Caledonian	3181	25.7%
Columbia-Presbyterian Med. Ctr.	5277	19.4%
Coney Island	1803	14.1%
*Elmhurst Hosp. Ctr.	3334	13.9%
*Flushing Hosp. Med. Ctr.	4005	23.9%

Name of Facility	Live Births	Cesarean Rate	Name of Facility	Live Births	Cesarean Rate
*Harlem Hosp. Ctr.	2916	20.3%	*St. Vincent Hosp. & Med. Ctr.	2306	20.8%
Interfaith Med. Ctr.	3335	17.0%			
Jamaica	1468	20.0%	St. Vincent's Med. Ctr. Richmond	2455	26.2%
*Kings Co. Hosp. Ctr.	5136	14.4%			
LaGuardia	2082	25.9%	Union Hosp. of the Bronx	824	29.2%
*Lenox Hill	4049	28.4%	University	2436	30.0%
*Lincoln Med. Ctr.	4794	18.9%	Victory Mem.	1024	47.6%
Long Island College	3045	24.4%	Woodhull Med. & Mental Hosp. Ctr.	3452	17.2%
*Long Island Jewish Med. Ctr.	3955	28.2%			
Lutheran Med. Ctr.	2492	26.8%	**Hospital Service Area 8:** Nassau and Suffolk Counties.		
*Maimonides Med. Ctr.	4164	16.5%			
Maternity Ctr.	211	0.0%	Brookhaven Mem.	1371	19.0%
*Methodist	2510	32.8%	*Central General	937	34.0%
Metropolitan Hosp. Ctr.	2092	20.1%	Central Suffolk	475	32.2%
*Montefiore Med. Ctr.	3453	20.4%	Community Hosp. W. Suffolk	1016	33.4%
*Mt. Sinai Med. Ctr.	4717	21.3%			
*New York	3454	27.3%	Franklin General	792	26.9%
*North Central Bronx	3264	9.3%	Glen Cove Community	759	25.7%
NY Infirmary-Beekman Downtown	1673	21.8%	Good Samaritan	2836	32.1%
			Huntington	1827	25.2%
*Our Lady of Mercy Med. Ctr.	2982	24.7%	*Mercy	2060	30.0%
			Mid Island	1453	31.9%
*Queens Hosp. Ctr.	2802	12.7%	*Nassau Co. Med. Ctr.	2936	20.1%
Roosevelt	1740	25.9%	*North Shore University	5284	29.9%
*State U. NY Hlth. Sci. Ctr. Brooklyn	2070	24.3%	South Nassau Community	1713	32.3%
			Southampton	536	27.6%
*Staten Island	3113	18.5%	Southside	2205	32.7%
St. John's Episcopal Hosp. S. Shore	1283	21.1%	St. Charles	1714	36.6%
			St. John's Episcopal	1151	33.2%
*St. John's Hosp. Queens	3257	26.7%	Syosset Community	1373	25.9%
*St. Luke's Hosp. & Woman's Div.	3061	23.5%	*University	2622	13.8%
			Winthrop University	3709	24.1%
*St. Mary's Hosp. Brooklyn	2290	16.9%	**STATE TOTALS**	**279738**	**23.7%**

Source: State of New York Department of Health, "Selected Health Statistics for Hospitals, Upstate New York", and New York City Department of Health, "Hospital Births by Mode of Delivery." Data on neonatal intensive care units from the American Hospital Association "1988 Guide to the Health Care Field."

North Carolina 1989

Name of Facility	Live Births	Cesarean Rate	Name of Facility	Live Births	Cesarean Rate
Alamance Co.	488	28.7%	Duplin General	397	23.4%
Albemarle	940	26.4%	Durham Co. General	2239	22.4%
Annie Penn Mem.	353	24.4%	Edgecombe General	764	19.4%
Anson Co.	270	20.4%	Forsyth Mem.	5642	25.8%
Ashe Mem.	46	13.0%	*Frye Regional Med. Ctr.	889	29.8%
Beaufort Co.	482	24.9%	Gaston Mem.	2160	18.0%
Betsy Johnson Mem.	292	32.9%	Grace	785	27.9%
Bladen Co.	116	21.6%	Granville	312	24.4%
Brunswick Co.	211	27.5%	Halifax Mem.	964	24.6%
Cabarrus Mem.	1281	26.1%	Haywood Co.	259	11.2%
Caldwell Mem.	415	27.7%	High Point Mem.	1903	28.0%
Cape Fear Mem.	439	26.2%	Hugh Chatham Mem.	212	30.2%
*Cape Fear Valley	4641	20.7%	Iredell Mem.	958	29.1%
Carteret General	510	31.8%	Johnston Mem.	505	19.0%
Catawba Mem.	1380	19.2%	Lenoir Mem.	839	28.2%
Central Carolina	841	22.4%	Lexington Mem.	566	26.9%
*Charlotte Mem.	4106	16.6%	Lincoln Co.	455	29.2%
Chatham	174	20.7%	Lowrance	144	18.8%
Chowan	409	25.4%	Lula Conrad Hoots Mem.	130	22.3%
Cleveland Mem.	1350	18.5%	Margaret R. Pardee Mem.	403	21.3%
Columbus Co.	673	17.2%	Maria Parham	674	26.4%
Community General	514	32.9%	Martin General	173	32.4%
Craven Regional Med. Ctr.	1101	23.0%	McDowell	328	29.0%
C.J. Harris Community	940	27.4%	Mem. Hosp. Ala. Co.	675	19.7%
Davis Community	455	27.7%	*Mem. Mission Hos. Wnc	3123	25.3%
*Duke University Med. Ctr.	2776	19.0%	Mercy Hosp. South	571	14.2%

Name of Facility	Live Births	Cesarean Rate	Name of Facility	Live Births	Cesarean Rate
Montgomery Mem.	231	22.1%	Rowan Mem.	1165	20.6%
Moore Regional	1308	37.8%	Rutherford	760	17.2%
Morehead Mem.	658	21.4%	Sampson Co. Mem.	582	22.2%
*Moses H. Cone Mem.	3643	28.1%	Scotland Mem.	939	22.5%
Mountain Park Med. Ctr.	38	39.5%	Sloop Mem.	104	15.4%
Murphy Med. Ctr.	139	30.9%	Southeastern General	1224	21.9%
Nash General	1413	22.9%	Spruce Pine Community	176	21.6%
*Naval	825	21.7%	Stanly Co.	487	25.7%
Naval Regional Med. Ctr.	993	19.4%	Tactical Hosp. USAF	412	20.4%
*New Hanover Mem.	2328	22.8%	Transylvania Community	264	13.6%
*North Carolina Mem.	2126	18.4%	Union Mem.	748	20.9%
Northern Hosp Surry Co.	538	11.0%	University Mem.	414	34.8%
Onslow Mem.	2255	22.8%	Valdese General	420	22.9%
Park Ridge	372	27.7%	*Wake Co. Med. Ctr.	3964	17.1%
*Pitt Co. Mem.	2691	30.4%	Washington Co.	97	28.9%
*Presbyterian	6737	28.1%	Watauga	841	30.4%
Randolph	488	18.6%	Wayne Co. Mem.	1322	15.3%
Rex	3749	25.5%	Wesley Long	1284	26.9%
Richmond Mem.	434	21.7%	Wilkes General	612	33.2%
Roanoke-Chowan	594	16.3%	Wilson Mem.	1285	31.1%
			Womack Army Community	2195	15.2%
			STATE TOTALS	**102128**	**23.5%**

Source: North Carolina Department of Environment, Health, & Natural Resources, Department of Human Resources, Divison of Health Services, "1989 Percent C-Sections by Hospital." Data on neonatal intensive care units from the American Hospital Association "1988 Guide to the Health Care Field."

North Dakota 1989

Name of Facility	Total Deliveries	Cesarean Rate	Name of Facility	Total Deliveries	Cesarean Rate
Carrington Health Ctr.	59	30.5%	Northwood Deaconess	36	5.6%
Cavalier Co. Mem.	65	18.5%	Pembina Co. Mem.	97	27.8%
Community Mem.	182	15.9%	Presentation Med. Ctr.	132	12.1%
County Mem.	40	27.5%	*St. Alexius Med. Ctr.	962	12.2%
Dakota	583	17.0%	St. Aloisius Med. Ctr.	41	9.8%
Good Samaritan	47	19.1%	St. Andrew's	39	0.0%
Grand Forks AFB	369	19.5%	St. Ansgar's	40	37.5%
IHS Hosp. Belcourt	94	8.5%	St. John's	567	16.2%
IHS Hosp. Fort Yates	45	0.0%	St. Joseph's Hosp. Dickinson	450	18.4%
Jamestown	317	18.0%			
Linton	63	27.0%	St. Joseph's Hosp. Minot	382	20.4%
McKenzie Co. Mem.	42	7.1%	*St. Luke's	1485	18.9%
*Medcenter One	715	19.0%	*Trinity Med. Ctr.	704	31.4%
Mercy Hosp. Valley City	137	13.1%	Union	47	8.5%
Mercy Hosp. Devil's Lake	355	25.1%	*United	1404	19.6%
Mercy Hosp. Williston	415	31.3%	Unity	76	18.4%
Minot AFB	489	19.8%	**STATE TOTALS**	**10479**	**19.4%**

Source: North Dakota State Department of Health "Cesarean Section Annual Report 1989." Data on neonatal intensive care units from the American Hospital Association "1988 Guide to the Health Care Field."

*indicates this facility has a neonatal intensive care unit

Ohio 1988

Name of Facility	Total Deliveries	Cesarean Rate	Name of Facility	Total Deliveries	Cesarean Rate
Akron City	3081	31.8%	Lancaster-Fairfield Community	942	30.3%
Akron General Med. Ctr.	1497	31.3%	Lawrence Co. General	88	37.5%
Allen Mem.	458	21.2%	Licking Mem.	850	23.9%
Alliance Community	322	18.6%	Lima Mem.	662	25.7%
Amherst	324	22.5%	Madison Co.	139	17.3%
Ashtabula Co. Med. Ctr.	391	23.5%	Mansfield General	1050	19.0%
*Aultman	2203	24.3%	Marietta Mem.	673	24.5%
Barberton Citizens	469	23.5%	Marion General	927	21.7%
Bellevue	71	22.5%	Mary Rutan	406	21.2%
Bethesda	759	28.3%	Marymount	870	23.3%
Bethesda Oak	3425	28.8%	Massillon Community	238	32.4%
Blanchard Valley	988	19.5%	McCullough-Hyde Mem.	461	19.7%
Bluffton Community	224	25.9%	Medina Community	569	29.5%
Brentwood	153	26.1%	Med. Ctr. Hospital	797	29.1%
Brown Co. General	271	11.4%	Mem. Hosp. Geneva	182	22.0%
Brown Mem.	103	23.3%	Mem. Hosp. Sandusky Co.	707	22.3%
Bucyrus Community	111	14.4%	Mem. Hosp. Union Co.	273	31.5%
Christ	4595	30.0%	Mercer Co. Jt. Twp. Community	606	15.3%
City	89	23.6%	Mercy Hosp. Lucas	412	29.4%
Clinton Mem.	365	20.0%	Mercy Hosp. Tiffin	383	19.1%
Community Hosp. Bedford	374	20.3%	Mercy Hosp. Willard Co.	129	25.6%
Community Hosp. Springfield	1386	20.9%	Meridia Euclid	1337	32.5%
Community Hosp. Williams Co.	509	23.8%	Meridia Hillcrest	2802	29.5%
Community Mem.	90	24.4%	Metrohealth Hosp. for Women	472	24.8%
Coshocton Co. Mem.	297	28.3%	Metrohealth Med. Ctr.	1042	26.1%
Cuyahoga Falls General	116	28.4%	*Miami Valley	2438	29.9%
Deaconess Hosp. of Cleveland	714	36.3%	Middletown Regional	731	18.3%
Defiance	445	22.2%	Morrow Co.	103	11.7%
*Doctors Hosp. North	659	34.6%	Mt. Carmel Med. Ctr.	2541	19.8%
Doctors Hosp. Stark Co.	373	39.9%	Mt. Sinai Med. Ctr.	982	29.1%
Dunlap Mem.	280	26.8%	*Ohio State U.	2401	24.9%
East Liverpool City	229	24.0%	Ohio Valley	543	19.2%
Elyria Mem.	827	24.8%	Our Lady of Mercy	1048	22.6%
*Fairview General	3744	23.8%	O'Bleness Mem.	359	23.4%
Fayette Co. Mem.	270	38.1%	Parkview	250	17.6%
Firelands Community Hosp. Decatur	797	26.1%	Parma Community General	1113	34.9%
Fisher-Titus Med. Ctr.	551	22.1%	Paulding Co.	116	15.5%
Flower Mem. & Lake Park	705	26.8%	Piqua Mem. Med. Ctr.	487	33.7%
Fostoria City	135	23.7%	*Riverside	680	38.5%
Ft. Hamilton-Hughes Mem.	1152	28.6%	*Riverside Methodist	4163	24.0%
Fulton Co. Health Ctr.	351	21.7%	Robinson Mem.	751	28.4%
Geauga	525	17.0%	Salem Community	531	28.8%
*Good Samaritan Hosp. Hamilton Co.	4611	29.5%	Samaritan Hosp. Ashland	437	28.4%
*Good Samaritan Hosp. Montgomery Co.	1502	22.6%	Scioto Mem.	746	25.3%
Good Samaritan Med. Ctr.	425	24.9%	Selby General	53	26.4%
*Grady Mem.	281	19.2%	Shelby Mem.	280	26.1%
Grandview Hosp. & Med. Ctr.	464	25.9%	Southwest General	1315	32.3%
*Grant Med. Ctr.	2708	26.8%	Stouder Mem.	409	33.0%
Greene Mem.	400	33.0%	St. Alexis Hosp. Med. Ctr.	96	13.5%
Guernsey Mem.	376	17.0%	St. Ann's	3034	23.6%
Hardin Mem.	135	21.5%	St. Charles	603	28.7%
Henry Co.	128	14.1%	*St. Elizabeth	2083	27.7%
Highland District	190	28.9%	St. Elizabeth Med. Ctr.	1630	21.8%
Holzer Med. Ctr.	535	35.5%	St. John & West Shore	814	23.1%
H.B. Magruder Mem.	59	23.7%	St. Joseph Hosp. & Health Ctr.	536	31.7%
Jewish Hosp. of Cincinnati	1101	33.2%	St. Joseph Riverside	492	35.6%
Joel Pomerene Mem.	550	19.3%	*St. Luke's Hosp. Cuyahoga Co.	1333	20.9%
Joint Township District Mem.	469	17.1%	St. Rita's Med. Ctr.	1571	20.6%
*Kettering Mem.	1900	26.1%	St. Thomas Med. Ctr.	532	25.8%
Knox Community	291	26.8%	*St. Vincent Med. Ctr.	978	19.6%
Lake East	1492	27.5%	*Timken Mercy Med. Ctr.	1047	27.3%
			*Toledo	3917	25.2%
			Trumbull Mem.	1035	33.2%
			Union Hosp. Association	567	27.3%

Name of Facility	Live Births	Cesarean Rate	Name of Facility	Live Births	Cesarean Rate
*University Hosp. of Cleveland	1843	25.4%	Wilson Mem.	295	15.3%
			Wood Co.	475	25.3%
*U. of Cincinnati	1209	27.5%	Wooster Community	725	15.4%
Van Wert Co.	267	31.8%	Wyandot Mem.	80	33.8%
Wadsworth-Rittman	352	22.4%	YHA Northside Med. Ctr.	716	29.7%
Warren General	135	41.5%	Youngstown Osteopathic	47	0.0%
Wayne	413	15.7%	**STATE TOTALS**	**118364**	**26.1%**

Source: Ohio Department of Health from hospital discharge data. Data on neonatal intensive care units from the American Hospital Association "1988 Guide to the Health Care Field."

Oregon 1988

Name of Facility	Total Deliveries	Cesarean Rate	Name of Facility	Total Deliveries	Cesarean Rate
Albany General	589	19.4%	Mercy Med. Ctr.	608	23.8%
Ashland Community	231	28.1%	Merle West Med. Ctr.	812	15.0%
Bay Area	639	32.2%	Mid-Columbia Med. Ctr.	307	24.8%
*Bess Kaiser	2097	20.0%	Mountain View	206	23.8%
Blue Mountain	72	25.0%	Newberg Community	181	23.2%
Central Oregon District	155	30.3%	North Lincoln	86	22.1%
Columbia Mem.	290	20.3%	Pacific Communities	212	25.9%
Coquille Valley	70	31.4%	Pioneer Mem. Hosp.	112	22.3%
Cottage Grove	198	18.7%	Prineville		
Curry General	70	14.3%	Portland Adventist Med.	1910	25.7%
Douglas Community	350	20.9%	Ctr.		
Dwyer Community	308	34.1%	Providence Med. Ctr.	863	23.5%
Eastmoreland General	135	29.6%	*Rogue Valley Med. Ctr.	1649	19.4%
*Emanuel	1928	30.7%	Salem	2784	19.6%
Forest Glen	41	19.5%	Seaside General	164	24.4%
Forest Grove Community	253	19.4%	Silverton	304	18.1%
Good Samaritan Med. Ctr.	2347	18.7%	*Sacred Heart General	2460	24.3%
*Good Samaritan	987	25.8%	St. Anthony	324	21.6%
Good Shepherd	354	15.8%	St. Charles Med. Ctr.	1010	27.4%
Community			St. Elizabeth Community	121	26.4%
Grande Ronde	368	17.9%	St. Helens	48	35.4%
Harney Co.	40	15.0%	St. Vincent	2400	17.5%
Holy Rosary	563	17.4%	Tillamook Co. General	156	31.4%
Hood River Mem.	232	18.1%	Tuality Community	719	21.7%
Josephine Mem.	742	14.2%	University	2779	20.4%
Kaiser Sunnyside Med. Ctr.	1405	13.3%	Valley Community	218	24.3%
Lake District	92	21.7%	Wallowa Mem.	39	28.2%
Lebanon Community	396	18.4%	Western Lane	103	19.4%
Lower Umpqua	97	15.5%	Willamette Falls	690	31.9%
McKenzie-Willamette	694	32.3%	Woodland Park	624	24.8%
McMinnville Community	471	17.6%	**STATE TOTALS**	**38103**	**22.0%**

Source: Oregon Department of Human Resources, Office of Health Policy, from hospital discharge data. Data on neonatal intensive care units from the American Hospital Association "1988 Guide to the Health Care Field."

*indicates this facility has a neonatal intensive care unit

Pennsylvania 1988

Name of Facility	Total Deliveries	Cesarean Rate	Name of Facility	Total Deliveries	Cesarean Rate
*Abington Mem.	3114	19.9%	*Hamot Med. Ctr.	1843	18.7%
*Albert Einstein Med. Ctr.	1478	19.4%	*Hanover General	791	20.2%
Allegheny General	1636	24.3%	*Harrisburg	3485	27.7%
Allegheny Valley	742	23.5%	Hazleton-St. Joseph Med.	688	20.6%
*Allentown Hosp.	3053	28.1%	Ctr.		
Association			*Holy Redeemer	1789	25.0%
Allentown Osteopathic	593	20.2%	Holy Spirit	576	30.9%
*Altoona	1414	27.3%	*Hosp. of Phila College of	564	42.9%
Andrew Kaul Mem.	253	24.9%	Osteo. Med.		
Armstrong Co. Mem.	636	33.5%	*Hosp. of U. of	3204	21.4%
Barnes-Kasson Co.	166	24.1%	Pennsylvania		
Berwick Hosp. Ctr.	365	29.0%	Hyman S. Caplan Good	1071	19.8%
Bloomsburg	498	18.5%	Samaritan		
Booth Maternity Ctr.	864	16.2%	Indiana	725	25.4%
Bradford	283	20.1%	Jameson Mem.	793	22.6%
Brandywine	858	17.0%	Jeanes	510	28.4%
*Bryn Mawr	1907	15.9%	Jeannette District Mem.	485	27.2%
Butler Mem.	983	21.9%	J.C. Blair Mem.	373	28.4%
Carlisle	926	20.8%	*Lancaster General	2636	23.1%
Centre Community	1194	17.6%	*Lankenau	2137	33.8%
Chambersburg	803	23.8%	Latrobe Area	980	25.7%
Charles Cole Mem.	355	16.6%	Lee	421	22.1%
Chester Co.	1849	24.0%	Lewistown	818	25.9%
Chestnut Hill	1349	22.7%	Lock Haven	399	17.3%
Citizens General	408	20.6%	Lower Bucks	1290	32.0%
Clarion	243	20.6%	*Magee Women's	9779	21.7%
Clearfield	394	30.7%	McKeesport	682	23.3%
Coaldale State General	82	35.4%	Meadville City	660	10.8%
Columbia	137	24.1%	*Med. College of PA	1991	19.2%
Community General	817	28.2%	Med. Ctr. Beaver	1531	27.8%
Community General	255	31.0%	Mem. Hosp. Bedford Co.	324	34.0%
Osteopathic			Mem. Hosp. Roxborough	335	27.2%
Community Hosp. Kane	80	23.8%	Mem. Hosp. Towanda	319	29.8%
*Community Hosp.	1060	28.5%	Mem. Hosp. York	551	19.4%
Lancaster			*Mercy Catholic Med. Ctr.	1805	28.5%
*Community Med. Ctr.	2053	29.8%	Fitzgerald		
*Conemaugh Valley Mem.	1101	28.3%	Mercy Hosp. Altoona	454	35.9%
Corry Mem.	319	25.1%	Mercy Hosp. Johnstown	328	19.2%
*Crozer Chester Med. Ctr.	2426	23.4%	*Mercy Hosp. Pittsburgh	767	16.9%
Delaware Co. Mem.	1196	23.6%	Mercy Hosp. Scranton	883	23.3%
Divine Providence Hosp.	375	22.9%	Mercy Hosp. Wilkes Barre	65	30.8%
Williamsport			Methodist	1518	24.4%
Doylestown	850	25.1%	Metropolitan Health Ctr.	100	20.0%
*DuBois Regional Med. Ctr.	819	34.8%	Metropolitan Hosp. Central	221	20.8%
Easton	869	25.5%	Div.		
Elk Co. General	191	41.4%	Metropolitan Hosp.	702	23.8%
Ellwood City	289	27.3%	Parkview		
Ephrata Community	678	19.5%	Metropolitan Hosp.	104	49.0%
*Episcopal	1653	15.3%	Springfield		
Evangelical Community	1069	19.1%	Meyersdale Community	94	13.8%
*Forbes Regional Health	1239	18.4%	Millcreek Community	216	10.6%
Ctr.			Monongahela Valley	364	29.1%
Frankford	1909	26.6%	Montefiore Hosp. Assoc. W.	294	37.8%
Franklin Regional Med. Ctr.	472	24.8%	PA		
Frick Community Hlth. Ctr.	642	21.3%	*Montgomery	782	21.4%
Fulton Co. Med. Ctr.	232	24.6%	Montrose General	91	11.0%
*Geisinger Med. Ctr.	1252	30.8%	Nason	152	23.7%
Geisinger Wyoming Valley	551	28.1%	*Nazareth	956	28.0%
Med. Ctr.			Nesbitt Mem.	2041	25.3%
Germantown Hosp. & Med.	761	27.7%	Neumann Med. Ctr.	272	32.7%
Ctr.			North Hills Passavant	1268	25.7%
Gettysburg	678	24.2%	North Penn	945	24.9%
Gnaden Huetten Mem.	367	31.3%	Northeastern Hosp. of Phil.	962	20.6%
Good Samaritan Hosp.	638	18.5%	Ohio Valley General	470	35.1%
Pottsville			Oil City Area Health Ctr.	488	21.1%
Grand View	1282	27.1%	Palmerton	104	26.9%
Greene Co. Mem.	275	23.3%	*Pennsylvania	4654	29.0%
Greenville Regional	672	29.3%	Philisburg State General	230	22.2%
*Hahnemann U	1868	17.8%	Phoenixville	1205	13.9%

Name of Facility	Total Deliveries	Cesarean Rate	Name of Facility	Total Deliveries	Cesarean Rate
Pocono	1001	27.9%	St. Joseph Hosp. Carbondale	288	26.4%
*Polyclinic Med. Ctr.	1769	21.7%	St. Lukes Hosp. Bethlehem	2184	21.8%
Pottstown Mem. Med. Ctr.	752	26.5%	St. Mary Hosp. Langhorne	1427	34.1%
Pottsville Hosp. & Warne Clinic	434	19.8%	*St. Vincent Health Ctr.	1768	25.2%
Punxsutawney Area	197	22.8%	Suburban General	468	29.5%
*Reading Hosp. & Med. Ctr.	2264	18.0%	Sunbury Community	240	22.5%
Riddle Mem.	954	29.2%	*Temple U.	2081	21.0%
Rolling Hill	1802	30.7%	*Thomas Jefferson U.	2930	20.8%
Sacred Heart Hosp. Allentown	991	27.1%	Titusville	162	34.0%
Sacred Heart Hosp. Norristown	679	23.9%	Tyler Mem.	314	26.1%
Sacred Heart Med. Ctr.	496	20.8%	Tyrone	105	53.3%
Sewickley Valley	948	17.2%	Union City Mem.	103	22.3%
Shadyside	380	22.6%	Uniontown	907	28.2%
Shamokin State General	94	17.0%	United Community	330	31.8%
Sharon General	744	16.9%	Warren General	486	21.8%
Soldiers & Sailors Mem.	414	22.0%	Washington	1012	13.2%
Somerset Community	456	22.4%	Wayne Co. Mem.	368	20.4%
St. Clair Mem.	1589	30.7%	Waynesboro	664	17.0%
St. Francis Hosp. & Med. Ctr.	664	29.4%	*Western Pennsylvania	1915	26.1%
St. Joseph Hosp. Lancaster	1595	20.6%	Westmoreland Hosp. Association	668	26.0%
St. Joseph Hosp. Reading	956	21.8%	Wilkes Barre General	518	19.3%
			Williamsport	1318	23.5%
			Windber	246	32.1%
			*York	2988	18.3%
			STATE TOTALS	**162475**	**23.9%**

Source: Pennsylvania Department of Health, State Health Data Center, Harrisburg, Pennsylvania. The Department specifically disclaims responsibility for any analyses, interpretations or conclusions. Data on neonatal intensive care units from the American Hospital Association "1988 Guide to the Health Care Field."

Rhode Island 1988

Name of Facility	Total Deliveries	Cesarean Rate	Name of Facility	Total Deliveries	Cesarean Rate
Kent	1505	23.4%	South Co.	405	25.9%
Landmark	785	20.4%	St. Joseph's	551	21.8%
Newport	885	26.6%	Westerly	648	27.0%
Pawtucket Mem.	681	30.8%	*Women & Infants	9095	20.9%
			STATE TOTALS	**14555**	**22.4%**

Source: Rhode Island Department of Health Epidemiology Unit, Family Health "Cesarean Section Data for Rhode Island Occurrence Births by Hospital 1988." Data on neonatal intensive care units from the American Hospital Association "1988 Guide to the Health Care Field."

South Carolina 1989

Name of Facility	Total Deliveries	Cesarean Rate	Name of Facility	Total Deliveries	Cesarean Rate
Abbeville Co.	116	31.0%	Clarendon Mem.	270	11.9%
Allen Bennett Mem.	244	31.6%	Colleton Regional	364	13.5%
Allendale Co.	111	0.0%	Conway	677	27.9%
Anderson Mem.	2049	22.7%	East Cooper Community	551	27.4%
Bailey Mem.	70	35.7%	Elliott White Springs Mem.	532	22.2%
Bamberg Co. Mem.	56	17.9%	Florence General	32	34.4%
*Baptist (Columbia) Med. Ctr.	3056	29.5%	Georgetown Mem.	776	25.3%
			*Greenville Mem. Med. Ctr.	4952	25.4%
Baptist (Easley) Med. Ctr.	356	18.0%	HCA Aiken Regional Med. Ctr.	951	22.8%
Beaufort Mem.	1180	27.5%			
Bon Secours St. Francis Xavier	875	21.7%	HCA Grand Strand General	830	17.1%
			Hilton Head	273	26.7%
Byerly	256	24.2%	Kershaw Co. Mem.	247	19.0%
Chester Co.	371	20.8%	Laurens District	253	29.6%
Chesterfield General	278	30.2%	Lexington Med. Ctr.	2165	22.4%

*indicates this facility has a neonatal intensive care unit

Name of Facility	Total Deliveries	Cesarean Rate	Name of Facility	Total Deliveries	Cesarean Rate
Loris Community	339	19.5%	Roper	1323	24.7%
Marion Mem.	317	30.6%	*Self Mem.	1879	26.7%
Marlboro Park	205	24.4%	*Spartanburg Regional Med. Ctr.	1827	20.5%
*Mary Black Mem.	1548	23.9%			
*McLeod Regional	2745	28.0%	St. Eugene Community	232	28.9%
Mullins	377	26.5%	Trident Regional Med. Ctr.	1649	22.1%
*Med. University S. Carolina Med Ctr.	2974	14.8%	Tuomey	1546	20.8%
			Upstate Carolina Med. Ctr.	305	25.2%
Newberry Co. Mem.	285	15.8%	Wallace Thomson	187	27.3%
Oconee Mem.	361	17.5%	Wilson Clinic	235	30.2%
Piedmont Med. Ctr.	1563	17.0%	**STATE TOTALS**	**46357**	**23.2%**
Regional Med. Ctr. Oburg	1597	17.7%			
*Richland Mem.	2972	23.8%			

Source: South Carolina State Budget and Control Board, Division of Research and Statistical Services, derived from hospital discharge data. Data on neonatal intensive care units from the American Hospital Association "1988 Guide to the Health Care Field."

Tennessee 1988

Name of Facility	Total Deliveries	Cesarean Rate	Name of Facility	Total Deliveries	Cesarean Rate
*Baptist Hosp. Memphis	5052	37.4%	John W. Harton	481	4.4%
Baptist Hosp. Nashville	4969	29.1%	*Johnson City Med. Ctr.	1631	22.1%
Baptist Hosp. Roane Co.	131	30.5%	Laughlin Mem.	501	15.6%
Baptist Hosp. Tipton	313	36.4%	Lewis Community	48	22.9%
Baptist Hosp. Union City	501	29.5%	Lewisburg Community	92	19.6%
Bedford Co. General	236	20.3%	Lexington Methodist	97	16.5%
Blanchfield Army	763	22.3%	Lincoln Regional	154	26.0%
Blount Mem.	816	27.9%	Livingston Regional	244	32.8%
Bradley Co. Mem.	1078	24.6%	Loudon Co. Mem.	157	22.3%
Bristol Mem.	494	21.1%	Madison	297	14.1%
Carthage General	66	12.1%	Maury Co.	1338	6.1%
City of Milan	42	11.9%	McNairy Co. General	309	29.4%
Clarksville Mem.	977	13.5%	Med. Ctr. Manchester	65	33.8%
Cocke Co. Baptist	255	16.1%	Methodist Hosp. Dyer	722	33.2%
Coffee Med.	67	31.3%	Methodist Hosp. McKenzie	236	15.3%
Cookeville General	962	15.8%	*Methodist Hosp. Memphis	1921	1.6%
Cumberland Med.	656	24.1%	*Methodist Hosp. North	539	3.0%
Dekalb General	92	27.2%	Methodist Hosp. Oak Ridge	948	28.6%
Donelson	686	13.4%	Methodist Hosp. Somerville	146	13.0%
*Erlanger Med. Ctr.	3449	24.3%	Middle TN Med. Ctr.	1480	25.6%
Franklin Co. Regional	509	29.3%	Moristown Hamblen	877	20.0%
Ft. Sanders Regional	1861	31.6%	*Nashville General	1396	11.7%
*G. W. Hubbard	423	18.7%	Nashville Mem.	450	30.0%
Gibson General	130	20.8%	Naval	461	14.8%
Goodlark	443	36.1%	Perry Mem.	45	44.4%
Hardin Co. General	35	31.4%	*Regional Med. Ctr. Memphis	6697	5.3%
Harriman City	181	16.6%	Rhea Co.	131	24.4%
Hawkins Co. Mem.	152	22.4%	River Park	349	15.8%
Haywood Park	241	19.1%	Scott Mem.	165	22.4%
HCA Athens Community	392	14.8%	Smith Co. Mem.	81	39.5%
HCA Crockett	352	28.7%	St. Francis	714	31.5%
HCA Hendersonville	448	31.9%	St. Joseph	671	1.3%
HCA Humboldt Cedarcrest	93	29.0%	St. Mary's Med. Ctr.	1893	25.8%
HCA Southern Hills Med. Ctr.	542	25.6%	St. Sanders Sevier	339	18.9%
HCA Stones River	36	5.6%	Summer Co. Mem.	590	16.9%
HCA Volunteer	261	37.2%	Sweetwater	136	21.3%
*HCA West Side	1904	25.7%	Sycamore Shoals	392	7.7%
Henry Co. General	106	26.4%	Takoma Adventist	216	21.8%
Highland	76	18.4%	Trinity	35	5.7%
Hillside	35	17.1%	U. of Tennessee Mem.	3209	31.4%
Holston Valley	1032	43.9%	University Med. Ctr.	402	22.1%
Humana E. Ridge	1435	33.0%	Vanderbilt U.	1366	24.2%
Humana McFarland	286	16.8%	White Co. Community	105	16.2%
Indian Path	254	36.2%	Whitwell Med. Ctr.	34	23.5%
Jackson Madison	2880	28.4%	Williamson Med. Ctr.	422	20.9%
Jellico Community	220	63.6%	**STATE TOTALS**	**68948**	**22.8%**
Jesse Hol. Jones	434	6.2%			

Source: Tennessee Department of Health and Environment. Data on neonatal intensive care units from the American Hospital Association "1988 Guide to the Health Care Field."

Utah 1988

Name of Facility	Live Births	Cesarean Rate	Name of Facility	Live Births	Cesarean Rate
Alta View	1313	25.2%	Jordan Valley Holy Cross	426	16.7%
American Fork	1123	16.0%	Kane Co.	57	17.5%
Bear River Valley	100	17.0%	Lakeview	1050	24.2%
Beaver Valley	71	28.2%	*LDS	4144	18.9%
Brigham City	533	22.9%	*McKay Dee	2953	17.7%
Castleview	456	17.5%	Pioneer Valley	646	17.0%
Central Valley Med. Ctr.	68	30.9%	Sanpete Valley	119	16.8%
Cottonwood	2803	21.6%	Sevier Valley	211	17.1%
Davis North Med. Ctr.	803	19.2%	St. Benedict's	1295	15.2%
Delta Community	94	20.2%	St. Marks	1934	25.5%
*Dixie Med. Ctr.	1121	22.3%	Tooele Valley	153	22.2%
Duchesne Co.	503	20.1%	*University of Utah	1897	24.1%
Fillmore	66	22.7%	*Utah Valley	3736	16.9%
Garfield Mem.	92	22.8%	Valley View	362	25.1%
Gunnison Valley	133	19.5%	Wasatch Co.	144	19.4%
Hill AFB	440	22.0%			
Holy Cross	2764	18.6%	**STATE TOTALS**	**31610**	**20.0%**

Source: Utah Department of Health, Bureau of Vital Records and Health Statistics. Note: tabulations limited to hospitals with cesarean rates of 15 per 100 live births or more. Data on neonatal intensive care units from the American Hospital Association "1988 Guide to the Health Care Field."

Vermont 1988

Name of Facility	Total Deliveries	Cesarean Rate	Name of Facility	Total Deliveries	Cesarean Rate
Brattleboro	497	17.3%	Northwestern Med. Ctr.	351	24.2%
Central VT	727	16.8%	Porter	420	10.5%
Copley	266	18.0%	Rockingham	53	18.9%
Gifford Mem.	385	17.1%	Rutland	801	24.0%
*Med. Ctr.(MCHV)	2725	18.3%	Southwestern Med. Ctr.	582	25.6%
North Country	290	13.4%	Springfield	289	32.2%
Northeast VT Regional	309	24.3%	**STATE TOTALS**	**7695**	**19.6%**

Source: Vermont Department of Health, Agency of Human Services, "Type of Delivery by Place of Birth." Data on neonatal intensive care units from the American Hospital Association "1988 Guide to the Health Care Field."

West Virginia 1989

Name of Facility	Total Deliveries	Cesarean Rate	Name of Facility	Total Deliveries	Cesarean Rate
Bluefield Community	563	26.8%	Reynolds Mem.	162	42.0%
*Cabell Huntington	1715	23.3%	Roane General	152	20.4%
Camden-Clark Mem.	550	32.4%	Stonewall Jackson Mem.	219	17.4%
Charleston Area Med. Ctr.	3158	23.7%	St. Joseph's Buchannon	290	24.1%
City	895	20.6%	St. Joseph's Parkersburg	836	21.3%
Davis Mem.	533	28.9%	St. Mary's	283	37.1%
Fairmount General	599	17.4%	Summers Co.	57	29.8%
Grant Mem.	127	14.2%	Summersville Mem.	222	12.6%
Jackson General	85	18.8%	Thomas Mem.	337	32.3%
Jefferson Mem.	240	30.4%	United Hosp. Ctr.	853	31.3%
Logan General	730	24.9%	Weirton Med. Ctr.	294	18.7%
Monongalta General	341	38.4%	Welch Emergency	253	19.8%
Ohio Valley Med. Ctr.	534	29.0%	Wetzel Co.	220	22.3%
Pleasant Valley	205	21.0%	Wheeling	1258	32.4%
Preston Mem.	110	16.4%	Williamson Mem.	155	49.7%
Princeton Community	470	34.3%	*WV University	780	29.6%
Raleigh General	1459	18.2%	**STATE TOTALS**	**18767**	**25.4%**

Source: West Virginia Health Care Cost Review Authority from hospital discharge data. Note: tabulations are for estimated 85% of 1989 non-Medicare data. Data on neonatal intensive care units from the American Hospital Association "1988 Guide to the Health Care Field."

*indicates this facility has a neonatal intensive care unit

Washington 1989

Name of Facility	Total Deliveries	Cesarean Rate	Name of Facility	Total Deliveries	Cesarean Rate
Auburn General	793	27.7%	Our Lady of Lourdes	631	23.1%
Ballard	407	20.4%	Overlake Hosp. Med. Ctr.	2436	23.0%
Cascade Valley	270	25.6%	Prosser Mem.	346	17.1%
Central Washington	1128	23.2%	Providence Centralia Mem.	512	14.8%
Columbia Basin	36	5.6%	Providence Hosp. Centralia	660	19.5%
Community Mem.	314	2.5%	Providence Med. Ctr.	1279	19.8%
Coulee Community	37	24.3%	Seattle		
Deaconess Med. Ctr.	1647	21.6%	Pullman Mem.	300	22.7%
*Evergreen General	2084	22.4%	Quincy Valley	37	8.1%
Forks Community	86	22.1%	*Sacred Heart Med. Ctr.	1940	16.8%
General Hosp. Everett	2604	19.3%	Samaritan	559	21.1%
Good Samaritan	1498	19.9%	Skagit Valley	747	24.4%
Grays Harbor Community	695	26.8%	Skyline	126	13.5%
Group Health Cooperative	1053	10.8%	Stevens Mem.	1644	18.3%
Group Health Eastside	1659	14.9%	St. Francis Community	974	22.8%
Harrison Mem.	1901	22.3%	St. John's	1378	21.1%
Highline Community	936	29.3%	St. Joseph Hosp. Belling	1603	19.2%
Highline Hosp. Riverton	204	44.6%	St. Joseph Hosp. & Health	1826	19.3%
Campus			Care Ctr.		
Holy Family	1353	12.2%	St. Joseph's Hosp. Chewe	31	22.6%
Island Hosp.	200	36.0%	*St. Mary Med. Ctr.	445	13.3%
Jefferson General	139	26.6%	St. Peter	1913	19.3%
*Kadlec Med. Ctr.	890	25.3%	Sunnyside Community	388	14.7%
Kennewick General	882	29.7%	*Swedish Hosp. Med. Ctr.	4003	23.6%
Kittitas Valley	265	19.2%	*Tacoma General	3462	28.0%
Klickitat Valley	83	19.3%	United General	312	21.2%
Lake Chelan Community	80	12.5%	U.W. Med. Ctr.	2168	22.0%
Lakewood General	559	22.7%	Valley General Hosp.	219	22.4%
Mason General	165	25.5%	Monroe		
Mid Valley	257	26.8%	Valley Hosp. Med. Ctr.	424	19.8%
Morton General	71	23.9%	Spokane		
Mount Carmel	281	14.9%	Valley Med. Ctr. Renton	2907	24.8%
Newport Community	30	10.0%	Vancouver Mem.	2275	17.6%
North Valley	100	16.0%	Virginia Mason	1432	19.6%
Northwest	2235	24.6%	Walla Walla General	377	8.8%
Okanogan Douglas Co.	151	16.6%	Whidbey General	311	22.5%
Olympic Mem.	615	21.8%	Whitman Community	34	23.5%
Othello Community	280	13.2%	*Yakima Valley Mem.	2636	16.6%
			STATE TOTALS	**66323**	**21.1%**

Source: Washington State Department of Health Comprehensive Hospital Abstract Reporting System, "Hospital Census Comparison by DRG." Data on neonatal intensive care units from the American Hospital Association "1988 Guide to the Health Care Field."

*indicates this facility has a neonatal intensive care unit

The Cutting Edge

The One Hundred and Seven Hospitals With the Highest Cesarean Rates (36% and Over)

State	Name of Facility	Cesarean Rate	Total Deliveries
Tennessee	Jellico Community	63.6%	220
Missouri	Bates Co.	55.0%	*40
Kentucky	Highland Regional Med. Ctr.	53.4%	472
Pennsylvania	Tyrone	53.3%	105
West Virginia	Williamson Mem.	49.7%	155
Pennsylvania	Metropolitan Hosp. Springfield	49.0%	104
California	Seneca	48.6%	72
New Jersey	St. James	48.5%	532
Florida	Hialeah	47.8%	1549
New York	Victory Mem.	47.6%	*1024
Arizona	Bullhead Community	46.3%	54
Florida	Mt. Sinai Med. Ctr.	45.2%	916
Washington	Highline Hosp. Riverton Campus	44.6%	204
New Jersey	Bayonne	44.6%	415
Tennessee	Perry Mem.	44.4%	45
Tennessee	Holston Valley	43.9%	1032
Maryland	Kent & Queen Anne's	43.2%	206
Florida	AMI Med. Ctr. Orlando	43.2%	368
New York	Westchester Co. Med. Ctr.	43.1%	*850
Pennsylvania	Hosp. of Phila. College of Osteo. Med.	42.9%	564
New York	Carthage Area	42.9%	*189
Florida	Plantation General	42.6%	1382
Florida	South Miami	42.6%	1620
Missouri	MO Baptist Hosp. Sullivan	42.3%	*168
West Virginia	Reynolds Mem.	42.0%	162
Florida	North Miami Med. Ctr.	41.6%	332
Ohio	Warren General	41.5%	135
Pennsylvania	Elk Co. General	41.4%	191
Florida	St. Anthony's	41.4%	304
New York	Mohawk Valley General	40.8%	*355
Minnesota	Virginia Regional Med. Ctr.	40.4%	*334
New Jersey	Meadowland Hosp. Med. Ctr.	40.3%	2018
Georgia	Dekalb General	40.2%	2731
New Jersey	Christ	40.2%	1201
California	Humana Hosp. San Leandro	40.1%	571
California	Northridge Hosp. Med. Ctr.	40.0%	2436
Ohio	Doctors Hosp. Stark Co.	39.9%	373
California	Tulare District	39.9%	803
Kentucky	Hazard App. Regional	39.9%	451
Florida	Mercy	39.8%	957
Nevada	Humboldt	39.6%	53
North Carolina	Mountain Park Med. Ctr.	39.5%	*38
Tennessee	Smith Co. Mem.	39.5%	81
Minnesota	Municipal Hosp. & Granite Manor	39.5%	*86
California	Nu Med Regional Med. Ctr.	39.4%	213
Florida	HCA Northwest Regional	38.9%	373
Maryland	Southern Maryland	38.8%	1432
California	Mercy Med. Ctr. Redding	38.6%	998
Ohio	Riverside	38.5%	680
Illinois	Mem. Hosp. Belleville	38.5%	1628
West Virginia	Monangalta General	38.4%	341
California	Circle City	38.4%	693
California	Med. Ctr. Tarzana	38.3%	2295
New York	Oneida City	38.3%	*368
Florida	Riverside Hosp. Pasco Co.	38.3%	682

New Jersey	Barnert Mem.	38.2%	1052
California	Huntington Mem.	38.2%	3920
Ohio	Fayette Co. Mem.	38.1%	270
California	Twin Cities Community	38.1%	459
Minnesota	Sleepy Eye Municipal	37.9%	*58
Pennsylvania	Montefiore Hosp. Assoc. W. Pa.	37.8%	294
North Carolina	Moore Regional	37.8%	*1308
Missouri	Barton Co.	37.7%	*114
Kentucky	Logan Co.	37.7%	204
California	Chinese	37.7%	276
Indiana	Community Hosp. Munster	37.6%	2468
Illinois	Rush North Shore Med. Ctr.	37.6%	306
Massachusetts	Martha's Vineyard	37.5%	160
Ohio	Lawrence Co. General	37.5%	88
Missouri	Reynolds Co.	37.5%	*40
North Dakota	St. Ansgar's	37.5%	40
Tennessee	Baptist Hosp. Memphis	37.4%	5052
California	Valley Presbyterian	37.4%	3047
California	El Centro Regional Med. Ctr.	37.4%	1092
California	Scripps Mem. Hosp. La Jolla	37.3%	2060
Tennessee	HCA Volunteer	37.2%	261
Georgia	Henry Co.	37.1%	429
Georgia	Perry Houston Co.	37.1%	307
West Virginia	St. Mary's	37.1%	283
Georgia	Gordon Co.	37.0%	335
California	Anaheim General	37.0%	470
Florida	AMI Palm Beach Gardens Med. Ctr.	37.0%	465
Indiana	Good Samaritan	36.9%	544
New York	Kingston	36.9%	*355
Indiana	Welborn Mem. Baptist	36.9%	981
Georgia	Jenkins Co.	36.8%	38
California	Bellwood General	36.8%	524
Georgia	Coliseum Park	36.7%	1421
New York	St. Charles Hosp. (HSA 8)	36.6%	*1714
Massachusetts	St. Joseph's	36.6%	601
New Jersey	Columbus	36.5%	1143
Tennessee	Baptist Hosp. Tipton	36.4%	313
Kentucky	Ephriam McDowell Mem.	36.4%	547
California	Foothill Presbyterian	36.4%	478
California	Mission Hosp. Regional Med. Ctr.	36.3%	2424
Ohio	Deaconess Hosp. Cleveland	36.3%	714
California	Santa Monica Hosp. Med. Ctr.	36.3%	2023
California	Inter-Community Med. Ctr.	36.3%	568
California	Corona Community	36.2%	824
Maine	North Cumberland	36.2%	94
Tennessee	Indian Path	36.2%	254
Tennessee	Goodlark	36.1%	443
New Jersey	Mem. Hosp. Burlington Co.	36.1%	2078
Kentucky	Our Lady of the Way	36.0%	253
Georgia	Mem. Hosp. Decatur Co.	36.0%	456
New York	White Plains Hosp. Med. Ctr.	36.0%	*1246
Washington	Island	36.0%	200

* These hospital cesarean rates were calculated using the number of live births, not the number of total deliveries. This method may slightly increase the hospital's cesarean section rate.

State Cesarean Section Rates for 41 States and The District of Columbia

State	Year	Cesarean Rate	Total Deliveries**	Unnecessary Cesareans***
Alabama	1988	26.0%	59647	8350
Arizona*	1989	20.6%	27105	2331
Arkansas	1988	24.7%	35022	4447
California	1987	25.0%	479902	62388
Colorado*	1987	19.4%	23058	1706
Connecticut	1989	22.6%	47558	5041
Delaware	1989	24.6%	11361	1432
District of Columbia	1989	26.5%	9732	1411
Florida*	1989	26.7%	95606	14054
Georgia	1988	24.9%	106171	13696
Hawaii	1989	21.2%	19123	1759
Idaho	1989	19.2%	15830	1139
Illinois	1988	22.4%	167400	17410
Indiana	1988	21.3%	80895	7524
Kansas	1988	26.6%	37819	5522
Kentucky	1988	23.4%	49969	5697
Maine	1989	21.5%	16292	1548
Maryland	1989	24.5%	65960	8245
Massachusetts	1988	24.4%	89433	11090
Michigan	1987	24.8%	140466	17933
Minnesota	1988	18.9%	65600	4526
Missouri	1989	23.4%	35663	4065
Nebraska*	1989	19.6%	10322	784
Nevada	1988	26.3%	13951	1995
New Hampshire*	1989	20.8%	8687	765
New Jersey	1988	27.9%	113382	18028
New Mexico	1988	19.2%	26686	1922
New York	1988	23.7%	279738	32729
North Carolina	1989	23.5%	102128	11745
North Dakota	1989	19.4%	10479	776
Ohio	1988	26.1%	118364	16689
Oregon	1988	22.0%	38103	3811
Pennsylvania	1988	23.9%	162475	19335
Rhode Island	1988	22.4%	14555	1513
South Carolina	1989	23.2%	46357	5192
South Dakota	1989	17.4%	11108	601
Tennessee	1988	22.8%	68948	7446
Utah	1988	20.0%	31610	2529
Vermont	1988	19.6%	7695	585
Washington	1989	21.1%	66323	6035
West Virginia	1989	25.4%	18767	2515
Wisconsin	1988	18.0%	70711	4243

* Indicates data for five or six months only; see state section in appendix for exact number.

** While we calculated most statewide cesarean section rates using the number of total deliveries, some states gave us the number of live births and not the number of total deliveries. Calculating cesarean rates using the number of live births may slightly affect a state's cesarean section rate.

*** In this report we use 12% as a proper c-section rate for a state; we designated as unnecessary those c-sections occuring above this 12% rate.

Appendix B

¶1. It shall be required of each physician and midwife providing obstetrical care to distribute to each maternity patient a brochure on maternity practices at the first prenatal visit. For patients who have not received prenatal care it shall be distributed by the hospital at the time of admission to the hospital or center. This brochure should also be available upon request to the general public from all hospitals in the state providing obstetric care. It shall be designed by the State Commissioner of Health with consumer participation and shall contain brief definitions and information on selected birth-related practices and procedures, as well as interpretation of rates, specified in subdivision two of this section.

¶2. This brochure shall include statistics relating to the annual percentage of maternity patients undergoing specific birth-related procedures at each hospital or birthing center in the state. [Note: may wish to substitute some geographical subdivision here in the larger states, such as health service area or block of counties], including but not limited to the following:

a) The annual rate of cesarean sections as a percentage of total deliveries.

b) The cesarean section rates for all individual physicians doing more than 20 deliveries per year at said hospital.

c) The annual percentage of women with one or more previous cesarean sections admitted for delivery who have a vaginal birth.

d) The annual percentage of deliveries by midwives.

e) The annual percentage of deliveries in birthing rooms.

f) The annual percentage of births utilizing continuous fetal monitoring 1) internal 2) external.

g) The annual percentage of vaginal births with episiotomies.

h) The annual percentage of women breastfeeding on discharge from the hospital.

i) A yes/no response to the question: Does this hospital use twenty-four rooming in of infants with mothers as the norm of care?

j) A yes/no response to the question: Does this hospital have a defined policy of confirming fetal distress originally detected on electronic monitoring with other tests?

k) A yes/no response to the question: Does this hospital or birthing center have a physician or midwife present in labor and delivery around the clock?

¶3. Compilation of the statistics set out in subdivision two of this Act shall be the responsibility of the Commissioner of Health. It shall be the responsibility of the hospitals and birthing centers to provide the Commissioner with information determined necessary to comply with the provisions of the Act.

¶4. Statistical information shall be presented in the most recent one year aggregate.

¶5. This Act shall take effect ____year after it shall have become a law.

Index

PUBLIC CITIZEN

Who We Are and What We Do

Public Citizen, known to many as "Nader's Raiders," is a non-profit organization based in Washington, D.C., with 95,000 members nationwide. Public Citizen represents citizens' interests through lobbying, litigation, research, and publications. Since its founding by Ralph Nader in 1971, Public Citizen has fought for consumer rights and for corporate and government accountability.

Public Citizen is active in the Congress, the courts, government agencies, and the media. In addition to our work on white collar crime and the savings and loan scandal, Public Citizen fights for campaign finance reform, congressional ethics, and limits on congressional pay raises. To prevent injuries and illness, we push for installation of air bags and other safety devices in cars, and we helped pass legislation protecting consumers against toxic wastes and pesticides. We also publish directories on unsafe or ineffective drugs, questionable doctors, and ratings of state health programs. Our attorneys have won sixteen victories in the U.S. Supreme Court since 1975.

Public Citizen does not accept government or corporate grants. Support funding comes generously from individual contributions and from the sale of publications.

Public Citizen has five components:

Congress Watch monitors legislation on Capitol Hill, documents, campaign financing abuses, tracks House and Senate voting records, and lobbies for the public interest.

Health Research Group fights for protection against unsafe foods, drugs, and workplaces, and for greater consumer control over personal health decisions.

Litigation Group brings precedent-setting lawsuits on behalf of citizens against the government, large corporations, and labor unions to enforce rights and ensure justice under the law.

Critical Mass Energy Project works for safe, efficient, and affordable energy.

Buyers Up is a group-buying organization that enables individuals to become more knowledgeable consumers and to exercise their economic leverage in the marketplace.

JOINING PUBLIC CITIZEN

We encourage you to become a member of
Public Citizen and to support our work.
With your annual membership contribution
of $20 or more, you will receive *Public Citizen*
magazine. This bimonthly publication will
keep you posted on Public Citizen's many pro-
jects and other important issues affecting you and
your famliy. With your membership contribution of $35 or
more, you will also receive an annual subscription to our monthly
Health Letter. This informative monthly guide will show you how
to lead a healthier and happier life.

Send your check or money order to:

Public Citizen Membership
2000 P Street N.W. - Suite 605
Washington, D.C. 20036

PUBLIC CITIZEN BOOKS FOR YOU AND YOUR FAMILY

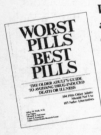

Worst Pills, Best Pllls This best-seller, which has sold
almost one million copies in the past two years,
exposes prescription drugs that are dangerous and
sometimes deadly for older adults. This important
reference book highlights 104 pills you should not
use and 183 safer alternatives. Authored by Public
Citizen physician Dr. Sidney M. Wolfe and the
Public Citizen Health Research Group (1989, 532
pages). Price $12.00, including postage.

Representing Yourself Do you need to spend hundreds,
and maybe even thousands of dollars on an attorney? Or
can you handle a routine legal matter yourself? This
informative publication tells you how to solve routine
legal problems without a lawyer, how to decide if you
do need a lawyer, and make sure you are adequately
represented. Chapters on buying and selling a house,
defective products, marriage and divorce, employee
rights, and many others. Authored by Kenneth Lasson
and the Public Citizen Litigation Group staff (reprinted 1987, 270
pages). Price: $12.95.

Send your check or money order for these books to:

Public Citizen Books
2000 P Street N.W. - Suite 605
Washington, D.C. 20036